Chronic Venous Insufficiency

CONTEMPORARY ENDOVASCULAR MANAGEMENT

Edited by Mark G. Davies and Alan B. Lumsden

The Contemporary Endovascular Management series is designed to be a focused, relevant, and timely review of the modern aspects of imaging and intervention in specific vascular beds. Each volume in the series addresses one vascular bed and equips readers with the current information necessary for vascular practice using a clear and easy-to-access format.

Volume 1 Chronic Venous Insufficiency

Volume 2 Venous Thromboembolic Disease

Volume 3 Dialysis Access: Creation and Maintenance
Forthcoming

Volume 4 Dialysis Access: Special Cases and Complications
Forthcoming

Please visit www.cardiotextpublishing.com for more information about this series.

Chronic Venous Insufficiency

CONTEMPORARY ENDOVASCULAR MANAGEMENT

Volume 1

editors

Mark G. Davies MD, PhD, MBA

Vice Chairman, Finance and Administration, Department of Cardiovascular Surgery; Program Director, Vascular Surgery Fellowship and Integrated Vascular Surgery Residency; Director of Research and Education, Methodist DeBakey Heart & Vascular Center, The Methodist Hospital, Houston, Texas; Senior Investigator, The Methodist Hospital Research Institute; Professor of Cardiovascular Surgery, Weill Cornell Medical College, New York, New York

Alan B. Lumsden MD

Chairman, Department of Cardiovascular Surgery; Medical Director, Methodist DeBakey Heart & Vascular Center, The Methodist Hospital, Houston, Texas; Professor of Cardiovascular Surgery, Weill Cornell Medical College, New York, New York

Daynene Vykoukal PhD assistant editor

Scientific Editor, The Methodist Hospital Research Institute, Methodist DeBakey Heart & Vascular Center, The Methodist Hospital, Houston, Texas

cardiotext

Minneapolis, Minnesota

Cardiotext Publishing, LLC
3405 W. 44th Street
Minneapolis, Minnesota 55410
USA

www.cardiotextpublishing.com

Any updates to this book may be found at:
www.cardiotextpublishing.com/titles/detail/9781935395096

Comments, inquiries, and requests for bulk sales can be directed to the publisher at:
info@cardiotextpublishing.com.

This book is intended for educational purposes and to further general scientific and medical knowledge, research, and understanding of the conditions and associated treatments discussed herein. This book is not intended to serve as and should not be relied upon as recommending or promoting any specific diagnosis or method of treatment for a particular condition or a particular patient. It is the reader's responsibility to determine the proper steps for diagnosis and the proper course of treatment for any condition or patient, including suitable and appropriate tests, medications, or medical devices to be used for or in conjunction with any diagnosis or treatment.

Due to ongoing research, discoveries, modifications to medicines, equipment and devices, and changes in government regulations, the information contained in this book may not reflect the latest standards, developments, guidelines, regulations, products, or devices in the field. Readers are responsible for keeping up-to-date with the latest developments and are urged to review the latest instructions and warnings for any medicine, equipment, or medical device. Readers should consult with a specialist or contact the vendor of any medicine or medical device where appropriate.

Except for the publisher's website associated with this work, the publisher is not affiliated with and does not sponsor or endorse any websites, organizations, or other sources of information referred to herein.

The publisher and the author specifically disclaim any damage, liability, or loss incurred, directly or indirectly, from the use or application of any of the contents of this book.

Unless otherwise stated, all figures and tables in this book are used courtesy of the authors.

Cover design by Brad Norr Design
Book design by Ann Delgehausen, Trio Bookworks

Library of Congress Control Number: 2011924294

ISBN: 978-1-935395-09-6

Printed in Canada

16 15 14 13 12 11 1 2 3 4 5 6 7 8 9 10

Contents

Part 4: Venous Malformations

Contributors

Editors

Mark G. Davies MD, PhD, MBA Vice Chairman, Finance and Administration, Department of Cardiovascular Surgery; Program Director, Vascular Surgery Fellowship and Integrated Vascular Surgery Residency; Director of Research and Education, Methodist DeBakey Heart & Vascular Center, The Methodist Hospital, Houston, Texas; Senior Investigator, The Methodist Hospital Research Institute; Professor of Cardiovascular Surgery, Weill Cornell Medical College, New York, New York

Alan B. Lumsden MD Chairman, Department of Cardiovascular Surgery; Medical Director, Methodist DeBakey Heart & Vascular Center, The Methodist Hospital, Houston, Texas; Professor of Cardiovascular Surgery, Weill Cornell Medical College, New York, New York

Contributors

Elizabeth Acquista MD Department of General Surgery, University of North Carolina, Chapel Hill, North Carolina

Javier E. Anaya-Ayala MD Department of Cardiovascular Surgery, Methodist DeBakey Heart & Vascular Center, The Methodist Hospital Research Institute, Houston, Texas

Jean Bismuth MD Methodist DeBakey Heart & Vascular Center, Division of Cardiovascular Surgery, The Methodist Hospital, Houston, Texas; Assistant Professor of Cardiovascular Surgery, Weill Cornell Medical College, New York, New York

Kevin G. Burnand MBBS, MS, FRCS Professor (emeritus), Department of Academic Surgery, St. Thomas's Hospital Campus, King's College London, London

Michael C. Dalsing MD E. Dale and Susan E. Habegger Professor of Surgery, Director of Vascular Surgery, Department of Surgery, Division of Vascular Surgery, Indiana University School of Medicine, Indianapolis, Indiana

Alan M. Dietzek MD, RPVI, FACS Clinical Associate Professor of Surgery, University of Vermont College of Medicine; Chief, Section of Vascular & Endovascular Surgery, Linda and Stephen R. Cohen Chair in Vascular Surgery, Danbury Hospital, Danbury, Connecticut

Angela N. Fellner PhD Research Specialist, E. Kenneth Hatton MD Institute for Research & Education, Good Samaritan Hospital, Cincinnati, Ohio

Peter Gloviczki MD Joe M. and Ruth Roberts Professor of Surgery, Division of Vascular and Endovascular Surgery, Gonda Vascular Center, Mayo Clinic, Rochester, Minnesota

Sofia Gonzalez-Morales MS Medical student, Universidad Panamericana, Mexico City, Mexico; Visiting Student at Methodist DeBakey Heart & Vascular Center, The Methodist Hospital, Houston, Texas

Nyla Ismail PhD Methodist DeBakey Heart & Vascular Center, The Methodist Hospital, Houston, Texas

Christof Karmonik PhD Research Scientist, Department of Neurosurgery, Methodist DeBakey Heart & Vascular Center, The Methodist Hospital, Houston, Texas; Assistant Professor of Physics in Radiology, Weill Medical College of Cornell University, New York, New York; Adjunct Assistant Professor of Computer Science, University of Houston, Houston, Texas

Joann M. Lohr MD, FACS, RVT Director of the Good Samaritan Hospital John J. Cranley Vascular Laboratory, Associate Program Director for the Vascular Surgery Residency at Good Samaritan Hospital, Good Samaritan Hospital, Cincinnati, Ohio

Francis Marshalleck MD Assistant Professor, Interventional Radiology, Indiana University School of Medicine, Riley Hospital for Children, Indianapolis, Indiana

Robert B. McLafferty MD, FACS Professor of Surgery, Division of Vascular Surgery, Department of Surgery, Southern Illinois University School of Medicine, Springfield, Illinois

Robert J. Min MD, MBA, FSIR, FACPh Chairman of Radiology, New York-Presbyterian Hospital/Weill Cornell Medical College, New York, New York

Colleen J. Moore MD Assistant Professor of Surgery, Department of Surgery, Division of Vascular Surgery, Southern Illinois University School of Medicine, Springfield, Illinois

Carolyn E. Munschauer BA Venous Institute of Buffalo, SUNY at Buffalo Department of Surgery, Buffalo, New York

Joseph J. Naoum MD, FACS Assistant Professor, Weill Cornell Medical College, New York, New York; The Methodist Hospital, Division of Vascular Surgery, Cardiovascular Surgery Associates, Houston, Texas

Peter Neglén MD, PhD Vascular Surgeon, The RANE Center at River Oaks Hospital, Flowood, Mississippi

Dušan Pavčnik MD, PhD Professor and Director of Research, Dotter Interventional Institute, Oregon Health & Science University, Portland, Oregon

Eric K. Peden MD Assistant Professor of Cardiovascular Surgery, Weill Cornell Medical College of Cornell University, New York, New York; Chief of Vascular Surgery, Department of Cardiovascular Surgery, Methodist DeBakey Heart & Vascular Center, The Methodist Hospital, Houston, Texas

Joseph J. Ricotta II MD, MS, FACS Assistant Professor of Surgery, Division of Vascular Surgery and Endovascular Therapy, Emory University School of Medicine, Atlanta, Georgia

Dipan J. Shah MD, FACC Assistant Professor of Medicine, Weill Medical College of Cornell University, New York, New York; Director, Cardiac Magnetic Resonance Imaging, Methodist DeBakey Heart & Vascular Center, The Methodist Hospital, Houston, Texas

Michael A. Vasquez MD, FACS, RVT Clinical Assistant Professor of Surgery, SUNY Buffalo Department of Surgery; Venous Institute of Buffalo, New York

R. Eugene Zierler MD Professor of Surgery, Division of Vascular Surgery, Department of Surgery, University of Washington School of Medicine; Medical Director, D. E. Strandness Jr. Vascular Laboratory, University of Washington Medical Center and Harborview Medical Center, Seattle, Washington

Acknowledgments

The editors would like to thank the following individuals for their kind contributions to the completion of this book: Yvette Whittier and Daynene Vykoukal, PhD, at The Methodist Hospital for organizational assistance, author relations, primary editing and manuscript assembly; Steve Korn, Mike Crouchet, Caitlin Crouchet, and Carol Syverson at Cardiotext Publishing for their roles in series development, content management and technical support; and Ann Delgehausen, Beth Wright, and Zan Ceeley at Trio Bookworks for their diligent execution of the publication and their contribution to the series designs and concepts. Without the time and effort of the contributors, no book can address its goals and we gratefully acknowledge the time and effort that each of the authors devoted to this project.

Mark G. Davies
Alan B. Lumsden

Introduction

Mark G. Davies

Recognition of venous disorders as a significant public health issue has increased awareness of venous problems among both the medical professions and the lay population. This awareness has resulted in greater attention to prevention, introduction of quality performance measures, and enhanced operative and pharmacological interventions, which have transformed the treatment of venous disease from a stepchild of several specialties into a robust subspecialty field in medicine. Venous problems may be divided into two categories, acute venous disorders and chronic venous disorders. This volume in the Contemporary Endovascular Management series provides a focused and timely review of the current state of the field in chronic venous disorders.

Chronic venous disease continues to be a common medical problem in Western Europe and the United States.[1] Reported prevalence ranges from 1% to 40% in females and from 1% to 17% in males. Estimates for varicose veins are higher, ranging from 1% to 73% in females and 2% to 56% in males. While many risk factors have been associated with chronic venous disease, the ones most commonly quoted are older age, female gender, pregnancy, family history of venous disease, obesity, and occupations associated with orthostasis. Chronic venous disease can be divided into primary and secondary disorders.

Primary chronic venous disorders, or those not associated with an identifiable mechanism of venous dysfunction, are among the most common venous problems.[2] Varicose veins without skin changes are present in about 20% of the population, while active ulcers may be present in as many as 0.5%. These problems arise from intrinsic structural and biochemical abnormalities of the vein wall that with progression lead to skin changes and ulceration. This progression arises from extravasation of macromolecules and red blood cells, leading to endothelial cell activation, leukocyte diapedesis, and altered tissue remodeling with intense collagen deposition. Patients may remain asymptomatic, or they may develop pain or swelling, skin changes, or a complication (thrombophlebitis, bleeding, ulceration). While physical exam allows for the identification of varicosities and saphenofemoral incompetence, venous duplex ultrasonography is the most common study used to define the function of the superficial and venous systems in the lower extremities. Primary venous disease is most often associated with truncal saphenous insufficiency. Until recently, these veins were treated with stripping of the saphenous vein and interruption and removal of major tributary and perforating veins. Currently, endovenous ablation techniques with radiofrequency, laser, or foam sclerotherapy are the norm. Sclerotherapy and cutaneous laser treatment are used in the management of telangiectasias; primary, residual, or recurrent varicosities without connection to incompetent venous trunks; and congenital venous malformations.

Secondary chronic venous disorders are those venous problems that occur following an episode of acute deep venous thrombosis.[3] Most occluded venous segments recanalize over the first 6 to 12 months after an episode of acute deep venous thrombosis, leading to chronic luminal changes and a combination of partial obstruction and reflux. These intrinsic changes lead to venous hypertension. The clinical manifestations of secondary chronic venous disease, including pain, venous claudication, edema, skin changes, and ulceration, are commonly referred to as postthrombotic syndrome. The diagnostic evaluation of secondary chronic venous disorders is similar to primary chronic venous disorders, although greater use of imaging and intervention to correct structural changes in veins is more common. In general, however, compression remains the primary treatment of chronic venous disorders and is essential for healing ulcers and minimizing recurrence. The efficacy of various adjuncts to ulcer treatment, including complex wound dressings and medications, have been variable. Although superficial venous surgery has not been demonstrated to improve ulcer-healing rates, it does decrease ulcer recurrence. Treatment of incompetent perforating veins remains controversial and appears to be appropriate for venous ulceration. With respect to venous obstruction, iliocaval angioplasty and stenting has emerged as the primary treatment for proximal iliofemoral venous obstruction, with surgical bypass assuming a secondary role.

References

1. Beebe-Dimmer JL, Pfeifer JR, Engle JS, Schottenfeld D. The epidemiology of chronic venous insufficiency and varicose veins. Ann Epidemiol. 2005;15(3):175-84.
2. Meissner MH, Gloviczki P, Bergan J, Kistner RL, Morrison N, Pannier F, et al. Primary chronic venous disorders. J Vasc Surg. 2007;46 Suppl S:54S-67S.
3. Meissner MH, Eklof B, Smith PC, Dalsing MC, DePalma RG, Gloviczki P, et al. Secondary chronic venous disorders. J Vasc Surg. 2007;46 (Suppl) S:68S-83S.

PART 1

Varicose Veins

A lack of rigor exists in the degree to which interventions for venous disease have been scientifically evaluated and evidence-based guidelines developed and followed. The professional societies have begun to tackle this problem, and a growing body of scientific investigation and practical classification systems now exist for developing best-practice protocols for the treatment of chronic venous insufficiency. With the recent expansion in venous therapies, evidence-based medicine will be necessary to allow appropriate delivery of care with a shrinking healthcare budget and resources. The rapid evolution and expansion of treatment in varicose veins has changed the field from an open inpatient procedure to a percutaneous therapy suitable for the office environment. This change in practice has been driven by the widespread introduction and competency in duplex ultrasonography and by a better understanding of the pathology of varicose veins. While duplex scanning has been effective in the extremities, the development of CTV and MRV has increased our understanding of both peripheral and central venous diseases and their association with venous incompetency. Both radiofrequency and laser-based systems provide equivalent results, and it appears that operator experience and patient selection are key to success. Sclerotherapy is evolving as an alternative to many of the catheter-based techniques but is still reserved for nonaxial varicose veins in the majority of practices. There is a remarkably low rate of true adverse reactions following all percutaneous therapies. However, many venous studies continue to suffer from short-term follow-up and small sample size, as well as an observational nature. These limitations tend to decrease the validity of assessments of outcomes for varicose vein recurrence and are the basis of the determinations of most insurance carriers. The evolution in the understanding of and therapy for venous perforator has had a fluctuating course. Open perforator surgery has evolved to SEPS and now to RFA or sclerotherapy. While restricted to therapies for advanced CVI, its widespread adoption is relatively low due to the conflicting reports and a general lack of evidence-based support to validate its use.

The understanding of and ability to image venous incompetence and the efforts to link these to clinical disease have advanced the field. Coupled to the introduction of less invasive therapies, the field is emerging as a patient-specific and disease-oriented intervention. An increase in evidence-based data is required to consolidate these initial positive advances.

CHAPTER 1

Overview of Therapy for Varicose Veins

Joann M. Lohr

Venous disorders are among the most prevalent medical conditions in the United States. An estimated 600,000 people per year have venous thromboembolism, a fact recently highlighted by the US Surgeon General's call to action to prevent deep vein thrombosis and pulmonary embolism.[1] In the United States, 35% of adults have some form of chronic venous insufficiency. More than one-third of men and women aged 18 to 64 years have varicose veins.[2] Venous ulceration is present in 4% of persons over the age of 65. The prevalence of this disorder results in a population-based cost of $1 billion per year, including 4.6 million workdays lost per year.

A variety of treatment options exists for varicose veins. Treatment may include high ligation and saphenous vein stripping with or without phlebectomy. Until recently, this vein stripping was the procedure most commonly performed by surgeons worldwide.

Many minimally invasive therapies have been introduced in recent years. Several of these modalities have been claimed to be as effective as surgery. These include radiofrequency or laser ablation of the great or small saphenous vein, a procedure that may be combined with phlebectomy, liquid sclerotherapy, or foam sclerotherapy. The Society for Vascular Surgery and the American Venous Forum have teamed up in an effort to develop practice guidelines to improve patient care for people who have venous diseases.

Randomized controlled clinical trials and observational studies showed that sclerotherapy was as effective as surgery, particularly in patients without incompetent perforating veins.[3] Sclerotherapy is well received by patients and is the preferred

Chronic Venous Insufficiency. Contemporary Endovascular Management series. © 2011 Mark G. Davies MD and Alan B. Lumsden MD, eds. Cardiotext Publishing, ISBN 978-1-935395-09-6.

initial treatment.[4] Patients who receive sclerotherapy are also less likely to require additional treatment.[5] Sclerotherapy gave better initial results,[6] but studies with longer follow-up duration suggested that the initial benefits declined over time.

A randomized controlled trial with a 10-year follow-up compared 6 treatment options (liquid sclerotherapy; high-dose liquid sclerotherapy; multiple ligations; stab avulsion; foam sclerotherapy; surgery (high ligation) followed by sclerotherapy). All treatments appeared equally effective in terms of recurrence, although the results from low-dose liquid sclerotherapy appeared to be less effective than those from high-dose liquid sclerotherapy and foam sclerotherapy, which were comparable to those from surgery.[7]

Many venous studies suffer from short-term follow-up and small sample size, as well as the observational nature of such studies. These limitations tend to decrease the validity of assessments of outcomes for varicose vein recurrence.

Short-term trials comparing endovenous laser ablation to standard ligation and stripping showed no difference between the 2 procedures at 3 months in terms of overall improvement and quality-of-life scores (36-Item Short Form Health Survey [SF-36]),[8] disease-specific quality of life (Aberdeen Varicose Vein Symptom Score [AVVSS]),[9] and symptoms (Venous Clinical Severity Score [VCSS]).[8] There was a slight increase in postoperative pain and bruising in the high ligation and stripping procedure.[8] Comparison of laser and radiofrequency ablation outcomes have, for the most part, been unable to detect a difference between the two procedures in terms of effectiveness and safety.[10] Saphenous vein occlusion at 2 weeks after the procedure is approximately 96% in both groups. Ultrasound examination of the saphenofemoral junction at a mean of 3 years postprocedure has shown no neovascularization in the groin. Marked symptom improvement was reported in most patients in both groups. When surgery is compared with all endoluminal ablation therapies (laser, radiofrequency, and foam), meta-analysis has shown that surgery leads to a nonsignificant reduction in the risk of varicose vein recurrence. All treatments for varicose veins are well tolerated and have no significant periprocedural adverse effects, particularly deep vein thrombosis and pulmonary embolism. Local complications are more common but, in general, minor.

Invasive treatments (surgical and endoluminal) are superior to conservative management in eliminating varicose veins and in decreasing recurrence rates. Liquid sclerotherapy, foam sclerotherapy, and endoluminal thermal ablation therapies have had short-term follow-up studies, making them unsuitable for assessing long-term outcomes. When compared to surgery, however, liquid or foam sclerotherapy and endoluminal thermal ablation therapy (laser and radiofrequency) are associated with faster return to work, shorter duration of disability, and less pain.

Randomized controlled clinical trials of newer and less invasive therapies, such as laser radiofrequency ablation and foam therapy, are needed so that their efficacy and safety can be compared to those of the standard procedure of ligation stripping and multiple phlebectomies.

These studies will need to stratify participants according to severity of symptoms. Long-term follow-up duration studies will be critically important. In the future, cost-effectiveness of these procedures will need to be analyzed. At present, surgery is the only treatment with long-term effectiveness data. The other, less invasive, treatments are associated with shorter disability and less pain, but only short-term effectiveness data are available.

Interest in venous diseases and their treatment options has increased dramatically in recent years, and it is hoped that answers to the questions these diseases and their treatments pose will be available in the near future.

References

1. Wakefield TW, McLafferty RB, Lohr JM, Caprini JA, Gillespie DL, Passman MA. Call to action to prevent venous thromboembolism. J Vasc Surg. 2009;49(6):1620-3.
2. Evans CJ, Fowkes FG, Ruckley CV, Lee AJ. Prevalence of varicose veins and chronic venous insufficiency in men and women in general population: Edinburgh Vein Study. J Epidemiol Commun H. 1999;53(3):149-53.
3. Hobbs JT. The treatment of varicose veins. A random trial of injection-compression therapy versus surgery. Br J Surg. 1968;55(10):777-80.
4. Chant AD, Jones HO, Weddell JM. Varicose veins: a comparison of surgery and injection-compression sclerotherapy. Lancet. 1972;2(7788):1188-91.
5. Beresford SA, Chant AD, Jones HO, Piachaud D, Weddell JM. Varicose veins: a comparison of surgery and infection/compression sclerotherapy. Five-year follow up. Lancet. 1978;1(8070):921-4.
6. Doran FS, White M. A clinical trial designed to discover if the primary treatment of varicose veins should be by Fegan's method or by an operation. Br J Surg. 1975;62(1):72-6.
7. Belcaro G, Cesarone MR, Renzo AD, Brandolini R, Coen L, Acerbi G, et al. Foam-sclerotherapy, surgery, sclerotherapy, and combined treatment for varicose veins: a 10 year, prospective, randomized controlled, trial (VEDICO trial). Angiology. 2003;54(3):307-15.
8. Rasmussen LH, Bjoern L, Lawaetz M, Blemings A, Lawaetz B, Eklof B. Randomized trial comparing endovenous laser ablation of the great saphenous vein with high ligation and stripping in patients with varicose veins: short-term results. J Vasc Surg. 2007;46(2):308-15.
9. Darwood RJ, Theivacumar N, Dellagrammaticas D, Mavor AID, Gough MJ. Randomized clinical trial comparing endovenous laser ablation with surgery for the treatment of primary great saphenous varicose veins. Br J Surg. 2008;95(3):294-301.
10. Ravi R, Rodriguez-Lopez JA, Trayler EA, Barrett DA, Dietrich EB. Endovenous ablation of incompetent saphenous veins: a large single-center experience. J Endovasc Ther. 2006;13(2):244-8.

CHAPTER 2

Chronic Venous Insufficiency

Comprehensive Treatment Guided by Investigation and Classification

Michael A. Vasquez and Carolyn E. Munschauer

Modern surgical practice is alive with protocols and classification instruments designed to focus myriad decision-making strategies on outcomes assessment. Whether attention is directed to procedural results, patient-reported outcomes, or both, these assessment methods serve to illuminate the path of surgical decision-making. The history of chronic venous disease therapy has paralleled treatment for other conditions,[1] developing technically and intuitively over time. Scientific investigation and practical classification systems have had important roles in the development of best-practice protocols for the treatment of chronic venous insufficiency. Assessment instruments include those that focus on the condition and those that focus on the perspective.

Chronic Venous Insufficiency. Contemporary Endovascular Management series. © 2011 Mark G. Davies MD and Alan B. Lumsden MD, eds. Cardiotext Publishing, ISBN 978-1-935395-09-6.

Generic and disease-specific instruments involve the assessment of disease states, the influence of disease states on the patient and community, and the effect of therapy on quality of life. Generic measurements are useful in various unrelated conditions, while disease-specific instruments are designed to reveal trends in the course and treatment of individual conditions. Recommendations have been made to include a generic and disease-specific assessment to fully measure quality of life.[2] Widely used generic instruments include 2 thorough assessment tools. The 36-Item Short Form Health Survey (SF-36) assesses physical functioning and mental well-being through examinations of limitations because of physical or emotional issues and the patient's perception of health.[3,4] The Nottingham Health Profile (NHP) measures the patient's perceived physical, emotional, and social effects from various disease states in a short assessment that has proven to be sensitive to variations in disease states.[3,4]

Disease-Specific Quality of Life

Several disease-specific quality-of-life measurements are available for use in chronic venous insufficiency. These are all designed to measure elements of venous disease and their influence on specific outcomes measures, including patient quality of life, economic effect, symptom resolution, and social issues. The Chronic Venous Insufficiency Questionnaire (CIVIQ) evaluates 4 aspects of disease, namely, pain and physical, social, and psychological effects. The second version of this instrument is equally weighted in all 4 dimensions and has been well validated.[3,5] The Venous Insufficiency Epidemiological and Economic Study (VEINES) comprises 2 parts, a quality-of-life assessment (VEINES-QOL) that estimates disease effect on quality of life and a symptom questionnaire (VEINES-Sym) that measures the prevalent symptoms.[3,6] The Aberdeen Varicose Vein Questionnaire (AVVQ) is a short (13-item) instrument that addresses the following salient features of venous disease: symptoms of pain and swelling and the presence of ulcers, the effect of varicose veins on daily activities (including cosmesis issues), and the use of conservative therapies (including compression stockings).[2,3] The Charing Cross Venous Ulceration Questionnaire (CXVUQ) is a patient-reported assessment of quality-of-life issues with venous ulcers. The instrument demonstrated validated consistency in a large patient cohort regardless of the ulcer therapy used.[3,7] The Specific Quality of Life and Outcome Response–Venous (SQOR-V) is a new survey designed to be used in clinical practice. This survey focuses on the patient's primary complaint and the relevance to venous disease. The emphasis is on symptoms, impairment of activities, appearance of the legs, and concerns about health risks. The questionnaire is completely patient driven and is undergoing validation of its English-language version.[3,8]

CEAP—Clinical, Etiologic, Anatomic, and Pathophysiologic

In addition to the patient-reported assessments, several physician-driven tools are used in evaluating the effects of chronic venous insufficiency and its therapies. These primarily have been used to classify the severity of the venous disease on presentation and, in some cases, to follow the outcomes of therapy. The CEAP classification was initially used as a common reporting method for diagnostic variables. It has demonstrated strong specificity for the symptoms and manifestations of chronic venous insufficiency, but its static nature makes it impractical for following the changes in disease states over time.[3,9,10] CEAP considers clinical, etiologic, anatomic, and pathophysiologic factors of venous disease to generate a patient classification at the time of diagnosis. While classifications may change over time in response to therapy or disease progression, higher initial classes may not reflect change in a timely manner. Clinical classes C_4 and C_5, which represent pigmentation changes and ulcer history, may be especially resistant to showing incremental improvements.[3] In 2004, a revision of CEAP was undertaken to refine the clinical class definitions and to improve reproducibility of observations.[9,11]

Revised Clinical CEAP Classes

C_0 No visible or palpable signs of venous disease

C_1 Telangiectasias or reticular veins

C_2 Varicose veins; distinguished from reticular veins by a diameter of 3 mm or more

C_3 Edema
C_4 Changes in skin and subcutaneous tissue secondary to CVD, now divided into 2 subclasses to better define the differing severity of venous disease:
- C_{4a} Pigmentation or eczema
- C_{4b} Lipodermatosclerosis or atrophie blanche

C_5 Healed venous ulcer
C_6 Active venous ulcer

Reprinted with permission from Elsevier from Revision of the CEAP classification for chronic venous disorders: Consensus statement by Eklöf et al.[11]

Venous Severity Scoring System

The Venous Severity Scoring system (VSS) was developed from clinical CEAP variables to be more sensitive to changes in patient disease status over time in response to treatment or disease progression. The following 3 elements of the VSS work together or individually to provide additional weight to factors considered important in the progression of venous disease: the Venous Disability Score (VDS), Venous Segmental Disease Score (VSDS), and Venous Clinical Severity Score (VCSS). The VDS extends the variables of CEAP to consider the effect of venous disease on the patient according to the level of work-based disability. The scoring scale relates to a traditional 8-hour workday, which underestimates the effect of venous disease on patients' usual activities.[3,12] The scale also considers the use of a "support device," which may be a more beneficial measure if clarified as compression therapy or as other treatments.[3,12-13] The VSDS evaluates venous reflux or obstruction and is calculated using data from duplex Doppler or phlebography. The VSDS draws on the anatomic and pathophysiologic elements of the CEAP score but has elicited criticism on reproducibility and ease of scoring.[3,12,13] The VCSS evaluates 9 elements of venous disease on a severity scale to derive a dynamic score. The VCSS reflects change in disease status due to progression or therapy owing to the construction of the scale. Each element of the scale is scored individually, allowing changes to be followed throughout the course of therapy. The VCSS is the only component of the VSS that is designed for use as a stand-alone scoring system. The method of scoring is similar to that of CEAP; the focus of CEAP is maintained, but sensitivity to longitudinal change is emphasized in the VCSS.[3,10,12-14] A revision of VCSS was recently completed that clarifies categories to reflect lessons learned from several studies.[10,14-17] (See table 2.1 on page 15.)

Although each of these assessment instruments contributes to quality-of-life measurement, the various categories and survey types make it difficult to choose the appropriate instrument for specific applications. Some investigators have recommended a combination of generic and disease-specific assessment tools, along with noninvasive testing, CEAP, and the VCSS for initial diagnostic classification and longitudinal assessment.[3,18-20] While this widespread approach to quality-of-life assessment may provide a thorough analysis of all contributing factors, it may be more than most clinicians want to undertake when planning an assessment protocol. Although the combination of generic and disease-specific instruments may not be crucial for complete quality-of-life assessment, the consideration of both patient-reported and physician-reported information may be.[3,8] The primarily clinical assessment of success elicited using a physician-generated instrument may provide an incomplete consideration of the patient's primary reason for seeking treatment.[3,8]

Global Assessment

Among 4 available validated disease-specific instruments are 2 that consider the overall effect of chronic venous disease (CIVIQ and VEINES), and 2 that address particular disease sequelae (AVVQ and CXVUQ). These patient-reported instruments are valuable in completing a thorough assessment of chronic venous disease. The CIVIQ evaluates overall quality-of-life issues, including physical, psychological, and social effects,[3] while the VEINES instrument is divided into 2 categories that measure symptoms and assess quality-of-life and psychosocial issues in light of disease states. The AVVQ also evaluates physical symptoms and social concerns but focuses specifically on varicose veins and their direct complications,[2,3] and the CXVUQ focuses on issues related to the presence of venous ulcers.[3] The recently completed SQOR-V may provide the most thorough disease-specific instrument, as it is designed to assess symptoms, cosmesis, influence on daily activities, and patient concerns regarding additional sequelae of chronic venous disease.[3,8]

Two physician-reported survey methods, CEAP and the VSS, are regularly used in chronic venous disease. Both have been widely studied and have been subjected to rigorous validation and revision. CEAP scores can be determined from the results of clinical evaluation and Doppler testing,[19] making it an easily quantifiable instrument in the diagnosis of chronic venous insufficiency. The main argument against CEAP as a stand-alone longitudinal measuring system lies in its static nature, which makes it resistant to revealing disease trends in response to treatment or progression.[13] The elements of the VSS have been used to study the effects of chronic venous disease from an elemental CEAP perspective. The VDS quantifies work-related disability, the VSDS relates noninvasive evaluation of obstruction and reflux to the level of disability, and the VCSS reports 9 salient features of chronic venous disease and their severity.[3,13] Although the components of VSS have all been used, terminology, scoring problems, and reproducibility have limited the use of the VDS and the VSDS.[3,10,13,14,20] The VCSS has been evaluated as a stand-alone scoring system and has shown promise in several studies.[3,10,13,14,17,20] The new VCSS revision should remain a strong clinical assessment instrument.[3,13]

Overall Evaluation

Much discussion has been given to the question of which instrument or combination of instruments will provide the best evaluation of patient quality of life and physician-assessed outcomes. In addition, protocols, quantification tools, and experiential assessments have been recognized as crucial in chronic venous disease management. Most of the patient-reported instruments have been validated in longitudinal studies of the effects of therapy or disease progression. The CIVIQ and AVVQ have been used before and after treatment to measure therapeutic effects. The VEINES has been used in long-term follow-up studies but focuses more on changing disease states and not directly on treatment effects. The CXVUQ has been useful in longitudinal research to report the effects of venous ulcers and the results of therapy.[3]

Physician-reported instruments have also been used in longitudinal studies. CEAP was originally designed as a tool for patient classification and management but was found to be static and inelastic to the effects of treatment or disease progression.[3,18,19] In 2004, CEAP underwent a revision designed to enhance its sensitivity to the effects of therapy.[9,11] Recently, this revised CEAP was used in the American Venous Forum's nationwide vein screening program. Although it was used only in a diagnostic application, it demonstrated good correlation with duplex Doppler studies performed in the same setting.[3] The VCSS has demonstrated value in longitudinal use,[3,10,13,14,17,20] and the revision will strengthen its position as a stand-alone assessment instrument.[3,13] The choice of instrument may depend largely on the way it is to be used in practice or research, as well as on the desired feedback. Reporting standards may involve surveys, patient-reported or physician-reported outcomes assessments, or the results of protocols or treatment plans. The value of data depends not only on the choice of instrument but also on the selection of elements to study and report. In this respect, experience is a valuable guide in the decision-making process. Rutherford states that "the results of therapy for vascular disease have little meaning if presented in isolation, no matter how uniform and valid the criteria used for reporting them."[20(p5)] Knowledge of the salient features of chronic venous disease, available therapies, and common elements of the patient population will guide the clinician in his or her choice of desired outcomes and assessment instruments.

Assessment and Management

When evaluating patients for chronic venous disease, several elements should be used to derive an appropriate clinical assessment and treatment plan. Eklöf et al[11] stratify this process into levels. Level 1 consists of the initial visit and examination, level 2 is noninvasive vascular laboratory testing, and level 3 comprises additional imaging or invasive studies. A detailed clinical examination is the first step in diagnosis and should be repeated at each reevaluation. The initial visit should also include assessment of venous disease manifestations (including edema, varicose veins, telangiectases, phlebitis, pigmentation and skin-quality changes, lipodermatosclerosis, venous stasis dermatitis, and ulcers). This objective assessment should be combined with a review of the patient's history that includes weight, smoking, pregnancies, physical activity, and family history of vein disease, along with relevant patient-reported symptoms (including pain, aching, tingling or burning, heaviness, and fatigue).[19,21-24] The somewhat subjective elements of clinical examination make diagnostic testing a useful objective measure.[24] Laboratory evaluations are important not only in assisting in the diagnosis of chronic venous insufficiency but also in identifying or excluding other conditions, including arterial disease, deep vein thrombosis, deep venous reflux, and venous obstruction.[24] While primary venous disease involves reflux, a sequelae of venous hypertension,[19,24,25] secondary chronic venous disease may involve reflux and an obstructive event.[24,25] The obstruction may be related to venous compression or the results of a deep vein thrombosis (postthrombotic syndrome).[25-27]

Imaging

Duplex Doppler is the usual first level of laboratory evaluation,[19,21] providing data on reflux (superficial or deep) and valvular incompetence, deep vein thrombosis, and obstruction,[19,28] but may be insufficient to demonstrate the hemodynamic significance of obstruction or reflux.[19] Invasive diagnostic methods, including venography and intravascular ultrasonography (IVUS), provide greater details about the hemodynamic significance of venous abnormalities.[19,24,28] Although not generally used in uncomplicated venous disease, venography is indicated in complex disease, multilevel disease, and obstructive disease.[24,25,28]

Obstructive causes of leg symptoms include deep vein thrombosis, postthrombotic syndrome, and nonthrombotic compressive phenomena (May-Thurner syndrome and nonthrombotic iliac vein lesions).[24-27,29-31] While the presence of these conditions can usually be elicited using duplex Doppler, the investigation of their contribution to the patient's symptoms and disease course may require additional testing. The presence of deep vein thrombosis should lead to further investigation into the age, size, and location of the clot, as well as the presence of recanalization.[19] Although contrast venography has traditionally been used to investigate thrombosis, recent advances in noninvasive imaging have led to increased use of cross-sectional applications, including computed tomography (CT) and magnetic resonance (MR) venography. Magnetic resonance venography has the added benefit of not requiring the use of contrast, while showing venous drainage and abnormalities in detail.[19] Both CT and MR venography are useful in evaluating other occlusive conditions, including May-Thurner syndrome and nonthrombotic iliac vein lesions (NIVL).[26,29-31]

Once an NIVL has been identified, treatment is guided by the severity of the resultant venous disease.[27] Symptoms of these lesions may mimic chronic venous insufficiency but may also consist of severe left leg swelling and pain that may interfere with normal activity.[27] In the past, the decision to treat these lesions was based on the results of venography. Over time, it has been noted that the standard views obtained using venography provide an incomplete diagnosis.[27,31] Recently, IVUS has been used to provide a more complete image of the nature of the lesion and can be combined with the placement of a stent to reduce the compressive effect on the iliac vein.[27,31]

While many assessment instruments are valid measures of disease progression,[3] not all are useful in predicting the course of disease or the effect of risk factors. The use of patient-generated symptom-based surveys may provide an indication of trends in symptom reporting following therapy or as the disease worsens but may not be singularly predictive of disease severity.[3] Physician-reported surveys, including CEAP and the VCSS, may be more accurate in predicting disease severity, the influence of risk factors, and the changing course of disease in response to therapy. This is largely due to the more objective nature of the assessment and to reliance on the results of the physical examination, especially with the CEAP classification.[3,11,19,22,24,25] Recent revisions to CEAP include a change to the "C" classification, an update of descriptors, and additional detail in classification and investigation.[11] These have lessened its static nature, making it suitable for use in chronic venous disease diagnosis and follow-up. The CEAP classification has also been shown to correlate well with disease-specific quality-of-life measurements, providing a positive relationship between physician observation and patient-reported severity measurements.[18]

The VCSS was designed as a longitudinal measure of salient features of venous disease and their severity at any point in the course of diagnosis and treatment.[14] Although not specifically designed to be a predictive instrument, it was used and validated in screening a population with a known thromboembolic risk.[10] In this study, the VCSS showed 2 areas of correlation. The results of the VCSS paralleled those of duplex Doppler imaging, scored using the VSDS and VDS. The ability of the VCSS to identify venous disease was assessed based on ultrasonographic scoring. In addition, in cases in which the VCSS was 0, there was a high likelihood (>97%) that no venous abnormality would be identified on Doppler examination.[10] The study by Meissner et al,[14] while not designed to test the predictive ability of the VCSS, found a strong correlation between the VCSS and CEAP scores in ranges of disease severity (ie, CEAP 0, CEAP 2–3, and CEAP 4–6). These studies show the potential of the VCSS as a predictive instrument in evaluating patients for chronic venous insufficiency.

Assessment of Therapy

The treatment of chronic venous insufficiency is multifactorial and depends on many variables. From conservative therapy (weight loss, leg elevation, and the use of compression hose) to direct intervention (open surgery, endovascular therapy, or a combination of the 2), the goals of therapy should be established and agreed on by the patient and the provider.[21,22,32] Patient-generated and physician-generated assessment instruments are useful for this.[17,22,32] At the time of diagnosis, each patient's unique symptoms, physical findings, and laboratory profiles should be considered to determine the most beneficial course of therapy. Other elements come into consideration when deciding on therapy, including insurance constraints and patient compliance with recommendations. Regardless of the initial choice of therapy, patients need to be aware that interventions for venous insufficiency are intended to treat the condition and to prevent its progression, not to provide a cure. Furthermore, all interventions will affect patient lifestyle, from wearing compression hose to practicing general leg hygiene following surgical interventions.[21] While the patient may seek treatment simply to remove unsightly and painful varicose veins, the surgeon understands that obliteration of refluxing veins may be the optimal choice for long-term relief and ultimate satisfaction.[32] Assessment instruments are valuable adjuncts in determining the direction of therapy. Frequently, investigators have used CEAP scoring to guide treatment decisions.[32-36] The use of these instruments has provided a useful perspective on the usual methods of diagnosis and treatment.

In one study,[17] our group looked at a large cohort of patients over 2 years to specifically evaluate VCSS changes during the first 4 months following ablation, the incidence and nature of complications, and factors implicated in treatment failure. CEAP was used at each visit for patient classification, and the VCSS was used and broken down into its components for analysis. This allowed us to analyze outcomes in terms of technical factors, to compare different techniques for ablation, and, possibly most importantly, to understand procedure outcomes in terms of patient expectations. As a result of this study, we were able to communicate better with patients about how their individual needs might be met using the procedure. All components of the VCSS began to decrease immediately after the procedure and continued to decrease for the 4-month follow-up period. Complications were mainly mild and self-limiting; none failed to resolve. When treatment failures were analyzed, we found volume of tumescent anesthesia, male sex, and younger age to be significant variables. Using the VCSS as the sum of its component parts allowed us to evaluate it as a stand-alone method of outcomes assessment. We found it to be useful in this patient cohort.

As the use of endovascular techniques has increased, an area of interest that has arisen is the management of adjunct procedures. With open ligation and stripping, other issues could be addressed in the same setting, including phlebectomy. With endovenous ablation, there are 2 schools of thought, namely, one that adjunct procedures should be performed in the same setting to address all issues and avoid reintervention, and another that adjunct procedures should be delayed to derive the maximum benefit from the initial ablation and obviate reintervention.[37]

Several studies have evaluated the merits of both approaches. Carradice et al[37] randomized patients to concomitant or sequential phlebectomy following endovenous ablation. They found that, although concomitant phlebectomy extended the time needed for the initial procedure, it reduced the need for staged procedures and improved patient quality of life. They used the VCSS, AVVQ, SF-36, and EuroQol instruments to evaluate the outcomes of the initial procedure, with the group receiving concomitant adjunct phlebectomy scoring significantly lower on the VCSS at 3 months. They found that "if patients do not undergo phlebectomy at the time of EVLT, it takes up to a year to see the same QoL benefits as those who have [concomitant phlebectomy]."[37(p373)] The authors recommend that the choice between sequential and concomitant phlebectomy should be made on a patient-by-patient basis after discussion of expectations, individual varicosities, and the patient's preferences about additional procedures and recovery time.

Welch[38] developed an algorithm to reassess residual varicosities after endovenous ablation. Over the course of follow-up in his patients, he noted that many varicosities that were visible before ablation shrink or disappear following the elimination of saphenous reflux. He demonstrated that, if the initial ablation is successful in addressing the origin of reflux, the patient's symptoms may improve to the point where he or she does not pursue adjunct phlebectomy.

The standard protocol in our group is to delay adjunct phlebectomy for at least 4 to 5 months following initial saphenous ablation.[39] We identified in a follow-up series of 320 patients (427 radiofrequency ablation [RFA] treated limbs) that the majority of the patients (69%) did not require reinterventions for persistent symptoms. Microphlebectomy was the most commonly performed reintervention, and 75% of these patients waited more than 150 days. Subsequent perforator treatment occurred in only 3% of these patients. Interestingly, limbs with higher initial CEAP and VCSS were significantly *less likely* to require further intervention than those with lower initial CEAP and VCSS. Many unnecessary procedures have been avoided through the use of this procedure.

The REVAS (recurrent varices after surgery) study by Perrin et al[40] followed patients presenting with recurrent varicosities after surgery for venous disease. They developed a classification system that works in conjunction with CEAP to identify the area, cause, source, and factors leading to recurrent varices. The information gained from a standardized classification allows collection of relevant data to assist in the decision-making and planning strategy for recurrent varices. The use of this system provides a uniform classification by which to evaluate recurrent varices. Surveillance and future therapy can be planned within a common framework, which facilitates discussion about concomitant vs. staged adjunct procedures.

Treatment of venous disease in its many forms is evolving. New techniques for recently discovered contributory factors are entering the surgical mainstream. The ability to present the results of these interventions in the same way as more established procedures would be beneficial to the provider and to the patient. Familiar and valid current classification systems may prove equally informative in providing a framework for assessing newer techniques. CEAP has undergone a recent revision to make it more sensitive to change in patient status and less static as a measurement device. The VCSS has been revised to increase its relevance as a measure of therapeutic outcomes and to eliminate some elements considered arbitrary.[3] The SQOR-V is a new instrument that is designed to measure patient-reported clinical objectives.[3,8]

CEAP and the VCSS have been used together in numerous studies and were shown to be effective in assessing the severity of venous disease.[41] The VCSS integrates well with the CEAP clinical score, as well as with the results of noninvasive imaging studies.[41] The main drawback with the original CEAP is the static nature of several of its elements, making it less responsive to longitudinal changes in disease progression.[11]

Updating CEAP

In 2001, a committee evaluated the clinical component of CEAP (the "C") to refine the consistency and reproducibility of the instrument in venous disease. Investigations had identified good external consistency but poor internal consistency, as well as good intraobserver reproducibility but poor interobserver reproducibility.[9] The impetus was to increase the accuracy of the clinical class to improve the consistency and reproducibility. This was accomplished by redefining clinical terminology to maintain consistency with the definitions used in the original document. The revisions refined the definitions of telangiectasias, reticular veins, varicose veins, and corona phlebectatica, with specific explanations of the appearance and location of each, including synonyms. Edema, pigmentation, eczema, lipodermatosclerosis, hypodermitis, white atrophy, and venous ulcer are similarly explained in terms of severity and disease significance. The classes are carefully explained in terms of the original CEAP document and the proposed changes.[9] These recommendations were revisited in 2004 when the American Venous Forum International Ad Hoc Committee for Revision of the CEAP Classification[11] began its work. The goal was to refine definitions of chronic venous disease, revisit the "C" class, add the descriptor "n" when no venous disease was identified, provide more information on the date of classification and the level of investigation, and introduce a simpler basic CEAP. These changes were not meant to transform CEAP into an instrument of longitudinal assessment but rather to strengthen its role as a descriptive instrument and to enable it to provide changing descriptions in response to changing disease states. The revisions involving the date of classification allow CEAP to be used repeatedly throughout the course of therapy to reflect disease state alterations. The level of investigation was added to classify disease diagnosis made at the office visit (level 1), the results of noninvasive laboratory testing (level 2), or the findings of invasive testing or complex imaging studies (level 3). A simpler basic CEAP was introduced to clarify some of the classification elements and to make the system readily accessible in clinical practice. The highest descriptive element is used for the "C" classification, and the "E," "A," and "P" are derived from the Doppler examination and are modified with "s," "p," and "d" descriptors for superficial, perforator, and deep. In this way, the relevant revisions to CEAP can be used in a format that allows straightforward, easily reproducible results. The complete version (advanced CEAP) may be most beneficial to researchers, as it allows patients to be grouped and subgrouped based on relevant elements and then reevaluated throughout treatment.[11]

CEAP was recently combined with the REVAS system to provide a classification for patients with chronic venous disease who have undergone an intervention and have recurrent varices. REVAS was designed to define true recurrences, veins with residual reflux, and varicosities resulting from disease progression. In the combined system, the site of recurrence, source of reflux, contributing factors, and cause are classified according to REVAS, while the clinical, etiologic, anatomic, and pathologic patterns are presented according to CEAP. The advanced CEAP classification was used to analyze subgroups of patients scored under REVAS. Before these 2 classifications were combined, there was no common platform for reporting information regarding recurrent varices. Combining REVAS and CEAP disseminates thorough information and allows appropriate reproducible classification of patients with recurrent varices following an intervention for chronic venous disease.[40]

Our group's experience using CEAP as a descriptive instrument was in combination with the VCSS.[17] In a large cohort of patients, we used CEAP and the VCSS from initial diagnosis through long-term follow-up to assess disease states and effects of therapy. CEAP scores were obtained at the first office visit to properly classify patients for an intervention and at each follow-up visit to track changes in classification. The VCSS was obtained before ablation and then at each follow-up visit. The VCSS and CEAP worked well together and in combination with ultrasonographic results to classify and track changes in venous disease throughout the course of therapy.

The VCSS is a physician-assessed measurement of the severity of 9 relevant hallmarks of venous disease. It has been validated in investigations evaluating the outcomes of venous therapy.[41] It has shown good correlation with the results of Doppler imaging and has been determined to be a good diagnostic tool for patients with symptoms of chronic venous disease.[10] Although it was originally presented as a component of the VSS, the VCSS has demonstrated relevance as a stand-alone scoring instrument for venous disease severity.[17] The benefits of the VCSS have been demonstrated, despite its limited use as a scoring instrument. Both benefits and shortcomings of the VCSS have been identified. It is acknowledged to provide treatment-driven information on venous disease but with ambiguity in the language of its clinical descriptors.

In 2007, through the American Venous Forum, an international ad hoc working group was created to revise VCSS (Table 2.1). The intention was to update the terminology, simplify the application, and clarify ambiguities. The additional objective was to protect the strengths of the VCSS, while acknowledging the limitations. Revisions to each of the clinical descriptors were made using, where applicable, quality-of-life language. The pain component now contains common patient symptoms (aching, heaviness, fatigue, soreness, and burning) that establish a venous origin. The effect on different types of daily activities is clarified. The varicose veins component has modified the vein size criterion to greater than or equal to 3 mm to maintain consistency with the revised CEAP. Telangiectasias

TABLE 2.1 **Revised VCSS Scoring Template**

	None (0)	Mild (1)	Moderate (2)	Severe (3)
Pain Pain or other discomfort (ie, aching, heaviness, fatigue, soreness, burning); presumes venous origin		Occasional pain or other discomfort (ie, not restricting regular daily activities)	Daily pain or other discomfort (ie, interfering with but not preventing regular daily activities)	Daily pain or discomfort (ie, limits most regular daily activities)
Varicose Veins "Varicose" veins must be ≥3 mm diameter to qualify		Few: scattered (ie, isolated branch varicosities or clusters); also includes corona phlebectatica	Confined to calf or thigh	Involves calf and thigh
Venous Edema Presumes venous origin		Limited to foot and ankle area	Extends above ankle but below knee	Extends to knee and above
Skin Pigmentation Presumes venous origin; does not include focal pigmentation over varicose veins or pigmentation due to other chronic diseases (ie, vasculitis purpura)	None or focal	Limited to perimalleolar area	Diffuse over lower 1/3 of calf	Wider distribution above lower 1/3 of calf
Inflammation More than just recent pigmentation (ie, erythema, cellulitis, venous eczema, dermatitis)		Limited to perimalleolar area	Diffuse over lower 1/3 of calf	Wider distribution above lower 1/3 of calf
Induration Presumes venous origin of secondary skin and subcutaneous changes (ie, chronic edema with fibrosis, hypodermitis); includes white atrophy and lipodermatosclerosis		Limited to perimalleolar area	Diffuse over lower 1/3 of calf	Wider distribution above lower 1/3 of calf

Table 2.1 continues on the following page

TABLE 2.1 **Revised VCSS Scoring Template (continued)**

Number of Active Ulcers	**0**	**1**	**2**	**3 or more**
Active ulcer duration (longest active)	N/A	<3 months	>3 months but <1 year	>1 year
Active ulcer, size (largest active)	N/A	<2 cm diameter	2–6 cm diameter	> 6 cm diameter
Use of Compressive Therapy	**(0)**	**(1)**	**(2)**	**(3)**
	Not used	Intermittent use of stockings	Wears stockings most days	Full compliance: stockings

From Vasquez MA, Rabe E, McLafferty RB, Shortell CK, Marston WA, Gillespie D, et al. Revision of the venous clinical severity score: venous outcomes consensus statement: special communication of the American Venous Forum Ad Hoc Outcomes Working Group. J Vasc Surg. 2010;52(5):1387-96. With permission from Elsevier.

and reticular veins remain without a score; however, corona phlebectatica (ankle flare) has been added to the mild category. The edema component presumes a venous origin and now reflects anatomic distribution and extent. Skin pigmentation has guideline criteria for anatomic distribution and extent and excludes nonvenous causes. Inflammation has been expanded to include more than just recent pigmentation changes or underlying infection. Erythema, cellulitis, venous eczema, and dermatitis have been incorporated, as well as anatomic distribution and extent. Induration has been modified to reflect more severe venous disease. Chronic edema with fibrosis, hypodermitis, white atrophy, and lipodermatosclerosis have been added. The ulcer categories have been refined to include size and duration to reflect the largest and longest active ulcers. The compressive therapy category led to the most discussion and has now eliminated leg elevation to reflect that the category comprises only the wearing of compression garments. This revised VCSS is currently undergoing field testing internationally.[42]

The SQOR-V is another assessment instrument for use in chronic venous disease that is undergoing validity testing. This is a patient-reported instrument that considers information specific to chronic venous disease. It addresses symptoms, cosmesis, effects of disease on daily activities, and concerns about the health risk of venous disease. The focus of the SQOR-V is on the main concern of the patient.[8] This differs from other instruments that focus on symptoms or the presence of particular signs of venous disease. The SQOR-V has been validated in Europe, and our group is using it in a study in combination with the VCSS to validate the English-language version and to assess its usefulness in conjunction with a physician-reported instrument.

Conclusion

As quoted in a chapter on venous disease, Meissner et al comment on the advantages of expanded outcomes assessments: "Bolstering clinical assessment by objective improvement in universally accepted venous tests could have a tremendous impact on venous outcomes assessment. However, this approach requires that the normal range for each venous test parameter be standardized, to allow separation of 'normal' from 'abnormal.' In addition, what constitutes a significant change in each of these parameters also needs to be established, to provide an objective basis for claiming improvement in response to an intervention. Finally, test protocols must be standardized and variability established for this approach to have universal application."[19(p20S)] This is an important consideration in designing and implementing assessment instruments in venous disease. If an instrument is to be valid, it must report meaningful information that can be readily interpreted and applied to various situations across the spectrum of diagnosis and treatment of chronic venous disease.

Our group, like many others over the past several years, has decided to follow our patient outcomes using the primarily physician-generated assessment instruments CEAP and the VCSS. The information we have gained from longitudinal follow-up of more than 2000 patients using these assessment methods has greatly influenced the way we approach the diagnosis and treatment of chronic venous disease. The experience gained from using the initial CEAP and the VCSS has helped us approach treatment options with increased information about patient symptom profiles and expectations. Longitudinal VCSS data have allowed us to evaluate each component over time and to devise strategies to address disease progression, recurrence, or persistent symptoms. We now delay adjunct procedures such as microphlebectomy for at least 4 to 5 months following ablation. The VCSS data indicated that varices improved or became less of a concern to the patient after 3 months. We expect that treatment protocols and options will continue to evolve based on clinical experience and the results of ongoing use of assessment instruments. The recent inclusion of the SQOR-V to assess the patient's most relevant issue will add an important dimension to clinical decision-making. Following our clinical outcomes gives us an objective lens to view what we do. It provides us the opportunity to compare our results to others in a more standardized fashion. We now have the tools we need to truly assess new treatment modalities and make up our own mind as to what is best for our practice and our patients. All we have to do is use them.

References

1. Bergan JJ, Yao JST, Flinn WR, McCarthy WJ. Surgical treatment of venous obstruction and insufficiency. J Vasc Surg. 1986;3(1):174-81.
2. Smith JJ, Garratt AM, Guest M, Greenhalgh RM, Davies AH. Evaluating and improving health-related quality of life in patients with varicose veins. J Vasc Surg. 1999;30:710-9.
3. Vasquez MA, Munschauer CE. Venous Clinical Severity Score and quality-of-life assessment tools: application to vein practice. Phlebology. 2008;23:259-75.
4. Wann-Hansson C, Hallberg IR, Risberg B, Klevsgård R. A comparison of the Nottingham Health Profile and Short Form 36 Health Survey in patients with chronic lower limb ischaemia in a longitudinal perspective. Health Qual Life Outcomes. 2004;2:e9-e20.
5. Launois R, Reboul-Marty J, Henry B. Construction and validation of a quality of life questionnaire in chronic lower limb

venous insufficiency (CIVIQ). Qual Life Res. 1996;5:539-54.

6. Lamping DL, Schroter S, Kurz X, Kahn SR, Abenhaim L. Evaluation of outcomes in chronic venous disorders of the leg: development of a scientifically rigorous, patient-reported measure of symptoms and quality of life. J Vasc Surg. 2003;37:410-9.
7. Smith JJ, Guest MG, Greenhalgh RM, Davies AH. Measuring the quality of life in patients with venous ulcers. J Vasc Surg. 2000;31:642-9.
8. Guex JJ, Zimmet SE, Boussetta S, Nguyen C, Taieb C. Construction and validation of a patient-reported outcome dedicated to chronic venous disorders: SQOR-V (Specific Quality of Life and Outcome Response–Venous). J Mal Vasc. 2007;32:135-47.
9. Allegra C, Antignani PL, Bergan JJ, Carpentier PH, Coleridge-Smith P, Cornu-Thénard A, et al. International Union of Phlebology Working Group. The "C" of CEAP: suggested definitions and refinements: an International Union of Phlebology conference of experts. J Vasc Surg. 2003;37:129-31.
10. Ricci MA, Emmerich J, Callas PW, Rosendaal FR, Stanley AC, Naud S, et al. Evaluating chronic venous disease with a new venous severity scoring system. J Vasc Surg. 2003;38:909-15.
11. Eklöf B, Rutherford RB, Bergan JJ, Carpentier PH, Gloviczki P, Kistner RL, et al. American Venous Forum International Ad Hoc Committee for Revision of the CEAP Classification. Revision of the CEAP classification for chronic venous disorders: consensus statement. J Vasc Surg. 2004;40:1248-52.
12. Rutherford RB, Padberg FT, Comerota AJ, Kistner RL, Meissner MH, Moneta GL. Venous severity scoring: an adjunct to venous outcome assessment. J Vasc Surg. 2000;31:1307-12.
13. Kakkos SK, Rivera MA, Matsagas MI, Lazarides MK, Robless P, Belcaro G, Geroulakos G. Validation of the new venous severity scoring system in varicose vein surgery. J Vasc Surg. 2003;38:224-8.
14. Meissner MH, Natiello C, Nicholls SC. Performance characteristics of the venous clinical severity score. J Vasc Surg. 2002;36:889-95.
15. Hartung O, Otero A, Boufi M, Decaridi G, Barthelemy P, Juhan C, et al. Mid-term results of endovascular treatment for symptomatic chronic nonmalignant iliocaval venous occlusive disease. J Vasc Surg. 2005;42:1138-44.
16. Masuda EM, Kessler DM, Lurie F, Puggioni A, Kistner RL, Eklöf B. The effect of ultrasound-guided sclerotherapy of incompetent perforator veins on venous clinical severity and disability scores. J Vasc Surg. 2006;43:551-7.
17. Vasquez MA, Wang J, Mahathanaruk M, Buczkowski G, Sprehe E, Dosluoglu HH. The utility of the Venous Clinical Severity Score in 682 limbs treated by radiofrequency saphenous ablation. J Vasc Surg. 2007;45:1008-15.
18. Kahn SR, M'lan CE, Lamping DL, Kurz X, Bérard A, Abenhaim LA; VEINES Study Group. Relationship between clinical classification of chronic venous disease and patient-reported quality of life: results from an international cohort study. J Vasc Surg. 2004;39:823-8.
19. Meissner MH, Moneta G, Burnand K, Gloviczki P, Lohr JM, Lurie F, et al. The hemodynamics and diagnosis of venous disease. J Vasc Surg. 2007;46(suppl S):4S-24S.
20. Rutherford RB. Presidential address: vascular surgery: comparing outcomes. J Vasc Surg. 1996;23:5-17.
21. Carr SC. Current management of varicose veins. Clin Obstet Gynecol. 2006;49(2): 414-26.
22. Chiesa R, Marone EM, Limoni C, Volonte M, Petrini O. Chronic venous disorders: correlation between visible signs, symptoms,

and presence of functional disease. J Vasc Surg. 2007;46:322-30.

23. Eklöf B, Perrin M, Delis KT, Rutherford RB, Gloviczki P. Updated terminology of chronic venous disorders: the VEIN-TERM transatlantic interdisciplinary consensus document. J Vasc Surg. 2009;49:498-501.
24. Meissner MH, Gloviczki P, Bergan J, Kistner RL, Morrison N, Pannier F, et al. Primary chronic venous disorders. J Vasc Surg. 2007;46(suppl S):54S-67S.
25. Meissner MH, Eklöf B, Coleridge Smith P, Dalsing MC, DePalma RG, Gloviczki P, et al. Secondary chronic venous disorders. J Vasc Surg. 2007;46(suppl S):68S-83S.
26. Neglén P, Thrasher TL, Raju S. Venous outflow obstruction: an underestimated contributor to chronic venous disease. J Vasc Surg. 2003;38:879-85.
27. Raju S, Neglén P. High prevalence of nonthrombotic iliac vein lesions in chronic venous disease: a permissive role in pathogenicity. J Vasc Surg. 2006;44:136-44.
28. Porter JM, Rutherford RB, Clagett GP, Cranley JJ Jr, O'Donnell TF, Raju S, et al. Reporting standards in venous disease. J Vasc Surg. 1988;8:172-81.
29. Neglén P, Hollis KC, Raju S. Combined saphenous ablation and iliac stent placement for complex severe chronic venous disease. J Vasc Surg. 2006;44:828-33.
30. Neglén P, Hollis KC, Olivier J, Raju S. Stenting of the venous outflow in chronic venous disease: long-term stent-related outcome, clinical, and hemodynamic result. J Vasc Surg. 2007;46:979-90.
31. Neglén P, Raju S. Intravascular ultrasound scan evaluation of the obstructed vein. J Vasc Surg. 2002;35:694-700.
32. Lurie F, Creton D, Eklöf B, Kabnick LS, Kistner RL, Pichot O, et al. Prospective randomized study of endovenous radiofrequency obliteration (closure procedure) versus ligation and stripping in a selected patient population (EVOLVeS study). J Vasc Surg. 2003;38(2):207-14.
33. Huang Y, Jiang M, Li W, Lu X, Huang X, Lu M. Endovenous laser treatment combined with a surgical strategy for treatment of venous insufficiency in lower extremity: a report of 208 cases. J Vasc Surg. 2005;42:494-501.
34. Kalteis M, Berger I, Messie-Werndl S, Pistrich R, Schimetta W, Pölz W, et al. High ligation combined with stripping and endovenous laser ablation of the great saphenous vein: early results of a randomized controlled study. J Vasc Surg. 2008;47:822-9.
35. Rasmussen LH, Bjoern L, Lawaetz M, Blemings A, Lawaetz B, Eklöf B. Randomized trial comparing endovenous laser ablation of the great saphenous vein with high ligation and stripping in patients with varicose veins: short-term results. J Vasc Surg. 2007;46:308-15.
36. Pittaluga P, Chastanet S, Guex JJ. Great saphenous vein stripping with preservation of sapheno-femoral confluence: hemodynamic and clinical results. J Vasc Surg. 2008;47:1300-5.
37. Carradice D, Mekako AI, Hatfield J, Chetter IC. Randomized clinical trial of concomitant or sequential phlebectomy after endovenous laser therapy for varicose veins. Br J Surg. 2009;96:369-75.
38. Welch H. Endovenous ablation of the great saphenous vein may avert phlebectomy for branch varicose veins. J Vasc Surg. 2006;44:601-5.
39. Vasquez MA, Wang J, Munschauer CE, Buczkowski G, Sprehe E, Dosluoglu HH. Adjunct procedures following radiofrequency ablation of the saphenous vein: incidence and timing. Presented American Venous Forum February 2009. Submitted J Vasc Surg.
40. Perrin MR, Labropoulos N, Leon LR Jr. Presentation of the patient with recurrent varices after surgery (REVAS). J Vasc Surg. 2006;43:327-34.

41. Kundu S, Lurie F, Millward SF, Padberg F, Vedantham S, Elias S, Khilnani NM, et al. Recommended reporting standards for endovenous ablation for the treatment of venous insufficiency: Joint Statement of the American Venous Forum and the Society of Interventional Radiology. J Vasc Surg. 2007;46:582-9.

42. Vasquez MA, Rabe E, McLafferty RB, Shortell CK, Marston WA, Gillespie D, et al. Revision of the venous clinical severity score: venous outcomes consensus statement: special communication of the American Venous Forum Ad Hoc Outcomes Working Group. J Vasc Surg. 2010;52(5):1387-96.

CHAPTER 3

Duplex Imaging of Varicose Veins

R. Eugene Zierler

The availability of endovenous treatment options, such as laser and radiofrequency ablation, has led to renewed interest in the objective evaluation of lower extremity varicose veins. While the superficial and deep veins can be imaged by magnetic resonance, computed tomography, and invasive contrast studies, from a practical point of view duplex scanning is the preferred method for venous imaging. This chapter reviews the role of duplex ultrasonography in the evaluation of varicose veins and chronic venous insufficiency.

Chronic Venous Insufficiency. Contemporary Endovascular Management series. © 2011 Mark G. Davies MD and Alan B. Lumsden MD, eds. Cardiotext Publishing, ISBN 978-1-935395-09-6.

Goals of Varicose Vein Imaging

Primary varicose veins are dilated and tortuous superficial veins that occur in the absence of any coexisting deep venous abnormalities, while *secondary* varicose veins are associated with obstruction or incompetence in the deep venous system. *Recurrent* varicose veins are those that reappear after treatment. Since the classification of varicose veins is an important consideration in planning therapy and predicting the outcome of treatment, the evaluation of varicose veins must include both the superficial and deep veins, as well as the perforating veins. The perforating veins may become primarily incompetent, similar to the superficial veins, or they may develop reflux secondary to deep venous obstruction. If the deep veins are normal by ultrasonography, a diagnosis of primary varicose veins is confirmed, and the results of intervention on the abnormal superficial veins should be favorable.

Based on these considerations, varicose vein imaging must address the following key points:

- The presence of obstruction or reflux in the deep veins of the lower extremity
- Great saphenous vein obstruction or reflux
- Small saphenous vein obstruction or reflux
- The location and extent of any branch varicose veins
- The locations of any incompetent perforating veins

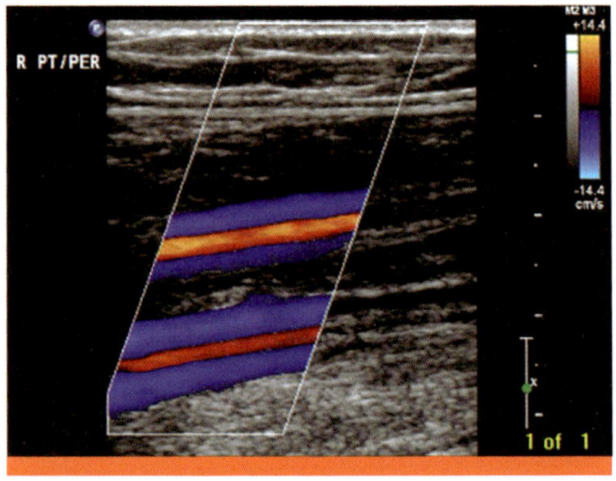

FIGURE 3.1 Longitudinal color-flow image of normal paired posterior tibial and peroneal veins (shown in blue) and arteries (shown in red).

Imaging Protocol

When a duplex scan is done for suspected acute deep vein thrombosis, the goal is to detect obstruction in the deep venous system. This is a component of the duplex examination for varicose veins, but the testing protocol must also include the superficial and perforating veins. In addition, a detailed evaluation for reflux in the deep and superficial veins must be performed.

Instrumentation

A standard duplex ultrasonography system with high-resolution B-mode imaging, pulsed Doppler spectral waveform analysis, and color-flow imaging is adequate for lower extremity venous scanning. Color-flow imaging facilitates the duplex examination by aiding in the rapid identification of arteries and veins, thus decreasing the overall time required, particularly for the tibial vessels (Figure 3.1). A variety of transducers is needed for a complete lower extremity venous duplex examination. Low-frequency transducers (2–3 MHz) are best for evaluating the inferior vena cava and iliac veins, while a higher-frequency transducer (5–10 MHz) is adequate in most patients for the lower extremity veins. The superficial veins can usually be imaged with high–frequency transducers. In general, the highest frequency transducer that provides adequate depth penetration should be used to obtain the best-quality images.

In addition to a duplex scanner, the standing reflux examination requires specially designed pneumatic cuffs and an automatic rapid cuff inflator. As will be discussed, this equipment provides a standardized stimulus for provoking reflux by rapid inflation and deflation of a cuff distal to the venous segment being evaluated.[1] This produces a physiologic stimulus similar to muscular contraction and relaxation.

Scanning Technique

Patients are generally scanned in the supine position with the head elevated 10° to 20° (reverse Trendelenburg position) and the leg externally rotated. However, the leg position should be varied as needed to provide access to the areas of interest, and a posterior approach with the patient prone can be useful for the popliteal, small saphenous, and muscular calf veins. The examination should include the inferior vena cava and iliac veins when clinically indicated. These segments are frequently obscured by bowel gas, but their status can be inferred based on the Doppler flow patterns in the external iliac and common femoral veins.

Deep Veins

The details of duplex scanning for acute deep vein thrombosis are discussed elsewhere in this book. Briefly, the deep venous segments from the distal external iliac veins to the distal tibial and peroneal veins are evaluated by longitudinal and transverse B-mode imaging, color-flow imaging, and Doppler spectral waveform analysis. Visualization of thrombus or incompressibility of a vein on B-mode imaging are the principal criteria for venous thrombosis (Figure 3.2). The absence of spontaneous flow, absence of respiratory phasicity, and absent or incomplete color filling in a venous segment are additional evidence for the presence of thrombus. Occasionally, focally increased flow velocities may be observed in a venous segment that indicate a site of intrinsic stenosis or extrinsic compression. The sensitivity and specificity of duplex scanning for diagnosis of symptomatic proximal deep vein thrombosis are in the range of 90% to 100%.[2-5] Ultrasound evaluation of the calf veins may be more difficult, with all 3 pairs of calf veins adequately visualized in 60% to 90% of studies.[5,6]

Superficial Veins

Varicose veins are, by definition, superficial veins, so the main purpose of the varicose vein evaluation is to determine the location and extent of superficial venous abnormalities. The principal veins of the medial superficial system of the leg are the great saphenous vein and the anterior and posterior accessory great saphenous veins. The great saphenous vein is located in the saphenous subcompartment of the saphenous fascia, which separates it from other veins in the superficial compartment.[5] This gives the appearance of an "Egyptian Eye" on transverse scanning of the great saphenous vein (Figure 3.3). The saphenofemoral junction is the confluence of the superficial inguinal veins—great saphenous, superficial circumflex iliac, superficial

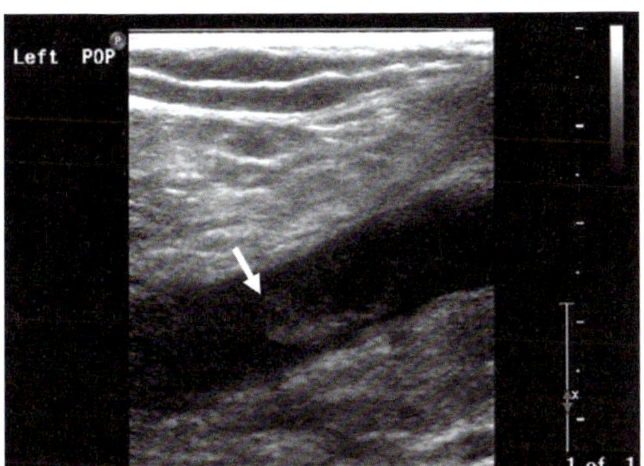

FIGURE 3.2 B-mode image of thrombus in a popliteal vein (see white arrow).

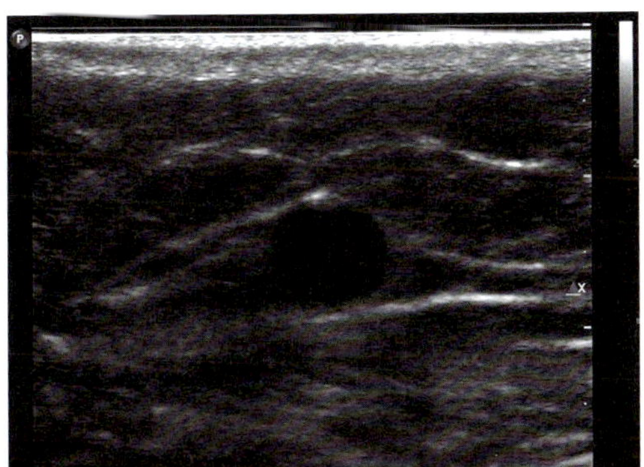

FIGURE 3.3 Transverse B-mode image of the proximal great saphenous vein. The layers of the saphenous fascia around the vein give the appearance of an "Egyptian Eye."

epigastric, and external pudendal—with the common femoral vein.

The small saphenous vein is the main superficial vein on the posterior aspect of the leg. It originates on the lateral side of the foot and joins the popliteal vein, most often just proximal to the level of the skin crease in the popliteal fossa. The intersaphenous vein (formerly referred to as the vein of Giacomini) is a variable branch that extends superiorly from the small saphenous vein near the saphenopopliteal junction to join with a posteromedial branch of the great saphenous system.

The great and small saphenous veins and their branches are scanned for evidence of thrombosis, wall-thickening, and varicosities. As for the deep venous evaluation, visualization of thrombus within the vein lumen or incompressibility on B-mode imaging are the key findings (Figure 3.4). Doppler spectral waveforms and color-flow imaging are used to document venous patency. Varicose veins are recognized as dilated, tortuous superficial veins that may appear in "nests" or "clusters" (Figure 3.5). If necessary, superficial vein diameters can be measured on a transverse view (Figure 3.6). When intervention is planned, the procedure is facilitated by marking the abnormal great and small saphenous veins and varicose branches on the skin.

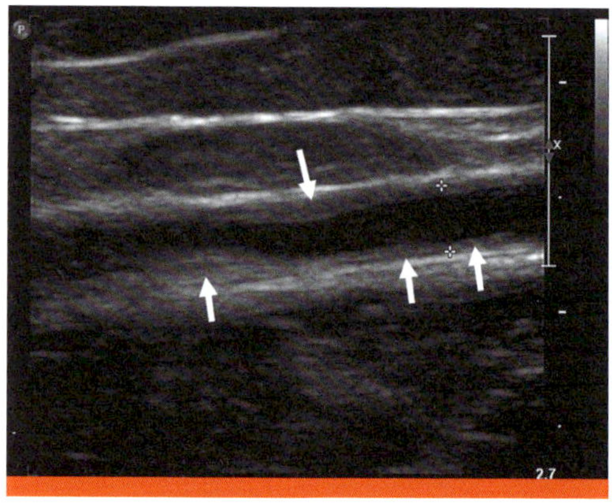

FIGURE 3.4 Longitudinal B-mode image of a great saphenous vein with mural thrombus and wall thickening (see white arrows).

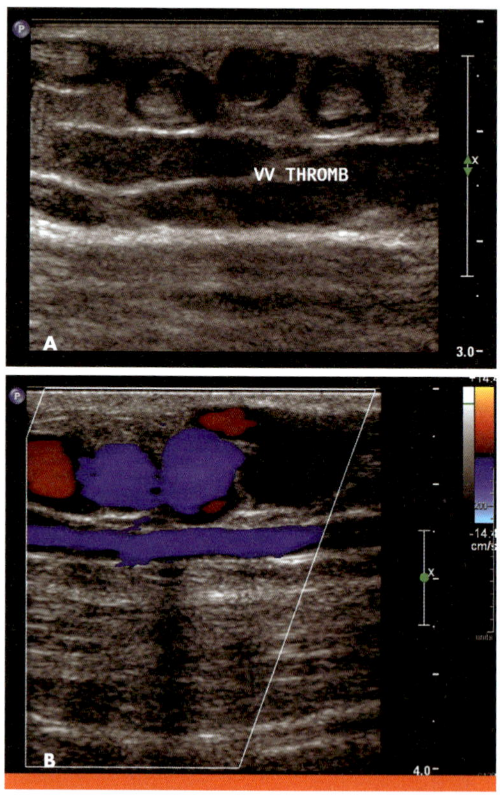

FIGURE 3.5 Cluster of great saphenous branch varicose veins. **A.** B-mode image shows varices in both transverse and longitudinal sections, with thrombus partially filling the lumen. **B.** Color-flow image confirms patency in some of the varicose branches.

Perforating Veins

The perforating veins pass through the muscular fascia and serve as conduits between the superficial and deep veins of the leg. Flow direction in the perforating veins is normally unidirectional from superficial to deep in the thigh and calf; however, bidirectional flow is considered normal in the perforating veins in the foot. When the perforating veins in the leg become incompetent, they dilate and allow high pressure in the deep veins

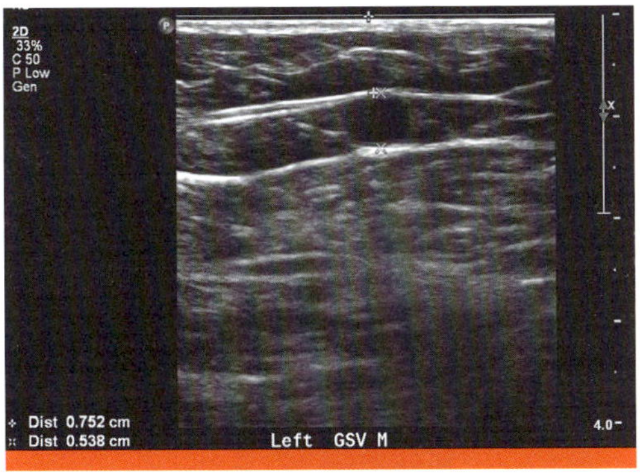

FIGURE 3.6 Diameter measurement of a left great saphenous vein at mid-thigh level. Electronic calipers on this transverse B-mode image indicate that the vein is 0.75 cm from the skin surface and is 0.54 cm in diameter.

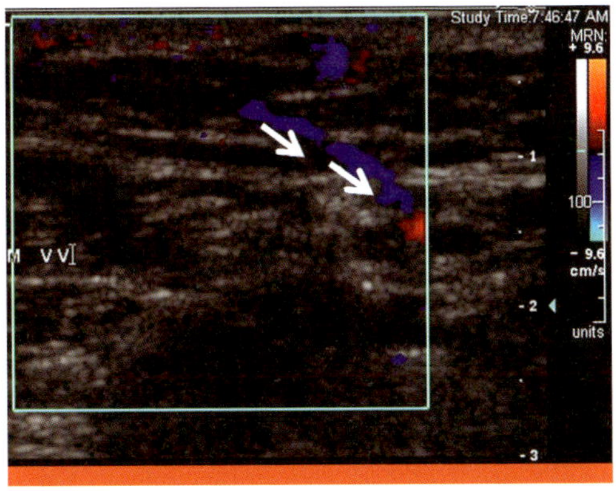

FIGURE 3.7 Color-flow image of a perforating vein. The vein is shown in blue passing through the muscular fascia, with flow direction from superficial to deep (white arrows).

to be transmitted to the superficial veins. This contributes to venous congestion in the superficial tissues, varicose veins, and eventually skin changes such as hyperpigmentation and ulceration. The most important perforating veins in the lower extremity are those on the medial side of the calf. These include the posterior tibial perforators, which connect the posterior accessory great saphenous vein and the posterior tibial veins, and the paratibial perforators joining the main great saphenous vein and the posterior tibial veins. Perforating veins in the adductor canal connect the great saphenous vein to the femoral vein in the distal medial thigh.

The perforating veins are visualized on duplex scanning as venous branches that penetrate the deep fascia. Color-flow imaging is particularly helpful in identification of perforating veins (Figure 3.7). Direction of flow within the perforators is determined by compression maneuvers, and reflux is defined as net flow from the deep to superficial veins. The number, size, and location of perforating veins is noted during the duplex scan, and these can be marked on the skin prior to intervention.

Reflux Evaluation

Successful interventions for varicose veins depend on eradication of all sources of reflux in the superficial venous system. Reliable identification of venous reflux depends on the method used to elicit reflux during testing. Historically, descending venography and ambulatory venous pressure measurements have been used to document the location and severity of venous reflux.[5] However, these methods are invasive and limited in their ability to precisely localize sites of valvular incompetence. Photoplethysmography (PPG) and air plethysmography (APG) are noninvasive techniques for assessing venous reflux, but these also provide mainly hemodynamic information and do not help to identify specific sites of reflux. Duplex scanning is the most clinically useful test for localizing sites of venous reflux and obstruction in the lower extremity. The combination of physiologic testing and duplex scanning provides complementary information on the overall severity and anatomic sites of venous disease.

Valsalva's maneuver and manual compressions of the leg with the patient supine have been compared with pneumatic cuff deflation in the standing position for eliciting venous reflux in the vascular laboratory.[1,7] The standing position is theoretically preferable for evaluating valvular incompetence because it simulates the physiologic conditions in which pathologic reflux occurs. These comparisons have shown that both Valsalva's maneuver and manual limb compressions can provoke reflux, but the results are variable and impossible to standardize or quantify. In addition, physiologic valve closure requires a reverse flow velocity of >30 cm/s.[8] Velocities of this magnitude are not reliably produced by manual limb compression, and they are only achieved in the most proximal levels of the lower limb by Valsalva's maneuver. Distal cuff deflation in the standing position provides a reproducible and quantitative method for assessing valvular incompetence by measuring the duration of venous reflux at various levels in the lower limb.

For the standing reflux examination, the patient is asked to stand with the leg being studied relaxed and their weight supported by the contralateral leg (Figure 3.8). This position is facilitated by using a platform with hand rails that allows the study leg to dangle, or having the patient hold on to a bed rail or other convenient support. Reflux can be evaluated at multiple levels in the leg, depending on the clinical status of the patient, with a pneumatic cuff placed immediately distal to the venous segment of interest. Typical segments tested include the common femoral, proximal great saphenous, femoral, popliteal, proximal small saphenous, posterior tibial, and peroneal veins. For each level, the cuff width should be approximately equal to the diameter of the limb to reliably compress the veins, particularly in the larger limb segments such as the thigh. A tapered thigh cuff (18–24 cm wide) is used for the common femoral, great saphenous, and femoral veins, while a smaller straight calf cuff (11–13 cm wide) is used for the popliteal, small saphenous, and tibial veins. A narrow cuff (7–8 cm) can be applied around the foot to assess the distal tibial veins.

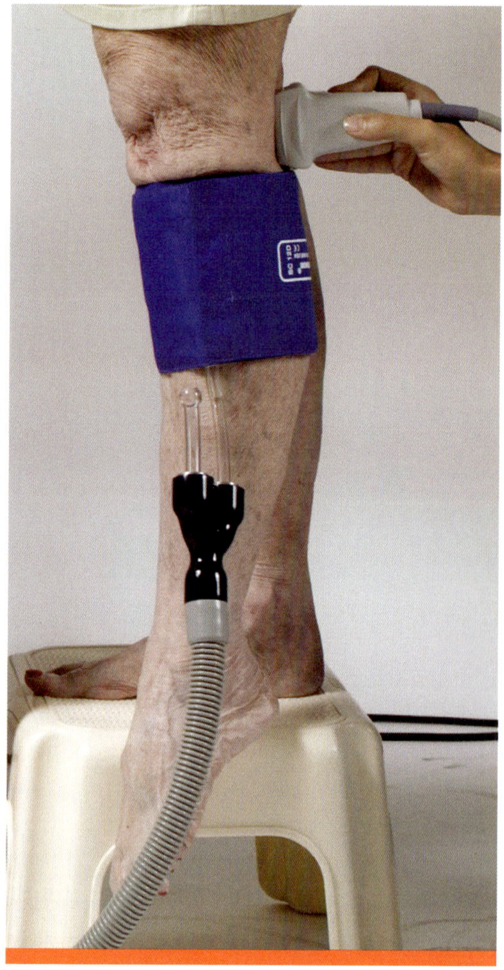

FIGURE 3.8 Standing reflux examination of the left leg. The patient is standing on a stool with body weight on the right leg and the left leg dangling. The duplex transducer and cuff are positioned for evaluating the popliteal vein segment. Photograph courtesy of D. E. Hokanson, Inc., Bellevue, WA.

For each measurement, the appropriate duplex transducer is placed 5 cm or less proximal to the cuff, with the venous segment imaged in a longitudinal view (Figure 3.8). The Doppler sample volume is placed in the lumen of the vein, and the venous flow pattern is monitored during cuff inflation and deflation by spectral waveform analysis. To compensate for the venous hydrostatic pressure in the standing position, maximal cuff inflation pressures are 80 mm Hg for the thigh, 100 mm Hg for the calf, and 120 mm Hg for the foot. An automatic cuff inflator is used to inflate the cuff over about 3 seconds, and then deflate it within 0.3 seconds. This rapid inflation/deflation sequence is necessary to simulate muscular activity and generate a sufficient reverse pressure gradient to assess venous reflux.

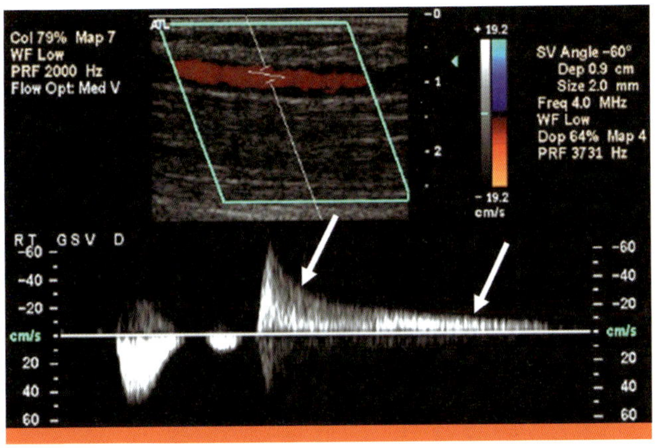

FIGURE 3.10 Doppler spectral waveform from a standing reflux examination of an incompetent great saphenous vein. There is a prolonged phase of retrograde flow (>0.5 second) following rapid cuff deflation (see white arrows).

The normal response to rapid distal cuff inflation and deflation in a competent venous segment is prompt valve closure with no prolonged phase of reflux flow (Figure 3.9). In general, valve closure normally occurs within 0.5 second or less, so reflux flow that persists for >0.5 second is usually indicative of valvular incompetence (Figure 3.10).[7] However, the duration of abnormal reverse flow may not be the same for all venous segments, and the thresholds for significant reflux listed in Table 3.1 have been suggested.[9]

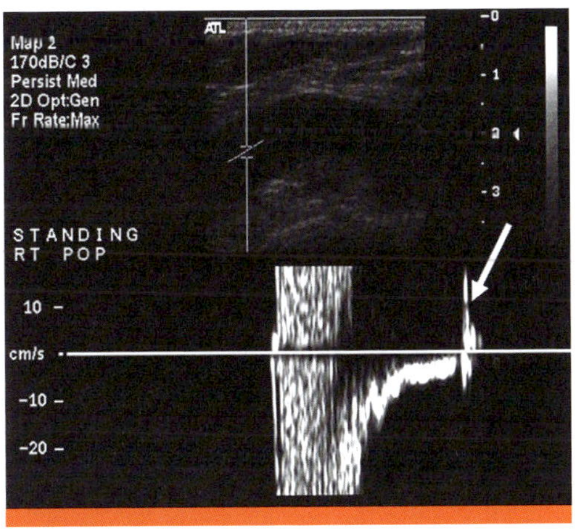

FIGURE 3.9 Doppler spectral waveform from a standing reflux examination of a competent popliteal vein. There is prompt valve closure and no prolonged retrograde flow on rapid cuff deflation (see white arrow).

TABLE 3.1 **Reflux Thresholds**

Venous Segment	Reflux Threshold (milliseconds)
Common femoral	>1000
Great saphenous	>500
Femoral	>1000
Popliteal	>1000
Small saphenous	>500
Tibial	>500
Perforators	>350

Thresholds for abnormal duration of reverse flow (valvular incompetence or reflux) in various lower extremity venous segments during the standing reflux examination. From Labropoulos N, Tiongson J, Pryor L, Tassiopoulos AK, Kang SS, Ashraf Mansour M, et al, 2003. With permission from Elsevier.

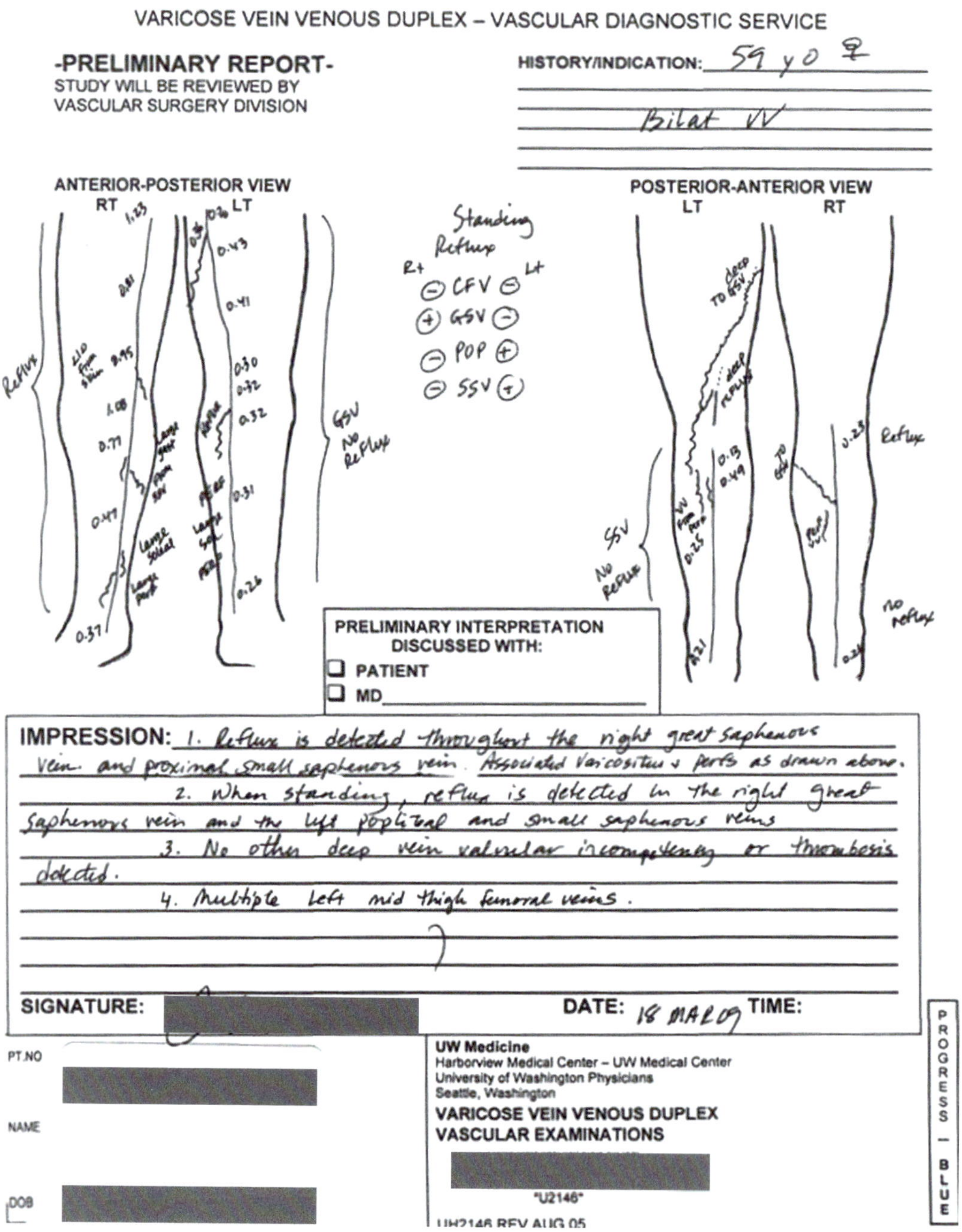

VARICOSE VEIN VENOUS DUPLEX – VASCULAR DIAGNOSTIC SERVICE

-PRELIMINARY REPORT-
STUDY WILL BE REVIEWED BY
VASCULAR SURGERY DIVISION

HISTORY/INDICATION: 59 y o ♀
Bilat VV

ANTERIOR-POSTERIOR VIEW
RT LT

POSTERIOR-ANTERIOR VIEW
LT RT

Standing Reflux
Rt Lt
⊖ CFV ⊖
⊕ GSV ⊖
⊖ POP ⊕
⊖ SSV ⊕

PRELIMINARY INTERPRETATION
DISCUSSED WITH:
☐ PATIENT
☐ MD

IMPRESSION: 1. Reflux is detected throughout the right great saphenous vein and proximal small saphenous vein. Associated varicosities & perfs as drawn above.
2. When standing, reflux is detected in the right great saphenous vein and the left popliteal and small saphenous veins.
3. No other deep vein valvular incompetency or thrombosis detected.
4. Multiple left mid thigh femoral veins.

SIGNATURE: DATE: 18 MAR 09 TIME:

PT.NO

NAME

DOB

UW Medicine
Harborview Medical Center – UW Medical Center
University of Washington Physicians
Seattle, Washington
VARICOSE VEIN VENOUS DUPLEX
VASCULAR EXAMINATIONS
"U2146"
UH2146 REV AUG 05

PROGRESS – BLUE

FIGURE 3.11 Example of a technologist worksheet from a varicose vein evaluation.

Varicose Vein Imaging and Outcomes

Figure 3.11 is an example of a technologist worksheet from a varicose vein evaluation in the vascular laboratory. The data recorded include all components of the examination—the deep veins, superficial veins, and perforating veins, as well as the standing reflux evaluation. Hand drawings are extremely useful for summarizing the test results and planning treatment. Clinical benefit from interventions for varicose veins depends on eliminating both the sources of venous reflux and the symptomatic varicosities. Since these abnormalities may be difficult to characterize by history and physical examination alone, identifying and localizing these abnormalities preoperatively should result in better outcomes.

In a review of 2036 lower limbs with primary varicose veins evaluated by duplex scanning, reflux was found at the confluence of the great saphenous vein with the common femoral vein in 1330 limbs (65%).[10] However, the presence of reflux at the level of the groin did not rule out other sources of significant reflux in that extremity. Reflux was noted in the popliteal fossa in 237 (11.6%) of the limbs. Most of these cases involved the confluence of the small saphenous vein with the popliteal vein, but reflux involving the intersaphenous vein and gastrocnemius veins was also observed. Incompetence was found in 238 perforating veins, with 85 (36%) of these located on the medial thigh.

The role of duplex scanning prior to varicose vein surgery was investigated in a randomized trial of 293 patients with 343 treated legs.[11] Preoperative duplex scanning was performed in 166 legs (group 1), and no preoperative imaging was done in 177 legs (group 2). In 44 of the legs from group 1 (27%), the duplex examination provided information that was not available from the clinical evaluation, and this resulted in a change in the surgical plan in 29 legs. After 2 months of follow-up, 14 legs in group 1 (8%) and 44 legs in group 2 (25%) were found to have superficial venous incompetence. At 2 years following surgery, there were 2 legs in group 1 (1%) and 14 legs in group 2 (8%) that required reoperations. Major incompetence was noted in 19 group 1 legs (11%) and 53 group 2 legs (30%). All the differences between group 1 and group 2 during follow-up are statistically significant. These findings support the conclusion that routine use of duplex scanning prior to interventions for primary varicose veins improves long-term outcomes. Duplex scanning is also helpful in determining the cause of recurrent varicose veins after treatment.

References

1. Van Bemmelen PS, Bedford G, Beach KW, Strandness DE. Quantitative segmental evaluation of venous valvular reflux with duplex ultrasound scanning. J Vasc Surg. 1989;10:425-31.
2. White RH, McGahan JP, Daschbach MM, Hartling RP. Diagnosis of deep-vein thrombosis using duplex ultrasound. Ann Intern Med. 1989;111:297-304.
3. Kearon C, Julian JA, Newman TE, Ginsberg JS. Noninvasive diagnosis of deep venous thrombosis. McMaster Diagnostic Imaging Practice Guidelines Initiative. Ann Intern Med. 1998;128:663-77.
4. Becker D, Philbrick J, Abbitt P. Real-time ultrasonography for the diagnosis of lower extremity deep venous thrombosis. Arch Intern Med. 1989;149:1731-4.
5. Meissner MH, Moneta GM, Burnand K, Gloviczki P, Lohr JM, Lurie F. The hemodynamics and diagnosis of venous disease. J Vasc Surg. 2007;46:4S-24S.

6. Atri M, Herba MJ, Reinhold C, Leclerc J, Ye S, Illescas FF, et al. Accuracy of sonography in the evaluation of calf deep vein thrombosis in both postoperative surveillance and symptomatic patients. Am J Roentgenol. 1996;166:1361-7.
7. Markel A, Meissner MH, Manzo RA, Bergelin RO, Strandness DE Jr. A comparison of the cuff deflation method with Valsalva's maneuver and limb compression in detecting venous valvular reflux. Arch Surg. 1994;129:701-5.
8. Van Bemmelen PS, Beach KW, Bedford G, Strandness DE Jr. The mechanism of venous valve closure. Arch Surg. 1990;125:617-9.
9. Labropoulos N, Tiongson J, Pryor L, Tassiopoulos AK, Kang SS, Ashraf Mansour M, et al. Definition of venous reflux in lower-extremity veins. J Vasc Surg. 2003;38:793-8.
10. Garcia-Gimeno M, Rodriguez-Camarero S, Tagarro-Villalba S, Ramalle-Gomara E, González-González E, Arranz MA, et al. Duplex mapping of 2036 primary varicose veins. J Vasc Surg. 2009;49:681-9.
11. Blomgren L, Johansson G, Bergqvist D. Randomized clinical trial of routine preoperative duplex imaging before varicose vein surgery. Br J Surg. 2005;92:688-94.

CHAPTER

4

The Role of Computed Tomography and Magnetic Resonance in Venous Imaging

Jean Bismuth, Dipan J. Shah, and Christof Karmonik

"As, year by year there is an increase in the number of patients operated upon in a more rational matter, so the demands upon x-ray examination of these patients have also risen. Under these circumstances it seems to be of great importance that a method of phlebography be worked out that would be as far as possible informative and reliable and, at the same time, simple of performance."[1]

Today these words remain as true as when they were first written in 1960 by the "godfather" of venography, Gunnar Bauer. The modalities available to image the venous system are abundant, including conventional direct venography, grayscale and Doppler ultrasonography and intravascular ultrasonography as well as magnetic resonance venography (MRV) and computed tomographic venography (CTV). Both MRV and CTV have revolutionized the way we look at the venous system because they readily and reliably demonstrate the structures in question. They allow for large fields of view (FOV), with cross-sectional images that provide superb soft tissue detail and levels of contrast that permit clear delineation between veins and adjacent structures. This is very valuable in identifying extra- or intraluminal filling defects that affect venous structures. Their usefulness becomes even more evident as vascular interventionalists continue to implant more and more devices in the venous system. The sizing and visualization of these devices is as important in the venous system as they are in the arterial. The impact of respiration, cardiac function, and Valsalva's maneuvers on the central venous

Chronic Venous Insufficiency. Contemporary Endovascular Management series. © 2011 Mark G. Davies MD and Alan B. Lumsden MD, eds. Cardiotext Publishing, ISBN 978-1-935395-09-6.

structures is quite pronounced and can profoundly affect the interpretation of venous anatomy. One must be cognizant of this fact when interpreting a diagnostic study. As much as possible, the aim should be in the direction of less invasive imaging. This can be successfully achieved with MRV and CTV, but each modality has its strengths and weaknesses.

It is the goal of this chapter to discuss these advantages and disadvantages and heighten the interest for both imaging techniques. For ease of use, CTV and MRV will be discussed in general terms first, followed by a description based on specific venous pathologies.

Imaging Performance

Some considerations are not readily differentiable between CTV and MRV. These include large FOV, tissue-contrast, and cross-sectional examination. Both can also be performed as indirect or direct venography. Direct venography implies that the limb of interest must be directly injected. This is seen in the situation in which a pedal vein is injected. A leg can also be studied indirectly by performing the contrast injection via an antecubital vein injection. The obvious advantage of injecting through an antecubital vein is avoiding a pedal injection, which can be quite painful and cause phlebitis. The obstacle in more indirect methods is determining the contrast arrival time. Most investigators probably subscribe to the "best guess" technique of determining imaging delay. When imaging the venous system, it is likely safer to err on the side of increased delay. Many variables affect the contrast travel time (ie, age, vascular/cardiac disease, point of injection), but generally one can allow 20 to 25 seconds for a healthy elderly patient, 25 to 35 seconds in patients with cardiac disease or aortic aneurysm, and finally, 40 to 50 seconds in severe cardiac failure.[2] These numbers are hardly absolute as there can be great variations. We have even developed some MRV protocols with delays of up to 40 minutes.

Indirect venography has another important advantage, namely the ability to visualize the pulmonary and systemic vessels concurrently.[3] Beyond these similarities, CTV and MRV each have their peculiarities, as described in the following 2 sections.

Computed Tomographic Venography

In the era of endovascular management of venous disease, computed tomographic venography (CTV) becomes extremely important. A majority of stents and filters being placed in the venous system are metallic and will as such cause flow voids on MRV, making CTV the study of choice. Importantly, CTV also allows for evaluation of the intrastent lumen.

Magnetic Resonance Venography

Magnetic resonance venography (MRV) is probably the modality that people generally avoid, as it often seems quite confusing with the multiple imaging sequence names that are available. However, when we evaluated what we believe to be a physicist's joke on physicians, we were able to utilize MRV as perhaps the most versatile imaging modality for the venous system. It is, of course, quite helpful if one has an MR physicist available to decipher MR language. In its simplest form, the following outline is a good way to explain MRV, as all sequences are minor variations of one another. They are also somewhat dependent on the equipment and software being used in a particular facility (Siemens, General Electric, Philips, Toshiba, etc).

I. Nonenhanced techniques
   A. Flow-independent sequences
      i. Spin echo imaging
      ii. Fast spin echo imaging
      iii. Single-shot turbo SE (HASTE, SSFSE)
   B. Flow-dependent sequences
      i. Time-of-flight imaging
      ii. Phase contrast imaging
II. Contrast-enhanced techniques

Other techniques that can further improve the yield of your MRV study are the application of breath-hold and cardiac gating protocols.

The remainder of this chapter delineates the distinct advantages and disadvantages of MRV and CTV as they pertain to particular clinical situations. We will attempt to give an overview of what we believe to be the most important clinical applications. This section does not claim to be exhaustive, but rather it gives some insight into how CTV and MRV can potentially be used.

Venous Thromboembolic Disease

There is mounting evidence that thrombolytic therapy for acute deep venous thrombosis (DVT) achieves a significantly better short- and long-term clinical outcome than conventional heparin/anticoagulation therapy.[4] Theiss et al showed that patients who presented 3 days, 1 to 2 weeks, and 3 to 4 weeks after the initial presentation of symptoms had complete or partial resolution of their deep venous thrombosis in 95%, 82%, and 69% of cases, respectively.[5] Therefore, thrombus delineation and staging become paramount. Acute venous thrombosis usually presents as a central filling defect within a dilated vessel, while a more chronic or subacute thrombosis will generally show a vessel with a diminutive caliber and variable collateralization. Herein lies the main difference between CTV and MRV, as far as thrombus is concerned. CTV does not have the ability to define the age of a thrombus. An acute thrombus can even be seen on a noncontrast study as a hyperdense mass within the lumen of the vessel or in a contrast study as a filling defect with indirect signs such as soft-tissue enhancement.[3] MRV, on the other hand, has been used to accurately stage a thrombus in a porcine model. This is based on changes in the oxygenation states of the hemoglobin over time, as well as changes in intracellular and matrix protein content and the hydration of cellular components.[6]

Duplex ultrasonography remains the gold standard for detection of DVT, but it has limitations. The studies can be time consuming and are highly technician dependent. Additionally, central veins, including the iliacs, can be challenging to define, and the study does not allow detection of pulmonary emboli (PE). CTV and MRV solve many of these issues in that they can visualize peripheral and central veins and the pulmonary vasculature for PE detection, as well as potentially delineating the cause for DVT (ie, May-Thurner, malignancy) and displaying the extent of collateralization. Duplex ultrasonography has been studied extensively and has been shown to have a high specificity and sensitivity, so in order to replace this study, MRV and CTV have to offer more than just concurrent imaging of the pulmonary vasculature; it needs to be a robust study in its specificity and sensitivity as well.

CTV has been studied quite thoroughly in the Prospective Investigation of Pulmonary Embolism Diagnosis (PIOPED II) study. Actually, the sensitivity and specificity of CTV and sonography were found to be equivalent in diagnosing or excluding DVT.[7] Furthermore, it was found that one could perform a CTV as discontinuous images (every 15.0 mm) as opposed to continuous (every 7.5 mm), while still maintaining a high degree of reliability. The kappa statistic showed good agreement ($\kappa = 0.75$), while reducing pelvic radiation by 75%.[8] Based on these results from the PIOPED II trial, the recommendations for low-, moderate-, and high-probability uses combined CTA/CTV as the initial radiographic study. In a moderate probability clinical assessment, the positive predictive value (PPV) was 92% and 90% for CTA and CTV, respectively. For a high-probability clinical setting, the PPV was 96% for CTA and CTV.[9] Should all patients suspected to have a VTE have a CTA/CTV? It is clear that patients who clinically are less likely to have a DVT have a lower PPV for CTV (57% for the low-probability group in PIOPED II), and therefore one should not resort to ordering a CTA/CTV on all patients with a suspicion of PE/DVT. The proportion of patients with a VTE who are diagnosed on the basis of a positive CTV is 14% on average, but remaining cost-effective should mandate being more restrictive.[10] When comparing MRV to contrast-enhanced venography, Laissy et al found that MRV was 100% sensitive and specific. The differences in sensitivity and specificity as compared to Doppler ultrasonography were nonsignificant, showing noninferiority of MRV.[11]

How then does MR compare to CT for not only diagnosing DVT, but also for the combined evaluation for a VTE and a DVT? In a meta-analysis, it was found that the pooled estimate of specificity and sensitivity were 94.8% and 91.5%, respectively. Furthermore, it was found that the sensitivity and specificity were equivalent for duplex ultrasonography and MRV.[12] Although the numbers are promising, they must be interpreted with caution, as multiple MR sequences were used and the data may therefore not be directly comparable. Nevertheless, investigators are obtaining good results with both nonenhanced and contrast-enhanced MRV for DVT detection, comparable to CTV.[13,14] As far as PE is concerned, a study examined 207 patients with combined studies for DVT/PE. Three thoracic sequences were evaluated (true-FISP, pulmonary perfusion, and thoracic angiography), and pulmonary perfusion was found to be the most robust with a sensitivity 93% to 100% and specificity 91% to 94%.[15] MRV detected DVT in 13 patients with a negative PE study or 17.1% more DVTs, as compared to ultrasonography. CT also showed similar diagnostic accuracy ($\kappa = 0.86$).[15-18] The conclusion must therefore be that MRA/MRV is equivalent to CTA/CTV. The issue for MR remains a question of sequences, and we would recommend a combination of time-of-flight (TOF) sequence and a T1 postcontrast sequence in the acute setting. We have used a TI-600 sequence with significant delays of up to 40 minutes, at which point the only intravascular structure that would be black on imaging would be thrombus. With this technique we have been able to differentiate bland thrombus from tumor thrombus (Figure 4.1).

Varicose Veins

Varicose veins (VV) are extremely common and are estimated to be present in some form in approximately 30% to 60% of adults in the world. The incidence is 13.5 per 1000 person years.[19,20] The general interest for this ailment has increased secondary to the development of less invasive treatment modalities. Currently, the most common diagnostic tool used for evaluation is duplex ultrasonography. This is primarily because ultrasonography is readily available and it provides solid information on the hemodynamics associ-

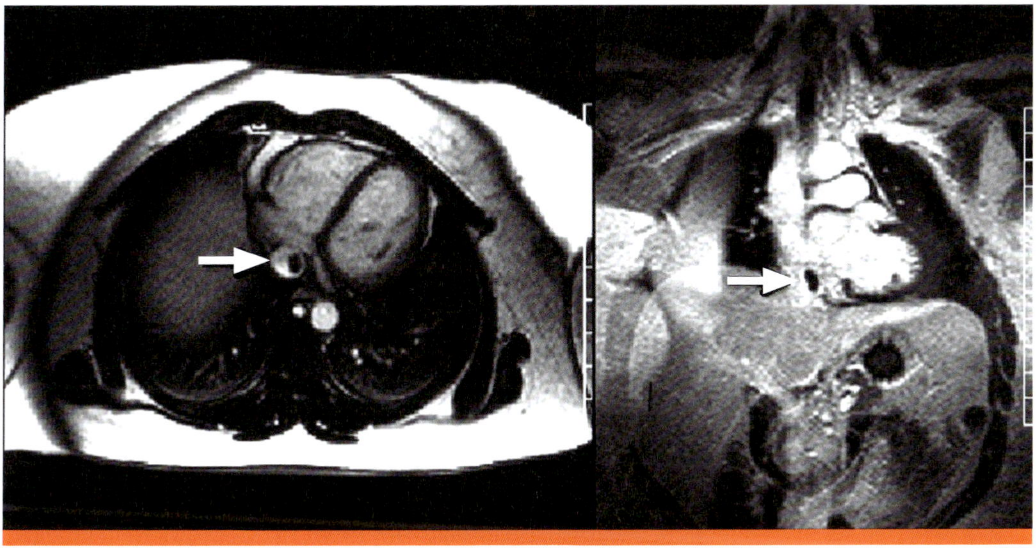

FIGURE 4.1 Delayed magnetic resonance venography for detection of thrombus.

ated with venous reflux. As always, ultrasonography remains technician dependent, and to provide successful management of the venous disease, preoperative evaluation must be able to uncover the root of the varicosities or ulcer (ie, secondary reflux, distribution of varicosity, and perforating veins).[21] Ultrasonography does have one significant limitation that could play a role in recurrence, however—namely, a limited field of view. CTV and MRV can potentially solve that limitation by having large fields of view, allowing visualization of the entire leg.

Lee et al showed in 100 consecutive patients that CTV performed with the patient in the supine position correlated well with ultrasonography findings (κ = 0.72). On CTV, the mean diameter of greater saphenous veins found insufficient at Doppler sonography was 7.0 mm and the mean diameter of greater saphenous veins found competent was 4.9 mm (P <0.001). The sensitivity and specificity of CTV to predict greater saphenous vein insufficiency was 98.2% and 83.3%, respectively.[21] All patients had indirect CTV with instillation of contrast via an antecubital vein and the scan delay was 3 minutes. Uhl et al found CTV particularly useful in mapping the reason for varicose vein recurrence.[22]

As already discussed, the successful management of VV is dictated by thorough preoperative evaluation, which is able to reveal all sources of reflux. Muller et al evaluated the use of direct contrast-enhanced MRV on the management of recurrent lower extremity VVs. Contrast was injected via a pedal arch vein, and veins were considered significant if they were measured as greater than 3 mm. MRV depicted significantly more incompetent veins, which affected management in 77% of legs evaluated. Surgical management of these incompetent veins confirmed MRV findings, and even more importantly 2 independent readers detected the same incompetent veins in all legs examined (κ = 1.00).[23] Likewise, Ruehm et al found direct MRV comparable to conventional contrast-enhanced venography, with a sensitivity and specificity for MRV of VVs of 94% and 96%, respectively.[24] Unenhanced techniques are also available for imaging of lower extremity veins. Edelman et al used signal targeting alternative radiofrequency and flow-independent relaxation enhancement (STARFIRE) to demonstrate the feasibility of MRV in the evaluation of lower extremity veins. The optimal inversion times (TI) were 900 and 1500 msec, because the signal intensity of blood vessels increases as the TI is shortened, as does the fat signal. This also means that fluid or edema will appear white, but this can easily be edited out.[25] The advantage of this technique is again its large FOV, while its major limitation is the lack of hemodynamic feedback.

Venous Malformations

Peripheral vascular malformations often require treatment as they enlarge, causing discomfort, ulceration, and deformity. They can affect the function of a limb. Their prevalence is estimated at 1.5% of the general population,[26] and venous malformations (VM) account for approximately half to two-thirds of all vascular malformations.[27] The management of these anomalies often requires multiple treatments, and it is imperative that accurate preoperative imaging be obtained to secure effective management. This is particularly true, as one needs to differentiate arteriovenous (high-flow) from venous (low-flow) malformations. Low-flow malformations can often be managed by direct percutaneous sclerotherapy, while high-flow malformations do well with transarterial embolization.

The evaluation of malformations is again limited for ultrasonography due to many of the same limitations already mentioned, namely small FOV, operator dependency, and restricted penetration. It is well established in the literature that low-flow lesions can be distinguished from high-flow ones.[28] One of the main attributes that differentiates arterial from venous malformations is flow voids. The absence of flow voids in conjunction with dilated venous spaces is consistent with VMs.[29] Differentiating venous from nonvenous malformations can be done using MRV criteria listed in Table 4.1. In general terms, low-flow malformations are generally of low intensity on T1 imaging while being of high intensity on T2 imaging; this is related to stagnant blood flow in abnormally dilated veins. Consequently, TOF gradient echo sequences are often of little value as flow in the VMs is usually too slow to be evaluated in this sequence. Delayed contrast-enhanced images are more likely to differentiate VMs from other low-flow malformations.[28] In one of the largest series in the literature, MRV was able to provide the correct diagnosis in

Table 4.1

Magnetic Resonance Venography Criteria for Assessment of Venous Malformation[28]

Characteristic	MRI Findings
1. Classification of malformation as high- or low-flow	• Presence or absence of flow voids • Presence or absence of large arterial feeding vessels
2. Description of malformation extent	• Focal • Multifocal • Diffuse
3. Identification of tissue layer involvement	• Skin • Subcutaneous • Muscle • Tendon • Bone

Adapted from Fayad LM, Hazirolan T, Bluemke D, Mitchell S. Vascular malformations in the extremities: emphasis on MR imaging features that guide treatment options. Skeletal Radiol. 2006;35(3):127-137. With kind permission from Springer Science + Business Media.

192 of 196 cases, for a sensitivity of 97.3%, specificity of 91.7%, positive predictive value of 98.7%, and negative predictive value of 84.6%. The protocols used in this series were spin-echo T1-weighted and fast spin-echo T2-weighted.[30]

Pelvic Varices

CTV and MRV can both be used as noninvasive tools to diagnose pelvic varices. They generally appear as dilated and tortuous parauterine tubular structures. One way to differentiate these structures from other pelvic structures is by their appearance, as they are isodense with other venous structures. Due to slow flow in these vessels, as with venous malformations, T1-weighted images often have signal loss, while T2-weighted images are often hyperintense or of mixed signal intensity.[31] The upper limit of normal for pelvic veins is 5 mm, with 8 mm clearly being abnormal and considered a varix.[32] Some arbitrary criteria were developed by Coakley et al to assist in the diagnosis of pelvic varices: (1) at least 4 ipsilateral dilated and tortuous parauterine veins, (2) at least one of these parauterine veins should measure >4 mm in diameter or the ovarian vein should measure >8 mm.[31] Asciutto et al used contrast-enhanced studies to evaluate pelvic varices and found that the sensitivity for detecting pelvic varices was 88%, 100%, and 91%, respectively, for ovarian, hypogastric, and pelvic plexus. Specificity was poor in this study.[33]

Central Venous Structures

Examination of the central venous structures can be critical to evaluate stenoses and occlusions, particularly in patients with superior vena cava syndrome and for the planning and follow-up of central venous and arteriovenous access. Prior papers have described evaluation by direct contrast-enhanced MRV showing excellent sensitivity and specificity of 100%, using conventional venography as a measure.[34-36] Kim et al found that the addition of a time-resolved angiographic maximum intensity projection (MIP) provided significant reader confidence and a sensitivity of 95%.[37] Administration of contrast can often become problematic, however, considering the recent reports of nephrogenic systemic fibrosis in patients with renal insufficiency after use of high-dose gadolinium-based contrast material.

MRV can successfully evaluate the central veins and differentiate between artifactual, benign, and malignant filling defects. Nevertheless, one must be careful as artifactual filling defects of the vena cava can lead to the most common misdiagnosis of clot or "pseudothrombosis." The most common reasons for a reading error are poorly enhanced blood, right heart failure causing reflux into vena cava with engorgement, and refluxing blood into hepatic branches from the renal vein.

For CTV, it is suggested that imaging of the central veins be performed after approximately 210 seconds, as this is the time when opacification was found to be most homogenous.[3] This delay in scanning is also very important because it is able to eliminate some potential flow artifacts, which can make thrombus detection very challenging. Gayer et al found that CTV was particularly useful in young patients with DVT, as at least 5% of these patients had central venous anomalies, which are commonly missed by the usual first-line imaging modality, ultrasonography.[38]

Dynamic MRV

In the section on venous malformations, we did not discuss the value of dynamic MRV

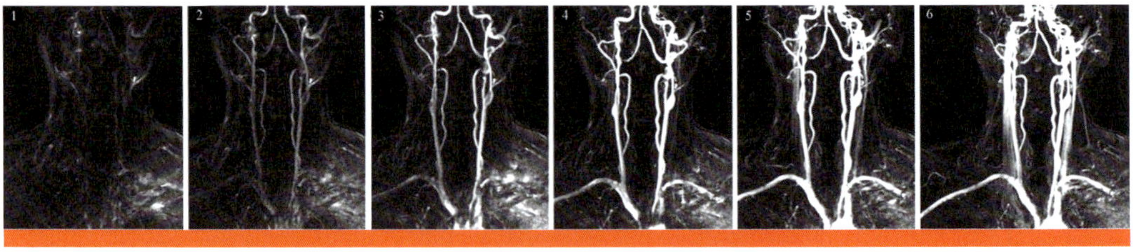

FIGURE 4.2 Time-resolved imaging of contrast kinetics (TRICKS), dynamic flow imaging from arterial to venous beds.

in the detection of AV malformations so that we may present them here. The advantage of dynamic MRV is seen in the contrast-enhanced imaging sequence TRICKS, where one is able to see the transition of contrast from the arterial to the venous side. This can serve as another way of determining the venous and arterial components of a malformation, and since it is contrast-enhanced, there will be no flow voids (Figure 4.2).

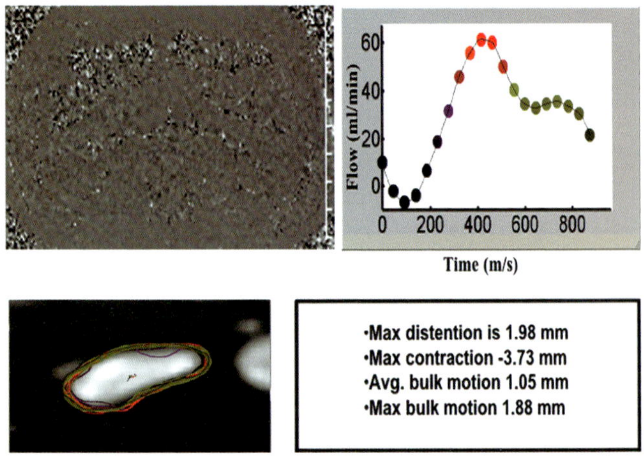

FIGURE 4.3 Phase contrast dynamic magnetic resonance venography of vena cava, with computational fluid dynamics (CFD). Gray-scale image is slice from which CFD measurements are determined.

The value of dynamic imaging in the venous system appears to be ever expanding as we continue to challenge the limits of endovascular therapy in venous disease. Murphy et al presented this concept very well with the use of intravascular ultrasonography (IVUS) to describe the movement of the inferior vena cava (IVC). In their paper, the IVC area changed significantly during the respiratory cycle, from 249 ± 23 to 310 ± 31 mm^2 (P = 0.01), while the IVC diameter significantly increased with Valsalva from 14.3 ± 4.1 to 19.6 ± 1.2 mm (P = 0.0001).[39] We can show the same motion in our dynamic phase contrast MR images (Figure 4.3). Our images were acquired during a breath hold, so we do not have the influence of respiration, nor do we have other parameters such as Valsalva or right-sided heart failure to affect the motion of the IVC. These parameters are well known to have a profound effect on the filling of the IVC, so would it not benefit our endovascular therapy if we took this fourth dimension into account? We believe it would. It could allow for more appropriate sizing of devices before implantation to prevent potentially catastrophic movement of devices.

Conclusion

MRV and CTV have proven to be robust alternative tools to evaluate the venous system. The key to success with these techniques is to understand where and how to use them. This is particularly true for MRV, in which a number of sequencing techniques can be used, each with a very specific role. Using CTV and MRV in some of the clinical situations noted in this chapter can be very straightforward and fruitful if one follows the simple indications outlined. Dynamic imaging adds a new dimension to venous imaging and can lend itself to understanding how movement influences implanted devices, as well as understanding how a number of parameters affect venous filling and hence, diameter.

References

1. Eklof B. The dynamic approach to venous disease—following in the footsteps of Gunnar Bauer and Robert Kistner. J Vasc Surg. 2005;42(2):369-76.
2. Zhang H, Maki JH, Prince MR. 3D contrast-enhanced MR angiography. J Magn Reson Imaging. 2007;25(1):13-25.
3. Rubin GD, Rofsky NM. CT and MR Angiography: Comprehensive Vascular Assessment. Philadelphia: Lippincott Williams & Wilkins; 2008.
4. Schweizer J, Kirch W, Koch R, Elix H, Hellner G, Forkmann L, et al. Short- and long-term results after thrombolytic treatment of deep venous thrombosis. J Am Coll Cardiol. 2000;36(4):1336-43.
5. Theiss W, Wirtzfeld A, Fink U, Maubach P. The success rate of fibrinolytic therapy in fresh and old thrombosis of the iliac and femoral veins. Angiology. 1983;34(1):61-9.
6. Corti R, Osende JI, Fayad ZA, Fallon JT, Fuster V, Mizsei G, et al. In vivo noninvasive detection and age definition of arterial thrombus by MRI. J Am Coll Cardiol. 2002;39(8):1366-73.
7. Goodman LR, Stein PD, Matta F, Sostman HD, Wakefield TW, Woodard PK, et al. CT venography and compression sonography are diagnostically equivalent: data from PIOPED II. Am J Roentgenol. 2007;189(5):1071-6.
8. Goodman LR, Stein PD, Beemath A, Sostman HD, Wakefield TW, Woodard PK, et al. CT venography for deep venous thrombosis: continuous images versus reformatted discontinuous images using PIOPED II data. Am J Roentgenol. 2007;189(2):409-12.
9. Stein PD, Woodard PK, Weg JG, Wakefield TW, Tapson VF, Sostman HD, et al. PIOPED II Investigators. Diagnostic pathways in acute pulmonary embolism: recommendations of the PIOPED II Investigators. Radiology. 2007;242(1):15-21.
10. Stein PD, Goodman LR, Sostman HD. In the era of multislice CT, do we still need leg ultrasonography to diagnose pulmonary embolism? Nat Clin Pract Cardiovasc Med. 2008;5(11):688-9.
11. Laissy JP, Cinqualbre A, Loshkajian A, Henry-Feugeas MC, Crestani B, Riquelme C, et al. Assessment of deep venous thrombosis in the lower limbs and pelvis: MR venography versus duplex Doppler sonography. Am J Roentgenol. 1996;167(4):971-5.
12. Sampson FC, Goodacre SW, Thomas SM, van Beek EJ. The accuracy of MRI in diagnosis of suspected deep vein thrombosis: systematic review and meta-analysis. Eur Radiol. 2007;17(1):175-81.
13. Ono A, Murase K, Taniguchi T, Shibutani O, Takata S, Kobashi Y, et al. Deep vein thrombosis using noncontrast-enhanced MR venography with electrocardiographically gated three-dimensional half-Fourier FSE: preliminary experience. Magn Reson Med. 2009;61(4):907-17.
14. Pedrosa I, Ngo L, Wei J, Schuster M, Mahallati H, Smith M, et al. Dynamic half-Fourier single-shot turbo spin echo for assessment of deep venous thrombosis: initial observations. Magn Reson Imaging. 2009;27(5):617-24.

15. Kluge A, Mueller C, Strunk J, Lange U, Bachmann G. Experience in 207 combined MRI examinations for acute pulmonary embolism and deep vein thrombosis. Am J Roentgenol. 2006;186(6):1686-96.
16. Kluge A, Gerriets T, Stolz E, Dill T, Mueller KD, Mueller C, et al. Pulmonary perfusion in acute pulmonary embolism: agreement of MRI and SPECT for lobar, segmental and subsegmental perfusion defects. Acta Radiol. 2006;47(9):933-40.
17. Kluge A, Luboldt W, Bachmann G. Acute pulmonary embolism to the subsegmental level: diagnostic accuracy of three MRI techniques compared with 16-MDCT. Am J Roentgenol. 2006;187(1):W7-14.
18. Ohno Y, Higashino T, Takenaka D, Sugimoto K, Yoshikawa T, Kawai H, et al. MR angiography with sensitivity encoding (SENSE) for suspected pulmonary embolism: comparison with MDCT and ventilation-perfusion scintigraphy. Am J Roentgenol. 2004;183(1):91-8.
19. Laurikka J, Sisto T, Auvinen O, Tarkka M, Laara E, Hakama M. Varicose veins in a Finnish population aged 40-60. J Epidemiol Commun H. 1993;47(5):355-7.
20. Makivaara LA, Jukkola TM, Sisto T, Luukkaala T, Hakama M, Laurikka JO. Incidence of varicose veins in Finland. Vasa. 2004;33(3):159-63.
21. Lee W, Chung JW, Yin YH, Jae HJ, Kim SJ, Ha J, et al. Three-dimensional CT venography of varicose veins of the lower extremity: image quality and comparison with doppler sonography. Am J Roentgenol. 2008;191(4):1186-91.
22. Uhl JF, Verdeille S, Martin-Bouyer Y. Three-dimensional spiral CT venography for the pre-operative assessment of varicose patients. Vasa. 2003;32(2):91-4.
23. Muller MA, Mayer D, Seifert B, Marincek B, Willmann JK. Recurrent lower-limb varicose veins: effect of direct contrast-enhanced three-dimensional MR venographic findings on diagnostic thinking and therapeutic decisions. Radiology. 2008;247(3):887-95.
24. Ruehm SG, Wiesner W, Debatin JF. Pelvic and lower extremity veins: contrast-enhanced three-dimensional MR venography with a dedicated vascular coil-initial experience. Radiology. 2000;215(2):421-7.
25. Edelman RR, Koktzoglou I. Unenhanced flow-independent MR venography by using signal targeting alternative radiofrequency and flow-independent relaxation enhancement. Radiology. 2009;250(1):236-45.
26. Eifert S, Villavicencio JL, Kao TC, Taute BM, Rich NM. Prevalence of deep venous anomalies in congenital vascular malformations of venous predominance. J Vasc Surg. 2000;31(3):462-71.
27. Breugem CC, Maas M, Reekers JA, van der Horst CM. Use of magnetic resonance imaging for the evaluation of vascular malformations of the lower extremity. Plast Reconstr Surg. 2001;108(4):870-7.
28. Fayad LM, Hazirolan T, Bluemke D, Mitchell S. Vascular malformations in the extremities: emphasis on MR imaging features that guide treatment options. Skeletal Radiol. 2006;35(3):127-37.
29. van Rijswijk CS, van der Linden E, van der Woude HJ, van Baalen JM, Bloem JL. Value of dynamic contrast-enhanced MR imaging in diagnosing and classifying peripheral vascular malformations. Am J Roentgenol. 2002;178(5):1181-7.
30. Lee BB, Choe YH, Ahn JM, Do YS, Kim DI, Huh SH, et al. The new role of magnetic resonance imaging in the contemporary diagnosis of venous malformation: can it replace angiography? J Am Coll Surg. 2004;198(4):549-58.
31. Coakley FV, Varghese SL, Hricak H. CT and MRI of pelvic varices in women. J Comput Assist Tomo. 1999;23(3):429-34.

32. Beard RW, Highman JH, Pearce S, Reginald PW. Diagnosis of pelvic varicosities in women with chronic pelvic pain. Lancet. 1984;2(8409):946-9.
33. Asciutto G, Mumme A, Marpe B, Koster O, Asciutto KC, Geier B. MR venography in the detection of pelvic venous congestion. Eur J Vasc Endovasc Surg. 2008;36(4):491-6.
34. Nael K, Laub G, Finn JP. Three-dimensional contrast-enhanced MR angiography of the thoraco-abdominal vessels. Magn Reson Imaging Clin N Am. 2005;13(2):359-80.
35. Oxtoby JW, Widjaja E, Gibson KM, Uzoka K. 3D gadolinium-enhanced MRI venography: evaluation of central chest veins and impact on patient management. Clin Radiol. 2001;56(11):887-94.
36. Tanju S, Sancak T, Dusunceli E, Yagmurlu B, Erden I, Sanlidilek U. Direct contrast-enhanced 3D MR venography evaluation of upper extremity deep venous system. Diagn Interv Radiol. 2006;12(2):74-9.
37. Kim CY, Mirza RA, Bryant JA, Whiting ED, Delong DM, Spritzer CE, Merkle EM. Central veins of the chest: evaluation with time-resolved MR angiography. Radiology. 2008;247(2):558-66.
38. Gayer G, Luboshitz J, Hertz M, Zissin R, Thaler M, Lubetsky A, et al. Congenital anomalies of the inferior vena cava revealed on CT in patients with deep vein thrombosis. Am J Roentgenol. 2003;180(3):729-32.
39. Murphy EH, Johnson ED, Arko FR. Evaluation of wall motion and dynamic geometry of the inferior vena cava using intravascular ultrasound: implications for future device design. J Endovasc Ther. 2008;15(3):349-55.

CHAPTER 5

Endovenous Radiofrequency Ablation of the Saphenous Vein

Mechanism of Action, Procedural Technique, and Review of Clinical Outcomes

Elizabeth Acquista and Alan M. Dietzek

Venous reflux produces hemodynamic changes including venous hypertension in the lower limb. This in turn can cause surface veins to distend and press against cutaneous sensory nerves, causing significant pain and discomfort for patients. Compression therapy, although effective at reducing short-term pain and discomfort, does not provide a cure for chronic venous reflux. Thus, the fundamental element of successful treatment of symptomatic superficial venous insufficiency in the lower extremities is to eliminate the sources of venous reflux. Treatments for chronic venous insufficiency are documented in historic, surgical literature dated from 450 BC in the writings of Hippocrates through Galen, Celsus, and de Chauliac and later recorded by Harvey and Weisman, who all advocated for compression of the lower extremity to cure ulcers. The sources of reflux most commonly emanate from the great and small saphenous veins, and it was Trendelenbourg who first published on the ligation of the great saphenous vein (GSV). Later, Moore developed the contemporary procedure for GSV ligation just distal to the saphenofemoral junction (SFJ). Most recently, these veins, when incompetent, were entirely removed from the venous circulation primarily with surgical stripping. Presently, endovenous radiofrequency ablation (RFA), also referred to as the closure procedure, a catheter-based endovascular intervention, offers a more effective, less morbid alternative for the treatment of superficial venous reflux. The indications for intervention and the imaging to document reflux have been illustrated in previous chapters.

Chronic Venous Insufficiency. Contemporary Endovascular Management series. © 2011 Mark G. Davies MD and Alan B. Lumsden MD, eds. Cardiotext Publishing, ISBN 978-1-935395-09-6.

Radiofrequency Vein Ablation Procedure

Although surgical removal of the saphenous vein is an effective, time-honored surgical procedure, it causes postoperative morbidity and carries a significant psychological burden to the patient. Endovenous RFA was first introduced into clinical practice in Europe in 1998 and in the United States little more than a year later. The objective of the less invasive endovenous radiofrequency vein ablation is to remove the refluxing saphenous vein from the circulation in a manner that minimizes patient discomfort, decreases postoperative morbidity, provides a good long-term outcome, and allows rapid return to normal activities. Since elimination of the refluxing saphenous vein from the circulation is the only goal of the procedure, judgment of RFA success can be assessed by duplex ultrasonography at any time postoperatively. Relief of patient symptoms, time to resume normal activities, postprocedure adverse events, and improvement in health-related quality of life are additional relevant measures of the procedure outcome, and these are linked to successful elimination of saphenous vein reflux.

The RFA procedure does not require a general anesthetic and can be performed using local tumescent anesthesia with or without conscious sedation. In the United States, it is usually performed in a physician's office or minor procedure room, although some surgeons prefer to perform the procedure on an outpatient basis in a day surgery center. While there are anecdotal reports of saphenous vein stripping being performed in an office setting, it is most commonly performed with general or regional anesthesia in a more formal operating room environment. The technical methodology of the endovenous RFA procedure is described in numerous publications and will be further elaborated upon here.[1,2]

The Closure system (VNUS Medical Technologies, San Jose, CA) consists of a radiofrequency (RF) generator and disposable catheters. The first-generation catheter (Closure PLUS) has collapsible bipolar electrodes (Figure 5.1). When deployed, the electrodes make direct contact with the luminal surface of the vein wall. RF energy is delivered through the electrodes into the vein, and the vein wall tissue resistance converts RF energy into thermal energy. With the RF energy activated, the catheter is slowly withdrawn to treat the desired length of vein. A thermocouple located on the electrodes monitors the temperature and provides feedback to the generator, which, in turn, controls the power delivery and the treatment temperature; the latter is set at either 85°C or 90°C. The thermocouple

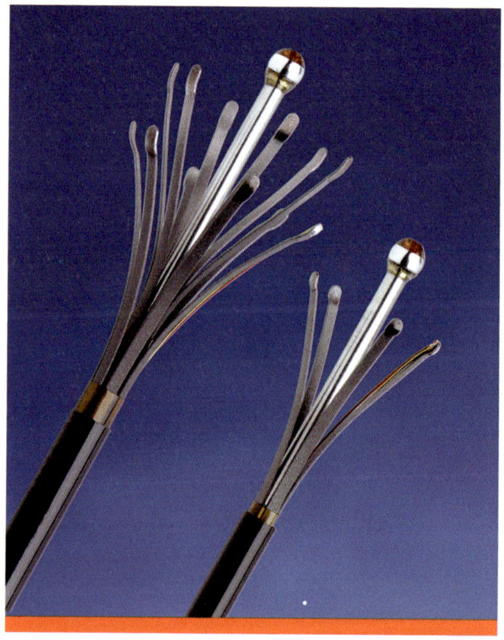

FIGURE 5.1 VNUS Closure PLUS catheter electrodes. VNUS product image copyright ©Covidien. Used with permission.

also monitors impedance, which gives an indication of how well the vein wall contact was established. These parameters are monitored during treatment to ensure that there is effective vein exsanguination and compression for adequate vein wall treatment instead of coagulating blood. Controlled energy delivery is a significant advantage of the RF technology and is believed to contribute to the favorable patient recovery profile when compared with an endovenous laser.

Since April 2006, a second-generation RF catheter (ClosureFAST [CLF]) has been in clinical use. ClosureFAST employs a segmental ablation technique by means of a catheter with a 7-cm coil (heating element) (Figure 5.2) at its terminus instead of the bipolar electrodes that were employed in the first-generation RF catheter. During energy delivery, the catheter remains stationary. The generator heats the catheter to 120°C for a period of 20 seconds. By conductive heat transfer, the vein wall segment in contact with the 7-cm heating element reaches a temperature of 100°C to 110°C. The catheter is then moved distally in 6.5-cm increments, thus achieving a 0.5-cm treatment overlap zone at each treated segment. Although there have been significant changes in the design, the CLF catheter maintains the temperature feedback loop and thus controlled energy delivery. Segmental ablation offers numerous advantages over past methods that employed continuous pullback, as done with prior generations of RF catheters and current laser fibers. By using higher temperatures and avoiding the variability in vein wall energy delivery inherent with continuous catheter pullback, vein occlusion efficacy is improved.[3,4] In addition, procedure times are significantly reduced vs. the first-generation RF catheter procedure times with catheter-in to catheter-out times averaging 16.4 minutes.[3] Early published experience with the segmental ablation catheter shows vein occlusion efficacy of 99.6% at 6- month follow-up compared to 89.2% with bipolar RF ablation using 85°C[3,4] (Figure 5.3). A recent presentation reported vein occlusion rates of 97% at 1 year with segmental ablation vs. 87% with bipolar RF ablation.[5]

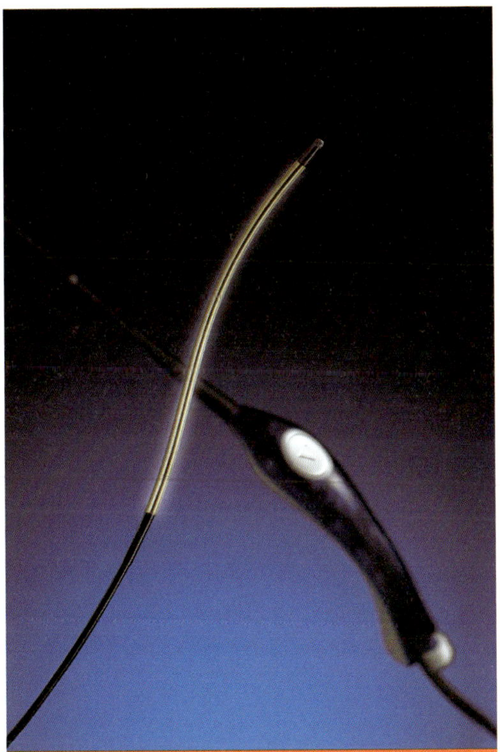

FIGURE 5.2 VNUS ClosureFAST catheter. VNUS product image copyright ©Covidien. Used with permission.

Evolution of Radiofrequency Vein Ablation

Endovenous RFA was introduced into clinical practice in Europe in 1998 and in the United States in 1999. Initially performed

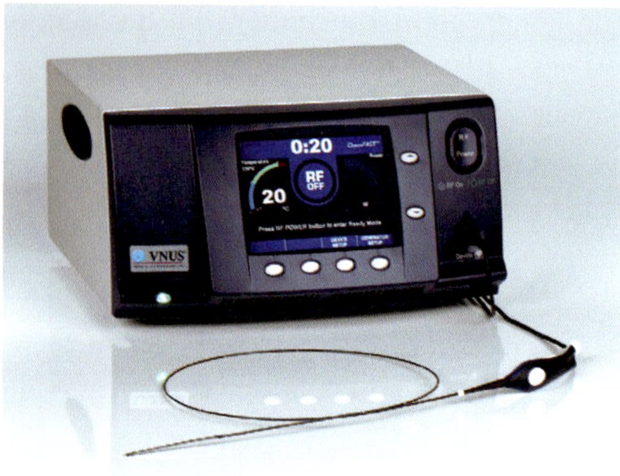

FIGURE 5.3 VNUS RFGPlus Radiofrequency Generator. VNUS product image copyright ©Covidien. Used with permission.

with high ligation of the saphenous vein and junctional tributaries, the procedure evolved to omit high ligation after demonstration that RF-ablated veins remained durably closed for 6 months after treatment. Since the adoption of endovenous RF ablation without high ligation, to the end of 2008, approximately 400,000 patients will have been treated in more than 40 countries.

Since 2000, more than 70 medical journal articles and 10 book chapters have been published on radiofrequency vein ablation. Some of the significant studies include 4 randomized trials comparing RFA to traditional vein stripping and ligation,[6-10] a comparative trial of RFA and laser vein ablation,[3,11] and 5 publications that reported results from a registry that followed RFA patients for 5 years after treatment.[12-16] An additional randomized trial of RFA versus endovenous laser ablation (RECOVERY Study), comparing postprocedural recovery and QOL parameters, was published earlier in 2009.[17] Other important reports include preclinical work that described the mechanism of vein occlusion and histopathology associated with RFA,[18,19] and sonographic studies that examined the course of the ablated GSV using serial ultrasonography scans of the treated GSV and tributary veins at 6, 12, and 24 months after treatment.[20,21]

It is easy to forget the controversy that emerged in 1999 when the RFA procedure changed from employing high ligation to being routinely performed without high ligation of the saphenofemoral junction. To determine whether high ligation contributed to patient outcomes, a study of the early experience with RFA compared patient outcomes using RFA with and without ligation of the SFJ and was published in 2000.[22] Once it was demonstrated that high ligation was not a requirement for successful patient treatment with RFA, tumescent local anesthesia (TLA) was incorporated into the procedures. Today, TLA is well understood as a standard and highly necessary component of successful endovenous thermal vein ablation, but it did not begin to be employed routinely with thermal ablation until the benefits were described in 2001.[23,24] Use of tumescent anesthesia augments external compression to significantly compress the treated vein onto the catheter, reducing the amount of blood in the vein and allowing energy to be more completely directed into the vein wall rather than to luminal blood. The result is enhanced, thermally induced collagen contraction, which reduces the risk of recanalization.[25] The use of TLA has also been instrumental in facilitating the performance of RFA procedures in an office setting, rather than in a hospital-based operating room or an outpatient surgery center. With the use of TLA, large amounts of dilute anesthetic, with low toxicity, can be utilized, resulting in an almost pain-free experience for the patient. In addition, the heat-sink effects of perivenous TLA reduces surrounding tissue injury, all but eliminates a risk of skin burn, and markedly reduces the incidence of temporary hypoesthesia.[24,25] With experience in the use of TLA and the RFA procedure, even large-diameter veins can be treated efficaciously.[15]

Mechanism of Vein Occlusion

Radiofrequency vein ablation delivers temperature-controlled energy directly to the vein wall in a manner designed to immediately contract the lumenal diameter and effect a fibrotic seal of the treated vein. Studies performed in the development of the RF ablation catheters and procedure demonstrated that heating collagenous tissue such as veins to temperatures greater than 60°C causes acute vein diameter reduction. Heating to higher temperatures of 85°C to 90°C causes maximum diameter reduction. Vein diameter reduction occurs primarily because of heat-induced collagen fibril shortening and thickening, and secondarily from subsequent inflammation of the vein wall. Heat denaturation of the collagen proteins after RF ablation was verified using polarized light microscopy to show loss of birefringence of the heated vein wall, and from scanning electron microscopy that showed shortening and thickening of the collagen fibrils.[18] The process of applying sufficient thermal energy to the vein wall to cause collagen contraction also generates a thermal injury to the vein wall, resulting in endothelial denudation, cellular injury, and a subsequent inflammatory response.

Within hours of RF treatment, the inflammatory response causes further thickening of the vein wall due to swelling of myocytes and other cellular components of the vein. This in turn further reduces the lumen. A small residual lumen may be present and filled with a small thrombus that organizes and fibroses in a matter of days (Figure 5.4). The residual lumen can be lessened if compression or preshaping of the vein are performed to remove most of the blood from the area under treatment. Compression is applied to the vein during RF energy delivery because collagen fibers constrict more aggressively under compressive loads, enhancing efficacy. Methods of applying compression to enhance vein-diameter reduction include external manual compression, an Esmark bandage, and most commonly, perivenous tumescent infiltration to increase local pressure in the saphenous fascial compartment.

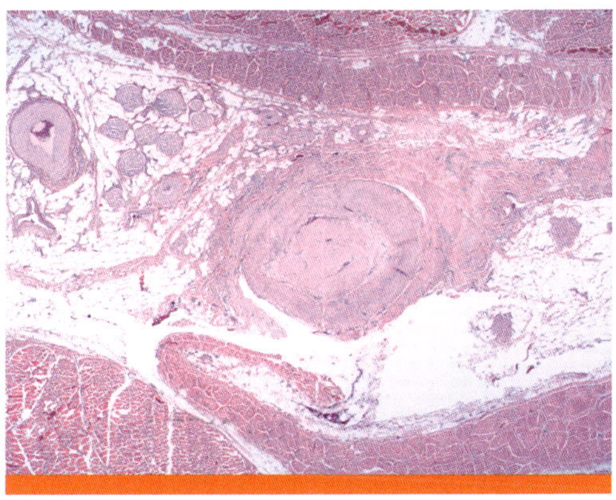

FIGURE 5.4 Goat saphenous vein at 12 weeks after ablation with VNUS ClosureFAST catheter. VNUS product image copyright ©Covidien. Used with permission.

Within days after RF ablation, light microscopy shows extensive fibroplasia in both the adventitia and former lumen of the vein as well as organized fibrotic thrombus. Fibroblasts provide the source of new collagen synthesis and are extensively distributed throughout the adventitia and fibrotic tissue that fills the former lumen 6 weeks after treatment.[18] Over the course of 12 months, as the fibrotically sealed vein is resorbed into surrounding tissue, further adventitial diameter contraction can be measured using serial ultrasonography.[3, 20]

Procedural Details: How We Do It

Approximately 15 minutes prior to the procedure, patients are brought into a changing room to change into a gown, and a small amount of nitropaste cream is applied by our medical assistant to the patient's leg above and below the knee. We have found that this prevents saphenous vasospasm prior to and during the procedure. Next, the patient is brought into the procedure room. The procedure room should have good lighting, preferably overhead, and be uncluttered and meticulously clean.

The table on which the procedure is performed should be well padded for patient comfort. Preferably, the table will be one with power and can be operated with foot controls. This allows the patient to be positioned as necessary during the procedure without the aid of an assistant and in the least possible amount of time. Most often we perform this procedure with the leg in the "frog-legged" position with a padded "bump" under the patient's knee to minimize discomfort.

The importance of ultrasonography in endovenous procedures cannot be overstated.

With duplex, the venous system is interrogated to answer several important procedure questions: optimal site for vein access and performance of vein access, vein tortuosity, diameter and tributary location, RF catheter position in relation to the saphenofemoral junction, the proper location for the application of tumescent anesthesia, and evaluation of the vein for successful closure immediately following the administration of RF treatment.

A vascular surgeon performing RFA procedures on a regular basis should become facile with performing his or her own duplex scanning. This is more time efficient than using a vascular technologist to perform imaging during the procedure. Furthermore, if you do not have a vascular lab in your office, it will become costly to use an itinerant vascular technologist if you do many endovenous procedures. If you have a noninvasive vascular laboratory in your office, it is not cost effective to take your technologist away from performing valuable noninvasive studies each time you do an RFA procedure. Learning to scan for this procedure is actually quite easy and can be learned in a minimal amount of time from a registered vascular technologist in your hospital or office if you have a vascular laboratory. Using a vascular technologist may require you to perform some RF procedures in your hospital operating room or ambulatory surgical center until you become comfortable scanning on your own. An additional benefit is that as you become more facile with performing duplex, you can expand your venous practice to include other procedures, including RFA of perforator veins and duplex-guided sclerotherapy. This may be well worth the investment of time.

Any standard-sized, good-quality, vascular ultrasound machine can be used to perform endovenous procedures. If procedure room space is an issue, however, then the use of a full-sized ultrasound machine may be untenable or uncomfortable for these procedures. In this circumstance or if you do not already have an ultrasound machine, we would recommend the use of one of the newer portable machines. In addition to utilizing a minimum of space, these machines can be moved from room to room with greater ease or from one office to another if you are performing endovenous procedures at multiple office sites. They are significantly cheaper than standard, hardware-driven, full-sized ultrasound machines, and image quality is more than adequate for endovenous procedures.

Vein access is the most technically challenging aspect of any endovenous procedure. It is performed under duplex guidance and therefore requires dual facility with a duplex probe, as well as good hand–eye coordination, the latter of which most vascular surgeons have mastered. Vein spasm can lead to unsuccessful and frustrating attempts at vein access, and all measures should be taken to avoid it. These measures begin when the patient first enters a doctor's office for the procedure. Minimizing patient anxiety and keeping the waiting and procedure rooms warm will lessen the chance of vein spasm. As mentioned previously, a small amount of nitropaste is applied to the patient's skin above and below the knee 15 minutes prior to the procedure. This helps to avoid vein spasm even after several unsuccessful attempts at vein cannulation. Too much nitropaste can result in hypotension and or headache, so caution should be taken when applying this medication.

Vein access is achieved with a 21-gauge micropuncture needle. Good duplex visualization of the vein to be accessed is critical to success. Long axis orientation of the duplex probe permits visualization of more vein wall surface area and thereby a greater target for vein access than a short-axis view and is my choice for most vein cannulations. Alternatively, a long-axis view visualizing both the needle and the vein wall simultaneously is harder to accomplish and requires slightly more skill if you are performing your own duplex. When the vein is close to the skin surface, vein access is most readily accomplished with the use of a short-axis view.

The vein is usually accessed below the knee versus above the knee so that the greatest length of vein proximal to the saphenous nerve is available for treatment. On occasion, vein access can prove to be quite difficult due to small vein size, tortuosity, or vasospasm subsequent to failed cannulation attempts or when proper preprocedure measures to prevent vasospasm have not been taken. Under such conditions, several steps can be taken to improve the chances for success. The easiest is to place the patient into reverse Trendelenberg to increase dilatation of the vein. If this is not helpful, then alternative sites for access should be examined. The first alternative site to evaluate is above the knee. If the vein appears disadvantaged at this area, then the saphenous vein at the ankle is often superficial and larger and is a suitable site for access. In the rare instance in which duplex-guided percutaneous vein access still cannot be achieved, a vein cutdown should be performed just below the knee. With duplex visualization, this can be done with a very small incision and in minimal time. No more than 10 to 15 minutes should be spent attempting percutaneous access; after this, common sense should prevail and a cutdown should be performed.

Once vein access has been accomplished, the Closure catheter is placed into the vein via the introducer sheath and most often passes unimpeded to the saphenofemoral junction. Not infrequently, the catheter's passage may be thwarted by vein tortuosity, a segment of diseased vein or a severe angle at the saphenofemoral junction. Forcibly pushing the catheter will be painful to the patient, may result in vein perforation, and will generally not succeed. Repositioning the extremity may adjudicate the difficult vein traversal. Gentle manual compression at the sight of catheter impedance may also resolve this problem, especially at the SFJ. If these measures should fail, then no time should be wasted before using a guidewire.

A .025 Teflon wire is utilized. This is the largest-caliber wire that will fit through the Closure catheter lumen. In uncommon instances in which this wire is not helpful, a second sheath is placed proximal to the area of vein tortuosity or disease, and 2 separate treatments are performed. Alternatively, and to save time, a .018 Terumo glide wire is almost always successful in crossing through difficult, tortuous, or diseased vein segments. This wire is not our first choice because it is significantly more expensive than the .025 Teflon wire.

The instillation of tumescent anesthesia causes the greatest patient discomfort. With the exception of difficult vein access, this is the most time-consuming portion of endovenous procedures. To minimize patient discomfort, injection of tumescent should be selected in advance and marked with an indelible marker. Local anesthesia, using 1% lidocaine is then injected at these sites with a 27-gauge needle. Bicarbonate is mixed with the lidocaine, in a 1:5 ratio to reduce its acidity and thereby reduce the pain and burning associated with this local anesthetic. On average, RFA surgeries require somewhere between 250 cc and 450 cc of tumescent solution, depending on the length of vein to be treated. The tumescent acts as a heat sump to prevent burning of the surrounding soft tissues and to adequately compress the vein onto the RF catheter. From a materials viewpoint, the simplest and least expensive way to achieve these volumes of tumescent is to use standard 20- or 30-cc syringes, refilled and injected multiple times along the course of the vein. With an average of 250 to 300 cc required for the procedure, this is time consuming and unpleasant for the patient. Use of a larger syringe in order to reduce the number of injections and procedure times requires much greater force for injection. Furthermore, the syringes are too large for the hands of most surgeons to use comfortably and repeatedly. An alternative is to use a powered pump for delivering large amounts of fluid under pressure in very little time and with a minimum of patient discomfort. The high pressure supplied by the pump causes the tumescent to travel rapidly around the saphenous vein along its course within the fascial envelope. As compared with hand injection, fewer injection sites are necessary to provide adequate tumescence for an entire extremity. A cost of several thousand dollars makes the powered pump a discretionary purchase for most. In our practice, we use a one-way valve syringe attached by IV tubing to a 500-cc bag of tumescent fluid. This allows several 20- to 30-cc injections to be performed at one site with one needle stick. The syringe is disposable and far less expensive than a powered pump. The necessary tumescent volume is delivered quickly and with minimum patient discomfort. There is little additional cost to perform the procedure with this syringe.

Once the infiltration of tumescent anesthesia is completed, the RF generator is initialized. The ClosureFAST catheter has a 7-cm heating element that is heated to 120°C by RF energy. By conductive heat transfer, the vein wall segment in contact with the 7-cm catheter heating element reaches a temperature of 100°C to 110°C. The generator heats the catheter for a period of 20 seconds. The catheter is then moved distally in 6.5-cm increments, thus achieving a 0.5-cm treatment overlap zone at each treated segment. Each vein segment is treated only once, except for the first segment, which is treated twice. There are otherwise no retreatments performed. Alternatively, Closure PLUS delivers RF energy from the catheter to the vein wall to achieve vein wall heating while the catheter is continually withdrawn. In our experience, the treatment time for a 45-cm vein with ClosureFAST is less than 3 minutes, and total procedure times are averaging less than 20 minutes. Postoperative bruising and pain are almost nonexistent and, as with Closure PLUS, patients are returning to their regular activities almost immediately.

Review of Clinical Outcomes

The morphologic and hemodynamic outcomes following RFA have been assessed using serial duplex ultrasonography scans, as described in detailed studies by Pichot and colleagues.[20,21] In these studies, the RFA-treated GSV showed progressive sonographic changes over time. Typically, occluded veins are initially hypoechogenic compared with the surrounding tissue. Over the course of 6 months, they become progressively more hyperechogenic and with further time, isoechogenic, indicating complete obliteration of the treated vein until it is incorporated into the surrounding tissue. In Pichot and colleagues' studies, approximately 60% of veins were hypoechogenic and 40% were hyperechogenic at 1 week. By 12 and 24 months, the treated GSV was isoechogenic in approximately 85% to 90% of treated limbs.[20,21] This sonographic disappearance of the RFA-treated great saphenous vein was also observed by Weiss in 90% of limbs at 2 years.[24] The most common sonographic observations at the SFJ was a short patent stump conducting antegrade tributary flow through the SFJ with an occluded or obliterated GSV trunk and an absence of neovacularization. Chandler and Bergan sought to define the role of ligation at the SFJ and junctional tributaries in their study that compared 60 limbs treated with high ligation plus RFA to 120 limbs treated with RFA and no ligation.[22] The authors concluded that no significant advantage or adverse effect existed with adding extended SFJ ligation to successful endovenous RF ablation of the GSV. GSV ablation with or without SFJ ligation yielded early reflux and varicose vein recurrence rates similar to those seen after high ligation and stripping, with significant and sustained improvement in symptoms and CEAP class. Together, these early studies showed that endovenous RFA eliminates the truncal reflux channel with minimal disturbance of the thigh soft tissue and the abdominal and pudendal superficial venous drainage. With junctional tributary drainage unimpeded, normal antegrade venous flow continues from branch veins, avoiding potential stimuli for neovascularization, which has been shown to be the most common cause of failure after traditional vein stripping and ligation.[26] The thermally contracted and injured truncal vein quickly becomes a fibrosed saphenous vein remnant that cannot participate in reflux.[18] The sonographic disappearance of the GSV in 85% to 90% of cases suggest that the majority of long-term failures are more likely to be due to disease progression rather than to recanalization of the saphenous trunk. To examine this hypothesis, the vein occlusion rate was examined over a course of 5 years in the Closure registry.

RFA treatment efficacy has been reported by various groups. Short- to mid-term efficacy was 90% to 96%.[9,12,27] The longest follow-up results are from the registry, which showed vein occlusion rates of 87% (102 of 117) and reflux-free rates of 84% (98 of 117) at 5 years, demonstrating the durability of the treatment.[16] Treatment efficacy on large veins was analyzed by Merchant and colleagues.[15] There were 39 veins with a diameter greater than 12 mm (maximum 24 mm) in the registry. The vein occlusion rate was 97.4% within 1 week and 96.2% at

6 months or 1 year. It is worthwhile to note that in the registry, the patients with longer follow-ups are those treated at the very early stage of the technology introduction. As discussed previously, the RFA procedure technique has improved over the years; consequently, the treatment efficacy has improved compared with earlier treatments.[3]

Partial occlusion or nonocclusion of treated veins constitutes anatomic failure, which can be due to initial incomplete treatment or subsequent recanalization of a short or long segment of the treated vein. Additionally, reflux into untreated junctional tributaries such as a residual anterior accessory vein can also contribute to recurrence. Irrespective of the presence of an anatomic failure, clinical improvement was often demonstrated in these patients, particularly when vein occlusion was partial.[13,16,25] For example, Merchant showed that 5 years after treatment, clinical symptom improvement was observed in 85% to 94% of limbs with complete occlusion and in 70% to 80% of limbs even with the occurrence of anatomical failure.[16]

In the RFA registry, approximately 85%, 79%, and 39% of limbs had pain, fatigue, or edema, respectively, before the procedure, which decreased to 29%, 7%, and 8%, respectively, within 1 week after the procedure. A further decrease in the percentage of symptomatic limbs was observed at 6 months, and the symptom improvement remained stable over 5 years. Pullback speed and body mass index were identified as risk factors for anatomic failure.[16] Clinical improvement was apparent even in anatomically failed patients. Another study by Vasquez that also utilized Venous Clinical Severity Scores (VCSS) to assess patient symptoms showed similar results. Symptom reduction as measured with VCSS decreased from 8.8 ± 3.7 in 648 limbs to 3.3 ± 1.6 in 479 limbs ($P < 0.0001$) followed at 6 months after RFA treatment.[25] Furthermore, 86% of limbs with ulcers achieved healing following RFA treatment ($P < 0.0001$). These results have established the short- and long-term treatment outcomes of RFA in eliminating saphenous reflux and alleviating patient symptoms.

The complication profile associated with RF vein ablation has been well characterized in numerous randomized trials, large multicenter reports, and several large, independent studies. As a standard protocol, patients treated with RFA are brought back within 72 hours of treatment for a venous duplex scan to document the presence of deep vein thrombosis or saphenofemoral junction thrombus extension into the femoral vein. The practice of routinely scanning all patients for thrombus is not followed with other treatment modalities such as traditional stripping, endovenous laser ablation, or foam sclerotherapy. As a result, asymptomatic and nonocclusive thrombus in the femoral vein or extending just beyond the GSV will be observed and documented with RFA but could be routinely missed with other treatment modalities that do not involve a routine posttreatment ultrasonography scan.

A review of 13 published reports on the rate of DVT associated with RF vein ablation shows the incidence of DVT ranging from a low of 0% in 6 reports totaling 290 limbs treated to a high of 16.4% from the initial 73 limbs treated at one academic center.[35] The author of the report with a high rate of DVT later wrote in a letter to the editor, "we do still believe in the benefits of the [RFA] technique and still continue to perform the technique. . . . When these deep venous thromboses have been encountered, they resolve with the outpatient administration of subcutaneous low-molecular-weight heparin."[37] The largest published series reporting on the rate of thrombosis included data from 32 centers participating in the Closure registry from 1998 to 2003, and showed 4 of 858 limbs (0.5%) with localized thrombus extending no more than 10% into the common femoral vein (CFV), and another 4 (0.5%) treated limbs with clot extending further into the CFV, including one pulmonary embolism. The second-largest published series is a single-center study by Vasquez showing a 0.15% rate of nonocclusive thrombus extension among 633 patients scanned routinely after RFA.[25] Reports from 4 prospective randomized controlled trials of RFA vs. vein stripping totaling 94 limbs treated with RFA showed no DVT or thrombus extension.[6-10] In a randomized trial of RFA using segmental ablation compared to 980-nm endovenous laser, the rate of DVT was 0% in 47 RFA-treated limbs whereas in the laser cohort 1 limb of 41 limbs treated with laser experienced a thrombus extension.[17] In comparison, a prospective study looking for DVT in patients following vein-stripping surgery resulted in a 5.3% DVT rate among 377 patients. Sixty percent of these were asymptomatic.[36]

The incidence and types of other adverse events reported with RF ablation have changed with the widespread use of tumescent anesthesia beginning in 2002. Prior to that time paresthesia rates as high as 14.5% were reported. At 4-year follow-up, the paresthesia rate declined to 2%.[15] With the use of perivenous tumescent anesthesia, the thermal load to adjacent nerves and the skin is reduced. This has resulted in reported paresthesia rates of 1.0% in 102 limbs at 6-month follow-up and a 0% rate of skin burns in 140 limbs.[24] A second series published in 2007 emphasized the use of volumetric TLA and also reported no skin burns and a paresthesia rate of 0.3% in 633 limbs followed for greater than 6 months.[25]

Randomized Trials of RFA vs. Vein Stripping or Laser Ablation

Endovenous RFA removes the incompetent vein from the circulation and provides an alternative to traditional vein stripping. The advantages of RFA over vein stripping are demonstrated in 4 randomized comparative trials. Rautio and colleagues reported significantly less postoperative pain, quantitated with a visual analog scale, in the RFA group than in the stripping group at rest ($P = 0.017$), on standing ($P = 0.026$), and on walking ($P = 0.036$). The most distinct differences were noted from days 5 to 14 postoperatively.[6] Sick leaves were also significantly shorter in the RFA group (6.5 ± 3.3 vs. 15.6 ± 6.0 days, $P < 0.001$), and physical function was restored faster in the RFA patients, measured with RAND-35 quality-of-life (QOL) questionnaires. All of the operations were successful, and the complication rates were similar between the 2 groups in this study. These patients were followed up at 3 years.[28] There was no difference in the average decrease in the Venous Clinical Severity Score (VCSS) and the Venous Disability Score (VDS) between the 2 groups. None of the RFA-occluded GSVs recanalized. The varicose vein recurrence rate was documented in 5 of 15 limbs (33%) in the RFA group and in 3 of 13 limbs (23%) in the stripping group, and the difference was not statistically significant ($P = 0.4$). Similarly, Stötter and colleagues reported significantly lower pain scores ($P = 0.014$) and lower discomfort scores ($P = 0.012$) in the RFA group vs. the stripping group within 6 weeks following the procedure in their randomized trial.[8] In another published report, RFA and vein stripping were compared in 16 patients with bilateral recurrent great saphenous vein reflux.[10] These patients were then randomly assigned to receive treatment with radiofrequency obliteration (RFO) on one leg and with vein stripping on the other. The RFO was faster (25 minutes vs. 40 minutes) and associated with significantly less postoperative pain and bruising and higher patient preference. It was concluded that Closure should be the treatment of choice for recurrent GSV reflux. The EVOLVeS (Endovenous Obliteration versus Ligation and Vein Stripping) trial is a multicenter prospective randomized trial sponsored by the manufacturer of the RF catheter. The early follow-up (4 months) focused on the comparison of procedure-related complications, patient recuperation, and QOL outcomes between the 2 treatment procedures.[7] The procedure impact on the hemodynamic and clinical outcomes was demonstrated through 1-and 2-year follow-up evaluations.[9] Patients with symptomatic varicose veins and GSV incompetence were randomized into either RFA or vein-stripping groups. RFA was performed on 44 limbs and stripping on 36 limbs. There were no differences between the groups in patient demographics, VCSS, or CEAP clinical class distribution before the treatment. The most significant differences seen between the 2 groups were on patient recovery. The mean time to return to normal activity was 1.15 days (95% confidence interval [CI] 0.05–2.34) for the RFA patients compared with 3.89 days (95% CI 2.67–5.12) (P = 0.02) for vein-stripping patients. Return to routine activities within 1 day was seen in 80.5% of RFA patients vs. 46.9% of patients who underwent stripping (P <0.01). Mean values for the time to return to work were 4.7 days (95% CI 1.16–8.17) in the RFO group and 12.4 days (95% CI 8.66–16.23) in the stripping group (P <0.05). Significantly fewer complications and adverse events were observed in the RFA group (P <0.05) through 3 weeks postoperatively, mostly owing to higher rates of tenderness, ecchymosis, and hematoma following vein stripping. The postoperative VCSSs were significantly better at 72 hours and 1 week for the RFA group, but the difference disappeared at later follow-up. The QOL surveys (CIVIQ2 [Chronic Venous Insufficiency Quality-of-Life questionnaire]) showed clearly superior patient QOL in the RFA patients, with the most significant differences observed in global, pain, and physical scores. The pain score improvement from pretreatment baseline was significantly better in the RFA patients than in the stripping patients at all of the follow-up time points to 2 years. The differences observed in global QOL scores were statistically significant at 72 hours and 1 week and surprisingly also at 1 year and 2 years. Clinical and hemodynamic outcomes were similar for both groups at 2 years. There were no differences in patient symptoms and signs and no differences in varicose vein recurrence rates. Duplex ultrasonography examination demonstrated 91.7% and 89.7% of limbs free of reflux in the RFA and vein stripping groups, respectively, at 2 years. Neovascularization was reported in 1 (2.8%) RFA limb and 4 (13.8%) stripped limbs (P >0.05).

Neovascularization is increasingly recognized as one of the principal causes of recurrence after vein stripping, in addition to technical failure and disease progression.[26,29-31] It occurs in more than 50% of the limbs with clinical recurrence and accounts for 85% of recurrent SFJ reflux.[26,30] Furthermore, 90% of observed neovascularization following vein stripping and ligation is evident at 2 years.[26,32] With RFA treatment, a low incidence of neovascularization was reported in the EVOLVes Trial and by Pichot and colleagues.[9,21] Pichot carefully studied 63 limbs with a detailed ultrasonography scan protocol and found no evidence of neovascularization at 2 years after RF treatment. Two major advantages of RFA thought to account for the low incidence of neovascularization are the absence of angiogenic stimuli such as an incision and surgical dissection of the groin and the preservation of junctional tributary veins and thereby normal physiologic abdominal wall drainage, resulting in minimal hemodynamic disturbance.

Recurrence can refer to either clinical recurrence or hemodynamic recurrence. The former is generally described as varicose vein recurrence, and the latter is often with SFJ or saphenous trunk reflux. Varicose vein recurrence rates after vein stripping have been reported between 20% and 40% at 2 to 5 years[26,30,32,33] and up to 70% by 10 years.[34] The varicose vein recurrence rate can, however, be affected by factors such as the completeness of varicosity removal at the time of initial surgery and the examiner's subjectivity. Recurrence of SFJ reflux is a more objective measure and provides important hemodynamic information that permits detection and prediction of clinical recurrence. It was reported that after vein stripping, 87% of limbs were free from reflux at 2 years, and 71% were reflux free at 5 years[26,29] compared with 88% at 2 years and 84% at 5 years after RFA.[4]

Two comparative trials of RFA and endovenous laser have been reported. Morrison reported his 2001 experience with pulsed 810-nm laser and RFA in 50 patients with bilateral disease, with each patient receiving laser in 1 limb and RFA in the other.[38]

Using a strict definition of complete vein occlusion this study resulted in statistically better (P <0.05) rates of primary vein occlusion for RFA, although both RFA and laser primary occlusion rates of 80% and 66%, respectively, were substantially lower than other reports. Pain and bruising were more common following laser than RF ablation. The Recovery Study was completed in 2008 and involved 87 limbs randomized to treatment by RFA with the ClosureFAST catheter or 980-nm endovenous laser.[17] This trial showed statistically fewer complications (P <0.021) and less pain (P <0.0001) with RF treatment compared to laser. Also, venous clinical severity scores and QOL measures were statistically lower in the ClosureFAST group up to 2 weeks following the procedures.

Conclusion

A review of all 4 published randomized trials comparing RFA to traditional vein stripping shows that for every clinical endpoint in which there was a finding of a statistical difference between the 2 therapies, the results favored RFA. Similarly, comparative trials of RFA and endovenous laser have also demonstrated a difference in outcomes that are statistically significant and favor RFA as a treatment modality. These studies show that temperature-controlled RFA treatment of saphenous vein reflux results in safe and effective vein occlusion, elimination of reflux, immediate quality-of-life improvement and fast recovery for the patient, allowing patients to return to normal activities in approximately 1 day. Five-year clinical follow-up has also established the durability of RFA in reducing patient symptoms and providing an effective long-term solution for the patient with venous reflux and varicose veins.

When performed appropriately, RFA is a highly safe and effective procedure with clinical outcomes that are equivalent to or in many instances favorable to vein stripping and laser ablation. The value of the preservation of competent junctional tributaries and the absence of neovascularization, the most common cause of long-term failure from conventional saphenous vein stripping surgery, have stood the test of time. As such, durable symptom improvement and mild patient recovery have become the hallmarks of the RFA procedure. The second-generation ClosureFAST RF catheter has demonstrated even greater efficacy when compared to the first-generation bipolar RF catheter. Using higher temperatures and segmental ablation, the procedure is now faster and easier to perform and delivers even more favorable outcomes for patients.

References

1. Roland L, Dietzek AM. Radiofrequency ablation of the great saphenous vein performed in the office: tips for better patient convenience and comfort and how to perform it in less than an hour. Perspect Vasc Surg Endovasc Ther. 2007;19(3):309-14.
2. Dietzek A. Endovenous radiofrequency ablation for the treatment of varicose veins. Vascular. 2007;15(5):255-61.
3. Proebstle T, Vago B, Alm J, Göckeritz O, Lebard C, Pichot O. Treatment of the incompetent great saphenous vein by endovenous radiofrequency powered segmental thermal ablation: first clinical experience. J Vasc Surg. 2008;47:151-6.
4. Merchant R, Pichot O, Closure Study Group. Long-term outcomes of endovenous radiofrequency obliteration of saphenous reflux as a treatment for superficial venous insufficiency. J Vasc Surg. 2005;42:502-9.
5. Dietzek AM. Two year follow-up data from a prospective, multicenter study of the efficacy of the ClosureFast catheter. Presented at the 35th Annual VEITH Symposium; 2008 Nov 19-23; New York.
6. Rautio T, Ohinmaa A, Perälä J, Ohtonen P, Heikkinen T, Wiik H, Karjalainen P, Haukipuro K, Juvonen T. Endovenous obliteration versus conventional stripping operation in the treatment of primary varicose veins: a randomized controlled trial with comparison of costs. J Vasc Surg. 2002;35:958-65.
7. Lurie F, Creton D, Eklof B, Kabnick LS, Kistner RL, Pichot O, et al. Prospective randomized study of endovenous radiofrequency obliteration (Closure) versus ligation and stripping in a selected patient population (EVOLVES study). J Vasc Surg. 2003;38:207-14.
8. Stötter L, Schaaf I, Bockelbrink A, Baurecht HJ. Radiofrequency obliteration, invaginated or cryostripping: which is the best tolerated treatment by the patient? Phlebologie. 2005;34:19-24.
9. Lurie F, Creton D, Eklof B, Kabnick LS, Kistner RL, Pichot O, et al. Prospective randomised study of endovenous radiofrequency obliteration (closure) versus ligation and vein stripping (EVOLVeS): two-year follow-up. Eur J Vasc Endovasc Surg. 2005;29:67-73.
10. Hinchliffe RJ, Ubhi J, Beech A, Ellison J, Braithwaite BD. A prospective randomised controlled trial of VNUS Closure versus surgery for the treatment of recurrent long saphenous varicose veins. Eur J Vasc Endovasc Surg. 2006;31:212-8.
11. Morrison N. Saphenous ablation: what are the choices, laser or RF energy. Semin Vasc Surg. 2005;18:15-8.
12. Kabnick LS, Merchant RF. Twelve and twenty-four month follow-up after endovascular obliteration of saphenous vein reflux—a report from the multi-center registry. J Phlebotomy. 2001;1:17-24.
13. Merchant RF, DePalma RG, Kabnick LS. Endovascular obliteration of saphenous reflux: a multicenter study. J Vasc Surg. 2002;35:1190-6.
14. Nicolini P, and the Closure group. Treatment of primary varicose veins by endovenous obliteration with the VNUS Closure system: results of a prospective multicentre study. Eur J Vasc Endovasc Surg. 2005;29:433-9.

15. Merchant R, Pichot O, Mayers KA. Four years follow-up on endovascular radiofrequency obliteration of saphenous reflux. Derm Surg. 2005;31:129-34.
16. Merchant R, Pichot O, for the Closure study group. Long-term outcomes of endovenous radiofrequency obliteration of saphenous reflux as a treatment for superficial venous insufficiency. J Vasc Surg. 2005;42:502-9.
17. Almeida JI, Kaufman J, Gockeritz O, Chopra P, Evans MT, Hoheim DF, et al. Radiofrequency endovenous ClosureFAST versus laser ablation for the treatment of great saphenous reflux : a multicenter, single-blinded, randomized study (RECOVERY study). J Vasc Interv Radiol. 2009;20:752-9.
18. Weiss RA, Goldman MP. Controlled radiofrequency-mediated endovenous shrinkage and occlusion. In: Goldman MP, Weiss RA, Bergan JJ, eds. Varicose Veins and Telangiectasias; Diagnosis and Treatment. 2nd ed. St. Louis: Quality Medical Publishing; 1999. p217-24.
19. Weiss R. A. Comparison of endovenous radiofrequency versus 810 nm diode laser occlusion of large veins in an animal model. Derm Surg. 2002;28:56-61.
20. Pichot O, Sessa C, Chandler JG, Nuta M, Perrin M. Role of duplex imaging in endovenous obliteration for primary venous insufficiency. J Endovasc Ther. 2000;7:451-9.
21. Pichot O, Kabnick LS, Creton D, Merchant RF, Schuller-Petrovic S, Chandler JG. Duplex ultrasound scan findings two years after great saphenous vein radiofrequency endovenous obliteration. J Vasc Surg. 2004;39:189-95.
22. Chandler JG, Pichot O, Sessa C, Schuller-Petrovic S, Osse FJ, Bergan JJ. Defining the role of extended saphenofemoral junction ligation: a prospective comparative study. J Vasc Surg. 2000;32:941-53.
23. Weiss RA. SUPT anesthesia for FR occlusion and EVLT procedures of the greater saphenous vein. Int Angiol. 2001;20 Supp 1-2.
24. Weiss RA, Weiss MA. Controlled radiofrequency endovenous occlusion using a unique radiofrequency catheter under duplex guidance to eliminate saphenous varicose vein reflux: a 2-year follow-up. Dermatol Surg. 2002;28:38-42.
25. Vasquez M, Wang J, Mahathanaruk M, Buczkowski G, Sprehe E, Dosluoglu HH. The utility of the Venous Clinical Severity Score in 682 limbs treated by radiofrequency saphenous vein ablation. J Vasc Surg. 2007;45(5):1008-14.
26. Jones L, Braithwaite BD, Selwyn D, Cooke S, Earnshaw JJ. Neovascularisation is the principal cause of varicose vein recurrence: results of a randomised trial of stripping the long saphenous vein. Eur J Endovasc Surg. 1996;12:442-5.
27. Kistner RL. Endovascular obliteration of the greater saphenous vein: the Closure procedure. Jpn J Phlebol. 2002;13:325-33.
28. Perala J, Rautio T, Biancari F, Ohtonen P, Wiik H, Heikkinen T, et al. Radiofrequency endovenous obliteration versus stripping of the long saphenous vein in the management of primary varicose veins: 3-year outcome of a randomized study. Ann Vasc Surg. 2005;19: 1-4.
29. Dwerryhouse S, Davies B, Harradine K, Earnshaw JJ. Stripping the long saphenous vein reduces the rate of reoperation for recurrent varicose veins: five-year results of a randomized trial. J Vasc Surg. 1999;29:589-92.
30. van Rij AM, Jiang P, Solomon C, Christie RA, Hill GB. Recurrence after varicose vein surgery: a prospective long-term clinical study with duplex junction reflux after ligation and stripping of the greater saphenous ultrasound scanning and air plethysmography. J Vasc Surg. 2003;38:935-43.
31. Fischer R, Linde N, Duff C, Jeanneret C, Chandler JG, Seeber P. Late recurrent saphenofemoral junction reflux after ligation and stripping of the greater saphenous vein. J Vasc Surg. 2001;34:236-40.

32. Dwerryhouse S, Davies B, Harradine K, Earnshaw JJ. Stripping the long saphenous vein reduces the rate of reoperation for recurrent varicose veins: five-year results of a randomized trial. J Vasc Surg. 1999;29:589-92.
33. Neglén P, Einarsson E, Eklöf B. The functional long-term value of different types of treatment for saphenous vein incompetence. J Cardiovasc Surg. 1993;34:295-301.
34. Campbell WB, Vijay Kumar A, Collin TW, Allington KL, Michaels JA. Randomised and Economic Analysis of Conservative and Therapeutic Interventions for Varicose Veins Study. The outcome of varicose vein surgery at 10 years: clinical findings, symptoms and patient satisfaction. Ann R Coll Surg Engl. 2003;85:52-7.
35. Hingorani AP, Ascher E, Markevich N, Schutzer RW, Kallakuri S, Hou A, et al. Deep venous thrombosis after radiofrequency ablation of greater saphenous vein: a word of caution. J Vasc Surg. 2004;40:500-4.
36. van Rij AM, Chai J, Hill GB, Christie RA. Incidence of deep vein thrombosis after varicose vein surgery. Br J Surg. 2004;9:1582-1585.
37. Hingorani AP. Letter to the editor. J Vasc Surg. 2005;41:374.
38. Morrison N. Saphenous ablation: what are the choices, laser or RF energy. SeminVasc Surg. 2005;18:15-8.

CHAPTER

6

Laser Ablation

Indications, Techniques, and Outcomes

Robert J. Min

Dr. Boné first reported on delivery of endovenous laser energy in 1999.[1] In 2001, a method for treating the entire incompetent great saphenous vein (GSV) segment was described by Min and Navarro.[2,3] Endovenous laser treatment, which received FDA approval in January 2002, creates nonthrombotic vein occlusion by delivering laser energy directly into the vein walls. Lasers with wavelengths of 810 nm, 940 nm, 980 nm, 1064 nm, 1320 nm, and 1470 nm have all been used with reported success. Over the past 10 years, reports of impressive clinical success and low complication rates have made the endovenous laser the treatment of choice for eliminating reflux in incompetent saphenous veins.

Chronic Venous Insufficiency. Contemporary Endovascular Management series. © 2011 Mark G. Davies MD and Alan B. Lumsden MD, eds. Cardiotext Publishing, ISBN 978-1-935395-09-6.

Subject Selection

Medical treatment of varicose veins should be contemplated when symptoms persist despite conservative methods such as gradient compression hose and exercise. Other indications may include treatment or prevention of complications arising from chronic venous hypertension such as bleeding, superficial thrombophlebitis, and damage to the skin. Relative contraindications for endovenous laser include inability to ambulate, acute deep venous thrombosis (DVT), general poor health, or pregnancy. Candidates with nonpalpable pedal pulses who cannot wear gradient compression may not be suitable for endovenous laser. More complex procedures with multiple access points may be required in subjects with nontraversable vein segments due either to thrombosis or to extreme tortuosity. Fortunately, these should all be identified on pretreatment history, physical, and venous duplex ultrasonography (DUS) evaluation.

Technique

Prior to treatment, abnormal venous pathways are mapped using DUS guidance, and the veins to be treated are marked on the overlying skin with the subject vertical. Additional important landmarks such as junctions, aneurismal vein segments, and areas of significant blood inflow from tributaries or perforators should be noted on the skin.

The subject is placed horizontal on the table such that areas to be treated are easily accessible to the operator. In general, subjects being treated for GSV, accessory saphenous vein (ASV), or thigh circumflex vein (TCV) reflux are placed supine or in the appropriate oblique position to expose the course of the target vein. When the small saphenous vein (SSV) is to be ablated, the subject is placed prone with feet hanging off the end of the table to relax the calf muscle and popliteal fossa. Treating an incompetent cephalad extension of the SSV (vein of Giacomini) or multiple sources of venous reflux may require repositioning and reprepping.

With rare exception, the target vein is entered directly or access is gained via one of its principal tributaries. Tributary veins are more prone to venospasm and may be more difficult to access. Entry via a tributary should be attempted only if the tributary is relatively straight and remains markedly enlarged in the horizontal position. The vein is usually punctured at, or just peripheral to, the lowest level of underlying reflux as determined by DUS. At this point, the vein diameter dramatically decreases just after it gives off a "refluxing escape" tributary and regains its competence. In many cases, GSV incompetence can occur segmentally. The reflux can completely spill out into a tributary vein and subsequently reenter the GSV at a lower level. In this case, one should access the lowest incompetent vein segment and attempt to treat all refluxing vein segments via one puncture; however, it is not uncommon that more than one puncture may be necessary.

The target vein is entered with either a 19-gauge or 21-gauge needle using realtime ultrasound guidance and single-wall technique. Utilizing reverse Trendelenburg positioning, keeping the procedure room warm, and minimizing the time the subject is waiting horizontally until access is obtained helps minimize shrinkage. Other ancillary procedures advocated by some practitioners to maximize vein size include a heating pad or a small amount of nitroglycerin paste at the access point. Non-GSV segments are particularly prone to venospasm and particular care must be taken when accessing a tributary vein or a non-GSV such as the ASV, SSV, or TCV.

A 5 Fr vascular sheath with distance markers is inserted over a guidewire into the vein and passed through the entire abnormal segment and into a more central vein. The laser fiber is inserted into the sheath and the sheath is pulled back, exposing a known length of the laser fiber tip. The sheath and fiber are withdrawn out of the deep veins and, using ultrasound guidance, positioned within the superficial venous system at the junction (Figure 6.1). The fiber is left in this position during tumescent anesthesia administration and will be repositioned just prior to delivery of laser energy. Confirmation of the position can be made by direct visualization of the red aiming beam through the skin.

Tumescent anesthesia utilizes large volumes of dilute anesthetic solutions, which makes treatment of long distances possible. Proper use of tumescent anesthesia should make endovenous laser painless without the need for intravenous sedation or general anesthesia. In fact, it can be argued that sedation adds risk to endovenous laser treatment by inhibiting subject feedback during

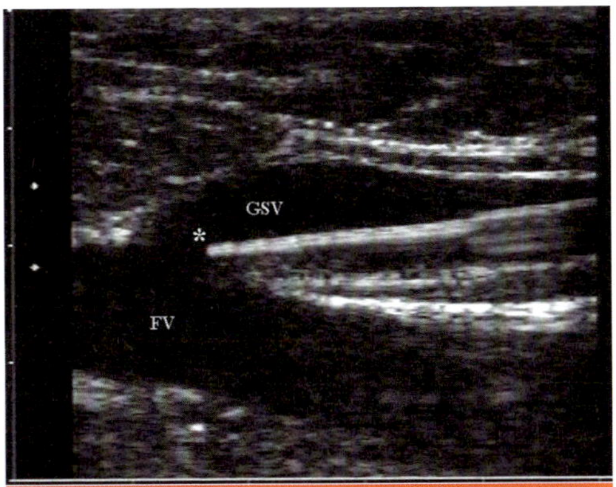

FIGURE 6.1 Under ultrasound guidance, the laser fiber is pulled out of the femoral vein (FV) and left in the GSV, as shown on this longitudinal image at the SFJ (subject's head is to the left). The fiber tip (*) will be repositioned after tumescent anesthesia delivery and prior to laser firing.

the procedure as well as delaying immediate postablation ambulation.

In addition to making treatment painless, tumescent anesthesia is used to maximize efficacy and safety of endovenous laser. Although venospasm may occur in portions of some accessed veins, proper delivery of tumescent fluid into the perivenous space is necessary to empty blood and ensures compression of the vein around the laser fiber. The goal is to maximize laser energy transfer to the vein walls from the laser fiber tip. Since blood is a chromophore for all laser wavelengths used for endovenous ablation, too much blood leads to inadequate vein wall damage. Occlusion by thrombosis results in eventual vein recanalization and treatment failure. After vein access is obtained and the vascular sheath inserted, Trendelenburg positioning, cooling the room, or chilling the tumescent fluid to induce venospasm also facilitates vein emptying.

The surrounding cuff of tumescent fluid may also serve as a protective barrier preventing harmful heating of nontarget tissues such as skin, nerves, arteries, or deep veins. Ultrasound is critical in guiding delivery of dilute lidocaine into the proper location between the target vein and adjacent nontarget tissues. One can imagine that delivery of fluid in the wrong plane could compress adjacent structures against the vein, exposing them to possible injury during laser energy delivery rather than separating and protecting them. This is particularly important when treating veins known to travel in close proximity to nerves and arterial branches such as the GSV below the knee, or the SSV. Injecting blindly or using highly pressurized devices to administer tumescent fluid, as is often done prior to liposuction, may be quicker, but such systems offer less control compared to hand injection. For this reason, it is preferred to deliver the tumescent anesthesia using hand pressure and a 1½-inch 25-gauge needle attached to a 20-mL syringe. For right-handed operators, the tumescent fluid is given from peripheral to central (Figure 6.2). Skin punctures are

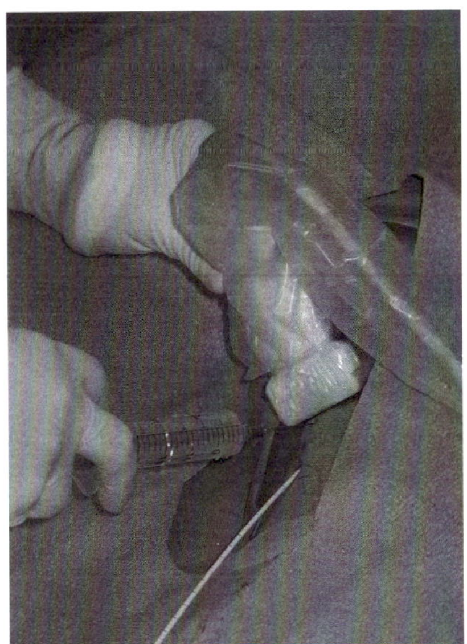

FIGURE 6.2 Tumescent anesthesia is delivered perivenously using ultrasound guidance.

required every 3 to 5 cm until the proper perivenous tissue plane is located. Once this occurs, fluid tracks more easily up and around the target vein, and longer distances can be covered with each needle puncture.

To treat a 45-cm segment of vein, approximately 100 to 150 mL of 0.1% lidocaine neutralized with sodium bicarbonate may be required. This mixture can be made by diluting 50 mL of 1% lidocaine in 440 mL of normal saline and adding 5 to 10 mL of 8.4% sodium bicarbonate. If larger volumes of tumescent anesthesia are anticipated to be necessary, a concentration of 0.05% lidocaine can be used effectively. These amounts of lidocaine are well within the safe doses of 4.5 mg/kg of lidocaine without epinephrine and 7 mg/kg with epinephrine. Lidocaine with epinephrine may be used to maximize venospasm and minimize bruising, but adequate and complete vein emptying can be achieved utilizing plain lidocaine.

Following tumescent anesthesia delivery, ultrasound in the transverse plane is used to check for completeness. Five to 10 mL of fluid surrounding the target vein, creating a separation from nontarget structures or from overlying skin, is sufficient (Figure 6.3). Proper delivery of tumescent may be particularly important when performing endovenous laser of certain veins such as the SSV near the saphenopopliteal junction (SPJ) or the GSV below the knee due to their close proximity to nerves or arteries. Checking with color Doppler following tumescent anesthesia delivery can be useful when assessing adequacy of separation of arterial branches from the target vein.

Because the laser fiber can move during tumescent anesthesia administration, the laser fiber is repositioned prior to delivery of laser energy. For the GSV, the fiber tip is positioned 5 to 10 mm peripheral to the saphenofemoral junction (SFJ), usually at or just below a competent superficial epigastric vein. When treating the SSV, seeing the fiber tip can be difficult due to venospasm and the acute angle taken by the SSV as it dives to join the popliteal vein. Following delivery of tumescent anesthesia, the laser fiber tip may be more easily visualized with ultrasonography. Accurate preprocedure marking of the SPJ is important, and when used with the red aiming beam enables precise positioning of the laser fiber. This red light should always be visualized, although dimming the room lights may be necessary in large subjects. Optimally, the laser fiber tip is placed 10 to 15 mm peripheral to the SPJ where the SSV turns parallel to the skin just below the popliteal fossa.

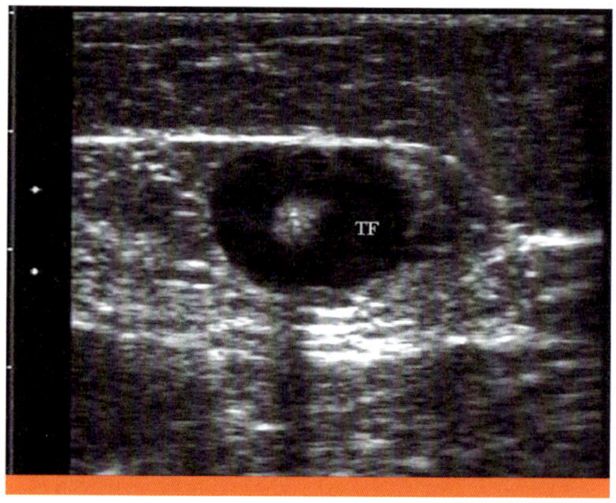

FIGURE 6.3 Transaxial ultrasound image of the vein walls compressed onto the laser fiber by a surrounding halo of tumescent fluid.

The vascular sheath and fiber are withdrawn together during laser activation. The minimum amount of energy required to result in nearly 100% durable vein closure seems to be an average of 70 J/cm throughout the treated segment.[4] This can be achieved by setting the laser at 14 W in "continuous mode" and withdrawing the laser fiber back at an average rate of 2 mm/sec. Although automatic catheter pullback

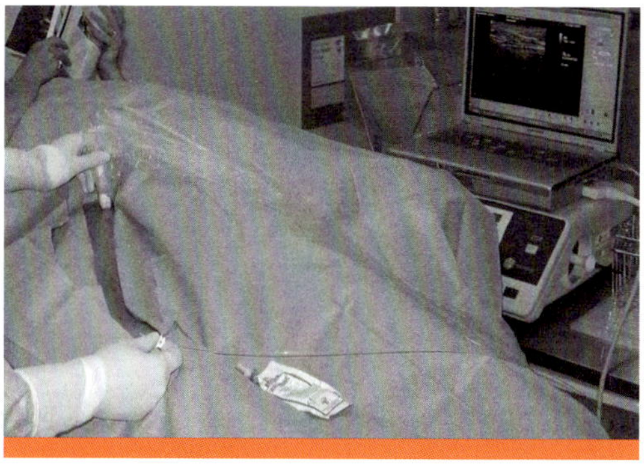

FIGURE 6.4 The laser is fired while the fiber and sheath are withdrawn. Distance markings on the vascular sheath and elapsed laser energy time on the laser console allow precise determination of linear energy delivery (J/cm).

devices are available, these are an unnecessary expense. Most manufacturers of endovenous laser ablation kits now provide marked vascular sheaths. Used in conjunction with the elapsed time display of the laser console, pullback rate is regulated (Figure 6.4).

Knowing pullback rate and wattage allows simple calculation and standardization of linear energy delivery in joules per centimeter. Manual withdrawal also allows laser energy delivery to be customized to the particular vein segment being treated, which enhances treatment efficacy and safety. For example, when treating the GSV, ASV, or TCV, higher laser energies are delivered to the most central portion of the vein, with the first 10 to 15 cm of the vein treated with 140 J/cm. This is achieved by withdrawing the laser fiber at a rate of 1 mm/sec. In general, the most central segment of the GSV is the most prone to treatment failure and is the least susceptible to venospasm. Thus, it is necessary to deliver proportionately larger amounts of tumescent anesthesia and greater laser energies to adequately treat this important portion of the vein. Higher laser energies may also be delivered in regions of blood inflow, such as near junctions with incompetent tributaries or refluxing perforators. When treating vein segments close to the skin, the SSV near the SPJ or the GSV below the knee, faster laser fiber withdrawal rates of approximately 3 mm/sec may be used to minimize the risk of injury to nontarget tissues.

Class II (30–40 mm Hg) gradient compression hose are placed on the subject immediately following endovenous laser treatment and worn for a minimum of 2 weeks at all times, except to sleep or shower. The purpose of gradient compression hose is to lower the risk of superficial thrombophlebitis in tributary varicosities that will tend to close once the underlying saphenous vein reflux is eliminated. Gradient compression, in addition to immediate ambulation following endovenous laser treatment, also increases the velocity of blood flow in the deep veins, reducing the likelihood of DVT.

Most subjects have significant improvement or resolution of pretreatment leg symptoms within a month following endovenous laser but require additional adjunctive procedures to completely eradicate the remaining varicosities and fully realize the treatment benefits. Sclerotherapy and ambulatory phlebectomy are the most commonly used techniques to accomplish this. The ideal timing of adjunctive procedures has been debated. Those practitioners who advocate waiting note that most subjects experience reduction in the size and fullness of associated varicosities, making ancillary treatments easier and more effective. Rarely, improvement is so dramatic and complete following endovenous laser ablation that additional procedures are not necessary. Proponents of performing adjunctive procedures at the same sitting as endovenous ablation cite decreased treatment sessions and lower risks of superficial phlebitis, particularly in large thigh varicose tributaries following elimination of the underlying reflux. Occasionally, treatment of nonsurface tributary veins or persistence of clinically significant perforator reflux require ultrasound-guided sclerotherapy with foam or strong liquid sclerosants.

Many subjects develop ecchymosis over the treated site due to puncture of the vein during access and administration of tumescent anesthesia. This is of no medical consequence and resolves within weeks following endovenous laser. Some subjects may experience mild discomfort over the treated vein beginning hours after the procedure and resolving within 24 to 48 hours. Many subjects also note delayed tightness and mild to moderate tenderness of the treated vein, particularly over the medial aspect of the lower thigh/knee. This sensation, described as a "pulling," usually starts after a few days, reaches a peak approximately 7 days following endovenous laser, and resolves by week 2 or 3. This delayed pain does not correspond to presence or degree of bruising and is most likely caused by transverse and longitudinal retraction of the vein as the acute inflammation transitions to cicatrisation. Most subjects feel better with gradient compression hose and ambulation. Occasionally, nonsteroidal anti-inflammatories may be necessary.

Outcomes

The technical success of endovenous laser is defined as a procedure with successful access, crossing the segment to be treated, proper administration of tumescent anesthesia, emptying the vein adequately, and delivery of sufficient laser energy to the entire incompetent vein. Anatomic success is based on permanent occlusion of the treated vein segments with successful elimination of related varicose veins. Figure 6.5 shows a right leg at baseline and following elimination of GSV reflux with endovenous laser and sclerotherapy of the associated varicosities.

Subject-reported outcomes such as health-related quality-of-life (HRQOL), treatment satisfaction, symptom relief, and side effects are other important factors in evaluating success.

In addition to clinical examination, DUS is essential following endovenous laser. Most practitioners perform DUS within 1 week following endovenous laser, at completion of treatment, and then yearly. DUS criteria for successful treatment are important to recognize. One week following endovenous laser, DUS imaging reveals a noncompressible vein, minimally decreased in diameter, with echogenic, circumferentially thickened vein walls, and no flow seen within the entire treated vein lumen upon color Doppler interrogation. Adequate treatment should result in occlusion due to vein wall injury with resultant inflammation. If present, intraluminal thrombus should be minimal and a secondary phenomena, not the primary cause of occlusion, which would result in recanalization. At 3 to 6 months' follow-up, DUS should demonstrate continued target vein occlusion with marked reduction in vein diameter. The vein should be absent or only a minimal residual cord visible upon DUS imaging at 1 year and beyond.[5,6]

Several investigators have reported outstanding success rates of endovenous laser ablation of the GSV.[7-15] These studies have consistently shown successful nonthrombotic occlusion of the saphenous vein in 90% to 100% of cases at 1 -to 7-year follow-up, with very rare recanalizations of previously occluded vein segments. Clinical improvement was noted in almost all

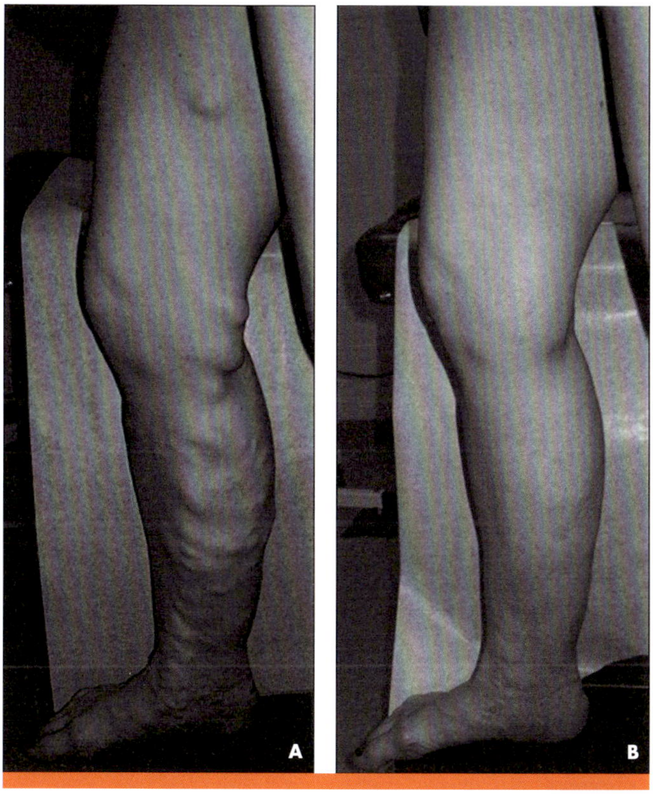

FIGURE 6.5 **A.** The pretreatment photograph demonstrates large right lower extremity varicose veins due to SFJ incompetence with GSV reflux. **B.** Three months following endovenous laser treatment of the incompetent GSV and sclerotherapy of associated varicosities, there is marked improvement in the appearance of the leg.

cases following successful saphenous vein occlusion. Subject acceptance was high, and adverse reactions were extremely rare, with heat complications such as DVTs, paresthesias, or skin burns virtually nonexistent.

The remarkably low rate of true adverse reactions following endovenous laser ablation compares favorably to other treatments of saphenous vein reflux such as surgery or other catheter-based procedures such as radiofrequency or chemical ablation. Complications related to endovenous techniques using radiofrequency have included skin paresthesias, skin burns, DVTs, and pulmonary emboli. Although liberal use of tumescent anesthesia has helped reduce the incidence of heat-related injury to adjacent nontarget tissues, there has been persistence of paresthesias (13%–15%), clinical phlebitis (2%–20%), thermal skin injury (4%–7%), and DVT (1%–16%) resulting from radiofrequency ablation.[16-19]

Although speculation exists regarding differences in success of endovenous laser vs. other treatment options, published literature directly comparing techniques is limited. The results of a recent meta-analysis and meta-regression analysis involving more than 60 studies concluded that endovenous thermal treatments of lower extremity varicosities were better at achieving anatomic success than surgery or ultrasound-guided foam sclerotherapy. It was also concluded that of the endovenous therapies, endovenous laser was determined to be more effective than radiofrequency ablation in obliterating insufficient veins. At 5 years, the pooled success rate of endovenous laser was 95.4%, compared to 79.9% for radiofrequency, 73.5% for ultrasound-guided foam sclerotherapy, and 75.7% for surgery.[20] A few studies have also shown that subjects treated with endovenous laser appreciated laser more than surgery because of fewer side effects and greater and faster improvements in HRQOL.[21,22]

Examination of treatment parameters has led to optimization of endovenous laser technique. Studies by Timperman[4,23] and Proebstle[24,25] have shown that the success of endovenous laser is dependent upon amount of laser energy, with treatment failures virtually nonexistent when at least 70 J are delivered per centimeter of treated vein. The vein reopenings seen within the first months following endovenous laser likely represent inadequate vein wall heating with thrombus recanalization. This is either because of excessively rapid pullback of the laser fiber or insufficient vein emptying, resulting in poor transfer of thermal energy to the vein wall. True recanalizations of treated veins can occur but appear to be uncommon. Initial vein wall diameter is unrelated to procedural success and there appears to be no size limit of vein that can be successfully treated with endovenous laser as long as adequate vein emptying is achieved. Veins with initial diameters in excess of 30 mm have been successfully closed with endovenous laser by several practitioners.

Some investigators have postulated that absorption of laser energy by blood plays a role in homogeneous distribution of thermal damage to the inner vein wall.[26] It is apparent from more recent scientific studies and mathematical calculations that steam formation from blood absorption is grossly inadequate to result in significant vein wall damage.[27,28] Fan and Rox-Anderson concluded that endovenous laser causes permanent vein closure through a high-temperature photothermolytic process at the point of contact between the vein and the laser fiber. They also calculated that steam production during endovenous laser, which occurs early in the photothermolytic process when temperatures reach 100°C, accounts for only 2% of applied energy dose, and is therefore unlikely to be the primary mechanism of action of thermal injury during the procedure.[29]

Performing endovenous ablation of the GSV without division of each of the tributaries at the SFJ goes against a fundamental rule in saphenous vein surgery; however, endovenous ablation procedures seem to have lower recurrence rates than surgical ligation and stripping. Staying out of the groin, preserving venous drainage in normal competent tributaries, and removing only the abnormal refluxing segments may not incite neovascularization often seen following surgical treatment. Although true recanalization of ablated saphenous veins is uncommon, recurrence of varicose veins is not. Even successful endovenous ablation does not entirely eliminate someone's propensity to develop venous insufficiency. This can occur from untreated portions of the saphenous vein, incompetent tributaries, perforator reflux, or worsening of veins during pregnancy. As durable and effective a technique that endovenous laser has proven to be, practitioners must counsel patients that venous insufficiency is a chronic condition.

References

1. Boné C. Tratamiento endoluminal de las varices con laser de Diodo. Estudio preliminary. Rev Patol Vasc. 1999;5:35-46.
2. Navarro L, Min R, Boné C. Endovenous laser: a new minimally invasive method of treatment for varicose veins-preliminary observations using an 810 nm diode laser. Dermatol Surg. 2001;27:117-22.
3. Min R, Zimmet S, Isaacs M, Forrestal M. Endovenous laser treatment of the incompetent greater saphenous vein. J Vasc Interv Radiol. 2001;12:1167-71.
4. Timperman PE, Sichlau M, Ryu RK. Greater energy delivery improves treatment success of endovenous laser treatment of incompetent saphenous veins. J Vasc Interv Radiol. 2004;15:1061-3.
5. Min RJ, Khilnani NM, Golia P. Duplex ultrasound of lower extremity venous insufficiency. J Vasc Interv Radiol. 2003;14:1233-41.

6. Khilnani NM, Min RJ. Duplex ultrasound for superficial venous insufficiency. Tech Vasc Interv Radiol. 2003;6:111-5.
7. Min R, Khilnani N, Zimmet S. Endovenous laser treatment of saphenous vein reflux: long-term results. J Vasc Interv Radiol. 2003; 14:991-6.
8. Proebstle TM, Gul D, Lehr HA, Kargl A, Knop J. Infrequent early recanalization of great saphenous vein after endovenous laser treatment. J Vasc Surg. 2003;38: 511-6.
9. Oh CK, Jung DS, Jang HS, Kwon KS. Endovenous laser surgery of the incompetent greater saphenous vein with a 980-nm diode laser. Dermatol Surg. 2003;29(11):1135-40.
10. Sadick NS, Wasser S. Combined endovascular laser with ambulatory phlebectomy for the treatment of superficial venous incompetence: a 2-year perspective. J Cosmet Laser Ther. 2004;6(1):44-9.
11. Perkowski P, Ravi R, Gowda RC, Olsen D, Ramaiah V, Rodriguez-Lopez JA, et al. Endovenous laser ablation of the saphenous vein for treatment of venous insufficiency and varicose veins: early results from a large single-center experience. J Endovasc Ther. 2004;11(2):132-8.
12. Min R, Khilnani N. Endovenous laser ablation of varicose veins. J Cardiovasc Surg. 2005;46(4):395-405.
13. Kabnick LS. Outcome of different endovenous laser wavelengths for great saphenous vein ablation. J Vasc Surg. 2006;43:88-93.
14. Ravi R, Trayler E, Barrett D, Diethrich EB. Endovenous thermal ablation of superficial venous insufficiency of the lower extremity: single center experience with 3000 limbs treated in a 7-year period. J Endovasc Ther. 2009;16:500-5.
15. Nwaejike N, Srodon PD, Kyriakides C. %-years of endovenous laser ablation (EVLA) for the treatment of varicose veins—a prospective study. Int J Surg. 2009;7:347-9.
16. Manfrini S, Gasbarro V, Danielsson G, Norgren L, Chandler JG, Lennox AF, Zarka ZA, Nicolaides AN. Endovenous management of saphenous vein reflux. J Vasc Surg. 2000;32:330-42.
17. Merchant RF, DePalma RG, Kabnick LS. Endovascular obliteration of saphenous reflux: a multi-center study. J Vasc Surg. 2002;35:1190-6.
18. Rautio TT, Perala JM, Wiik HT, Juvonen TS, Haukipuro KA. Endovenous obliteration with radiofrequency-resistive heating for greater saphenous vein insufficiency: a feasibility study. J Vasc Interv Radiol. 2002;13:569-75.
19. Hingorani AP, Ascher E, Markevich N, Schutzer RW, Kallakuri S, Hou A, et al. Deep venous thrombosis after radiofrequency ablation of greater saphenous vein: a word of caution. J Vasc Surg. 2004;40:500-4.
20. van den Bos R, Arends L, Kockaert M, Neumann M, Nijsten T. Endovenous therapies of lower extremity varicosities: a meta-analysis. J Vasc Surg. 2009;49:230-9.
21. De Medeiros CA, Luccas GC. Comparison of endovenous laser treatment with an 810 nm laser versus conventional stripping of the great saphenous vein in subjects with primary varicose veins. Dermatol Surg. 2005;31:1685-94.
22. Mekako AI, Hatfield J, Bryce J, Lee D, McCollum PT, Chetter I. A nonrandomized controlled trial of endovenous laser therapy and surgery in the treatment of varicose veins. Ann Vasc Surg. 2006;20:451-7.
23. Timperman PE. Prospective evaluation of higher energy great saphenous vein endovenous laser treatment. J Vasc Interv Radiol. 2005;16:791-4.
24. Proebstle TM, Krummenauer F, Gul D, Knop J. Nonocclusion and early reopening of the great saphenous vein after endovenous laser treatment is fluence dependent. Dermatol Surg. 2004;30:174-8.

25. Proebstle TM, Moehler T, Herdemann S. Reduced recanalization rates of the great saphenous vein after endovenous laser treatment with increased energy dosing: definition of a threshold for the endovenous fluence equivalent. J Vasc Surg. 2006;44: 834-9.
26. Proebstle TM, Sandhofer M, Kargl A, Gul D, Rother W, Knop J, et al. Thermal damage of the inner vein wall during endovenous laser treatment: key role of energy absorption by intravascular blood. Dermatol Surg. 2002;28;596-600.
27. Mordon SR, Wassmer B, Zemmouri J. Mathematical modeling of endovenous laser treatment (ELT). BioMedical Engineering OnLine. 2006;5:26;http://www.biomedical-engineering-online.com/content/5/1/26.
28. Mordon SR, Wassmer B, Zemmouri J. Mathematical modeling of 980 nm and 1,320 nm endovenous laser treatment. Lasers Surg Med. 2007;39:256-65.
29. Fan CM, Rox-Anderson R. Endovenous laser ablation: mechanism of action. Phlebology. 2008;23:206-13.

CHAPTER 7

Recommendations for Sclerotherapy of Spider Veins, Reticular Veins, and Varicose Veins

Joann M. Lohr and Angela N. Fellner

Generalized indications for intervention on varicose veins include general appearance, aching pain, leg heaviness, easy leg fatigueability, superficial thrombophlebitis, external bleeding, ankle hyperpigmentation, lipodermatosclerosis, atrophie blanche, or history of venous ulcer.[1] Varicosities of the lower extremity can be classified into 3 groups. Group 1 consists of spider bursts and telangiectatic veins, which normally have a competent saphenous system. Group 2 are mild to moderate varicosities in which the saphenous system is competent. Group 3 are moderate or marked varicosities with an incompetent saphenous system.[2]

Vessels can be further subclassified into types. Type 1, spider veins or telangiectasias, are 0.1 to 1.0 mm in diameter and are red to cyanotic (Figure 7.1). Type 1A, with telangiectatic matting vessels, are <0.2 mm in diameter and tend to be red (Figure 7.2). Type 1B, communicating telangiectasias, are type 1 veins in direct communication with the varicose veins of the saphenous system (Figure 7.3). Type 2 is a mixture of telangiectatic and

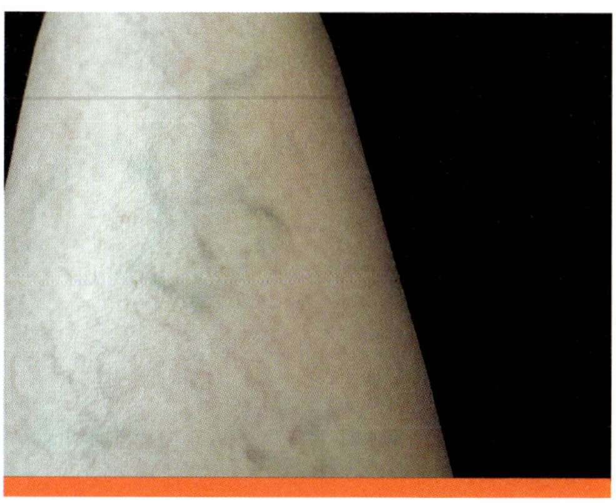

FIGURE 7.1 Type 1 vessels. Spider veins or telangiectasias are 0.1–1.00 mm in diameter and are red to cyanotic.

Chronic Venous Insufficiency. Contemporary Endovascular Management series. © 2011 Mark G. Davies MD and Alan B. Lumsden MD, eds. Cardiotext Publishing, ISBN 978-1-935395-09-6.

varicose veins with no direct communication with the saphenous system (Figure 7.4). They can be 1 to 6 mm in diameter and are cyanotic to blue. Type 3, nonsaphenous varicose veins (reticular veins), are 2 to 8 mm in diameter and are blue to green (Figure 7.5). Type 4, saphenous varicose veins, are usually more than 8 mm in diameter and blue to blue-green (Figure 7.6).[3,4]

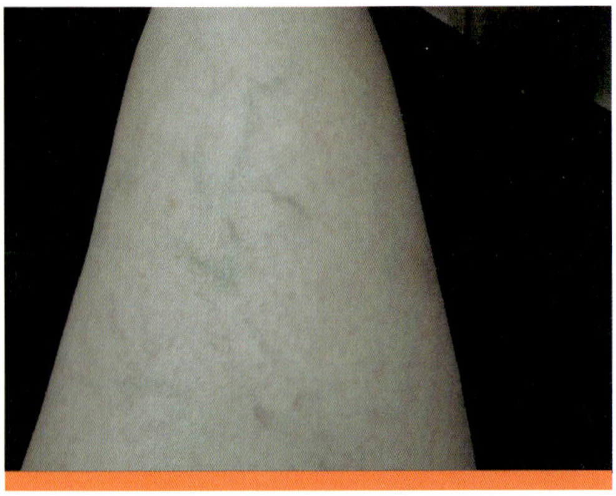

FIGURE 7.2 Type 1A vessels with telangiectatic matting are <0.2 mm in diameter and tend to be red.

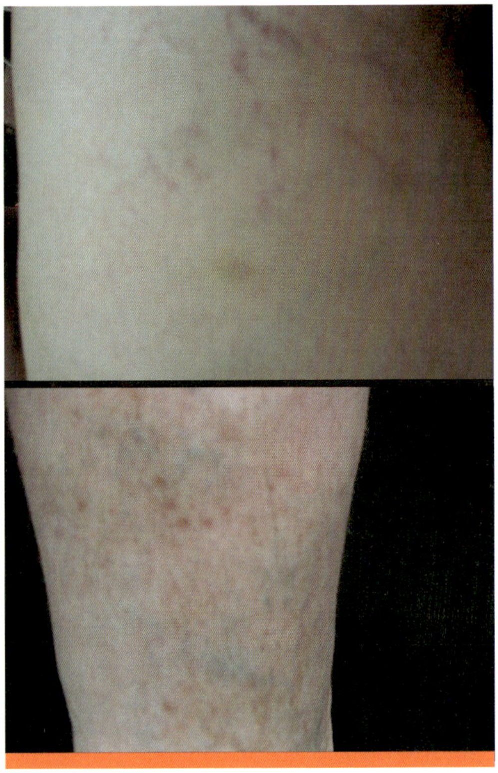

FIGURE 7.4 Type 2 vessels are a mixture of telangiectatic and varicose veins with no direct communication with the saphenous system.

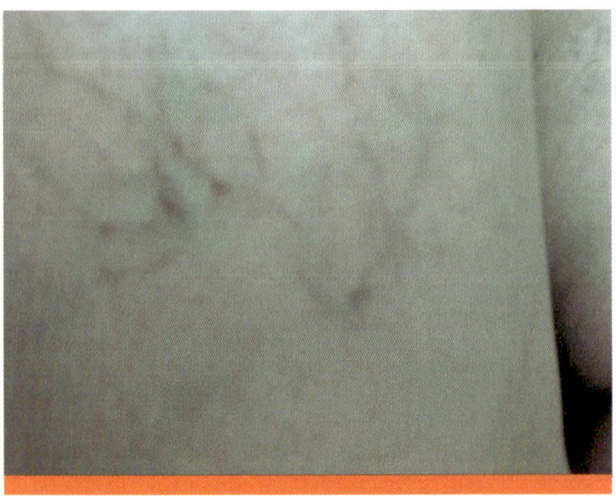

FIGURE 7.3 Type 1B vessels, communicating telangiectasias, are type 1 veins in direct communication with the varicose veins of the saphenous system.

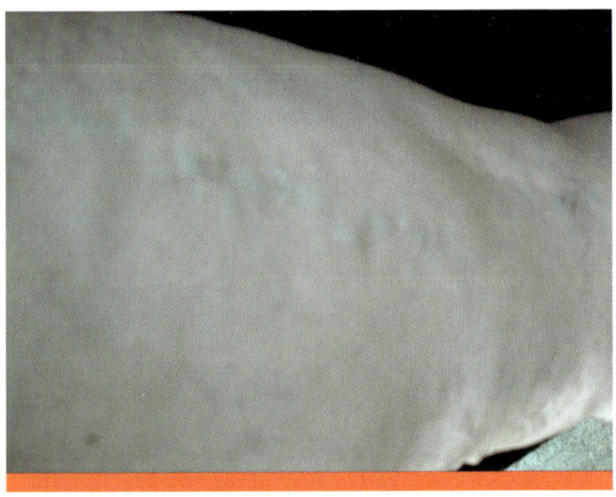

FIGURE 7.5 Type 3 vessels are nonsaphenous varicose veins (reticular veins) that are 2–8 mm in diameter and are blue to green.

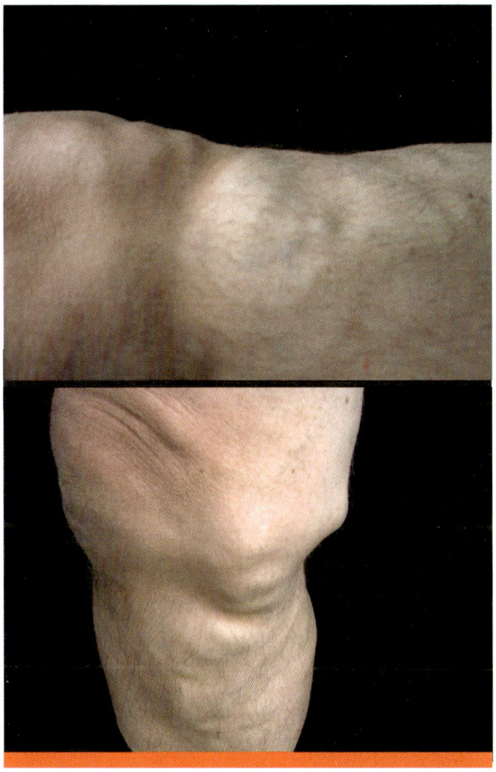

FIGURE 7.6 Type 4 vessels are saphenous varicose veins, which are usually more than 8 mm in diameter and are blue to blue-green.

Guidelines for the Treatment of Varicose and Telangiectatic Leg Veins

Location and site help determine treatments for varicose veins. Conservative treatments for varicose, reticular, and venous telangiectatic veins include compression (eg, bandaging, support hose, external compression devices), diet, exercise, leg elevation, good skin hygiene, weight loss, and medication. Endovenous and interventional therapies include sclerotherapy, laser or light therapy, and endovenous obliteration of the saphenous vein. Surgical options include ambulatory phlebectomy or stab avulsion phlebectomy, ligation and stripping, and transilluminated powered phlebectomy (TIPP).[5]

When considering treatment of varicose veins by sclerotherapy, absolute contraindications for sclerotherapy include patients with acute deep vein thrombosis, acute infections including cellulitis, allergies to sclerosant solutions, bedridden or immobile patients, patients with blood dyscrasias or thrombophilias, patients who are breastfeeding, cancer patients undergoing active chemotherapy, pregnancy, and uncontrolled diabetes. Anyone who has peripheral artery disease should be approached with caution. Caution should also be used in women who are on oral contraceptives or hormone replacement therapy.[5]

Successful sclerotherapy requires creating realistic expectations and selecting appropriate treatment options for the individual setting. This requires appropriate preoperative evaluation, valve assessment, informed consent, setting realistic patient expectations and goals, and having treatment sessions that are patient friendly (eg, warm room, shorts to be worn for comfort and modesty). Photographs are taken for records using a black background and standardized techniques, injection sites are compressed, legs are elevated, stockings are added, and microthrombectomy is also used to decrease pigmentation. We perform reflux perforator mapping evaluation with the patient in the upright or semiupright position. Manual squeeze as well as inflation cuff technique is utilized. Normal valve closure time is defined as less than 0.5 seconds' duration, borderline is between 0.5 and 1.0 second, and anything greater than 1 second is considered abnormal.[6]

When considering sclerotherapy for treatment of varicose veins, the skin of patients who are considering treatment should be evaluated. Fitzgerald's skin classifications are important to note as different skin types are at increased risk for pigmentation, as shown in Table 7.1.[7]

Evaluation of Sclerotherapy Outcomes

To evaluate sclerotherapy, we want to evaluate and grade our results. We use a 4-point scale to quantify pain duration, where 0 = no pain, 1 = short duration (<2 min), 2 = moderate duration (2–10 min), and 3 = prolonged duration (>10 min). Additionally, we also want to monitor for immediate local reactions including pain, inflammation, swelling, allergies, and pain duration. Immediate systemic reactions can include dizziness, nausea, vomiting, dyspnea, cardiac manifestations, hypotension, fainting, asthma, skin allergies, and anaphylactic shock. These should all be graded using the 4-point scale, where 1 = none, 2 = mild, 3 = moderate, 4 = severe.

Delayed local reactions may also occur. These may include local vein thrombosis (presence or absence should be noted), ecchymosis (measured in cm^2), and necrosis (measured in cm^2). Again, these may be graded using a 4-point scale, where 1 = none, 2 = mild (<1 cm^2), 3 = moderate (1–2 cm^2), and 4 = severe (>2 cm^2). Results can be standardized.

Hyperpigmentation should also be noted. A standardized brown scale is useful, and here we have used paint sticks to grade the pigmentation and to standardize the observations between technicians and treatment sessions. Here, 1 = deep brown, 2 = light brown, 3 = tan, and 4 = no pigmentation.

The presence or absence of neovascularization should also be noted.

TABLE 7.1 **A Classification of Skin Phototypes Based on Susceptibility to Sunburn in Sunlight, Tanning Ability, and Skin Cancer Risk**

Skin Phototype	Sunburn Susceptibility	Tanning Ability	Skin Cancer Risk	No. of Standard Erythema Dose* Required for Minimal Erythema
I	High	None	High	1–3
II	High	Poor	High	
III	Moderate	Good	Low	3–7
IV	Low	Very good	Low	
V	Very low	Excellent	Very low	7–12
VI	Very low	Excellent	Very low	

*A standard erythema dose is equivalent to an erythemally effective radiant exposure of 100 J/mL. Approximately 3 standard erythema doses are required to produce just perceptible or minimal erythema in unacclimatized skin of the most common Caucasian and northern European skin types.

From Wolff K, Goldsmith LA, Katz SI, et al. Fitzpatrick's Dermatology in General Medicine, 7th ed. New York: McGraw Hill Medical; 2008:810. With permission of the McGraw-Hill Companies, Inc.

Efficacy is defined as the disappearance of varicosities and is graded on a 5-point scale, where 1 means the varicosities are worse than before, 2 means they are the same as before, 3 means a minority of varicosities have disappeared, 4 means a majority have disappeared, and 5 means they have completely disappeared. Secondary efficacy corresponds to "overall clinical improvement" and encompasses vein disappearance, hyperpigmentation, and neovascularization. On a 10-point scale, 0–2 = poor, 3–4 = fair, 5–6 = moderate, 7–8 = good, and 9–10 = excellent. Patient satisfaction is graded on a 4-point scale, where 1 = unsatisfied, 2 = moderately satisfied, 3 = satisfied, and 4 = very satisfied. Efficacy allows the scoring and grading by both the patient and the clinician. This method of evaluation allows reproducibility by standardizing observations and thereby decreasing variability in patient assessment.

Sclerosing Agents

There are 3 categories of sclerosing solutions: detergent sclerosing solutions, hypertonic sclerosing solution, and the caustic chemical sclerosing solution. The potency of the sclerosing solution should be matched to the vein size and diameter. Suggested potency and vein dimensions are given in Table 7.2.[8] Care should be taken to not use too high a concentration for the vein size treated, or the likelihood of complication increases. Retreatment with a more concentrated solution, if needed, is a better approach.

The sclerosing solutions all work after being placed in the vein and released. In the early stage, the endothelial cells are affected, with minimal organizing thrombosis. In the

TABLE 7.2 **Relative Potency of Sclerosing Solutions**

Vein Diameter (mm)	Sclerosing Solution
< 0.4	Glycerin 70% Chromated glycerin 50% Polidocanol 0.25% Sodium tetradecyl sulfate 0.1% Hypertonic saline 11.7% Sclerodex Ethanolamine oleate 2% Polyiodinated iodine 0.1% Polidocanol 0.5% Sodium morrhuate 0.25%–0.3%
0.6–2.0	Chromated glycerin 100% Sodiun tetradecyl sulfate 0.25% Polidocanol 0.75% Polyiodinated iodine 0.5%–1.0% Ethonalamine oleate 5% Hypertonic saline 23.4% Sodium morrhuate 1.0%–2.5%
3–5	Polidocanol 1%–2% Sodium tetradecyl sulfate 0.5%–1% Sodium morrhuate 5% Polyiodinated iodine 2%
>5 Perforators Saphenofemoral/ popliteal injections	Polidocanol 3%–4% Sodiun tetradecyl sulfate 2%–3% Polyiodinated iodine 3%–12%

From Goldman MP, Bergan JJ. Sclerotherapy: Treatment of Varicose and Telangiectatic Leg Veins, 3rd ed. St. Louis: Mosby; 2001:174. With permission from Elsevier.

late stage, there is thrombosis and cord formation. Ideally the treated vessel progresses directly from damaged endothelium to a fibrous cord, avoiding the thrombotic phase (Figure 7.7).[9]

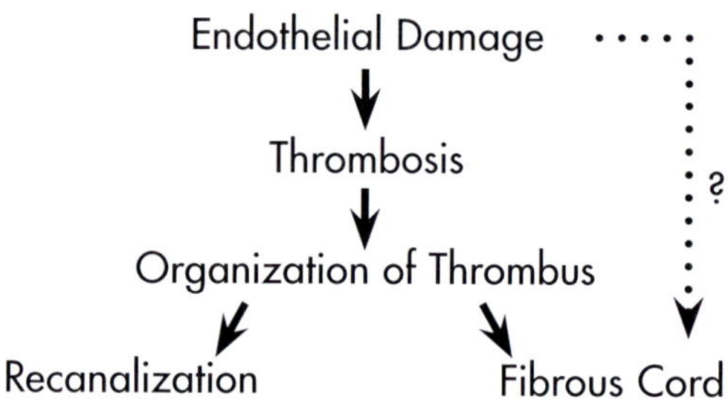

FIGURE 7.7 Chain of events occurring after sclerotherapy. Ideally, the treated vessel will progress directly from damaged endothelium to a fibrous cord. However, some degree of intravascular thrombosis usually occurs. From Goldman MP, Bergan JJ. Sclerotherapy: Treatment of Varicose and Telangiectatic Leg Veins, 3rd ed. St. Louis: Mosby; 2001:170. Copyright Elsevier.

Sclerotherapy can extravasate in a variety of different ways, including through multiple needle holes in the vein or along the needle after its slight withdrawal, extravasation of the sclerosing solution along the needle shaft itself, extravasation from the injection with the needle bevel both in and outside of the vein, or extravasation through excessive destruction of the vein wall itself.[10]

Complications of sclerosing agents include pigmentation, allergic reaction, necrosis, and pain. Different solutions in different concentrations are known to have different complication profiles as noted in Table 7.3.[11]

Avoiding overinjection can decrease complications, especially pigmentation, and can decrease the amount of matting that may occur. Early microthrombectomy may be of benefit to decrease the amount of pigmentation.[12] Pigmentation may be defined

TABLE 7.3 **Summary of Complications of Sclerosing Agents**

Solution	Pigmentation	Allergic Reaction	Necrosis	Pain
Sodium morrhuate	++	++	+++*	+++
Sodium tetradecyl sulfate	++	+	++*	+
Ethanolamine oleate	+	++	++*	++
Polidocanol	+	+	+*	0
Hypertonic saline	+	0	+++*	+++
Sclerodex (+ 0% saline 5% dextrose)	+	0	+	++
Chromated glycerin	0	+	0	++
Polyiodinated iodine	++	+	+++*	+++

Minimal +, Moderate ++, Significant +++, Concentration-dependent*

From Goldman MP, Bergan JJ. Sclerotherapy: treatment of varicose and telangiectatic leg veins, 3rd ed. St. Louis: Mosby; 2001:231. With permission from Elsevier.

as any brown-black staining of the skin that occurs after sclerotherapy. Persistent pigmentation is defined as that which remains after 1 year. Pigmentation most likely results from a combination of incontinence of melanin pigment and hemosiderin deposition. Defects in iron storage and metabolism may also be found in some patients who develop pigmentation. The incidence of pigmentation is multifactorial, including solution type and concentration, technique, gravitational and other intravascular pressures, innate tendency toward cutaneous pigmentation (total body iron stores/altered iron transport and storage mechanisms, innate enhanced histamine release or hypersensitivity and vessel fragility), postsclerotherapy treatment (graduate compression), vessel diameter, and concomitant medications.[7]

Insurance coding for various sclerotherapy purposes includes the diagnostic code, noninvasive testing code, and sclerotherapy treatment code.[13] These are listed in Table 7.4.

TABLE 7. 4 **Insurance Coding for Various Sclerotherapy Services**

Diagnostic	**Noninvasive Testing**	**Sclerotherapy Treatment**
Spider veins (448.1)	Doppler venous unilateral (93965)	Cosmetic procedure (A9370)
Elective/cosmetic procedure (V50.1)	Doppler venous unilateral (93965-50)	Spider—face (36469)
Varicose veins (454.9)	Doppler arterial (93922)	Spider—nonface (36468)
Varicose vein with inflammation (454.1)	Duplex examination —unilateral, limited (93971)	Varicose vein —single unilateral (36470)
Leg pain (729.5)	Duplex examination —bilateral, complete (93970)	Varicose vein —single bilateral (35470-50)
Leg edema (782.3)	Photoplethysmography —unilateral (93965)	Varicose vein —multiple unilateral (35471)
Leg ulcer—chronic (707.1)	Photoplethysmography —bilateral (93965-50)	Varicose vein —multiple bilateral (35471-50)
Chronic venous insufficiency (459.81)		Sclerotherapy tray (A4550)
Thrombophlebitis, leg (451.2)		Sodium tetradecyl sulfate (J3490)
Hematoma complicating a procedure (998.12)		Compression bandages (A4460)
Lymphedema (457.1)		Compression stockings —knee high (A4500)
		Compression stockings —thigh high (A4495)
		Puncture aspiration of hematoma (10160)

From Goldman MP, Bergan JJ. Sclerotherapy: Treatment of Varicose and Telangiectatic Leg Veins, 3rd ed. St. Louis: Mosby; 2001:231. With permission from Elsevier.

Foam Sclerosing Agents

One of the new areas of development is sclerosing agents that are made of foam. Several types of foam are possible. The foam may be a froth generated from simple mixing of air with a detergent solution with bubbles that range from millimeters (eg, generated by the Orbach method), foam that is a generation of a foam with bubbles having a diameter of greater than 100 μm (eg, the Monfreux method), minifoam in which bubbles range from 50 to 100 μm, or microfoam, in which the bubbles are smaller than 50 μm.[14]

Liquid sclerosants are mixed with blood in the vein being treated, resulting in inactivation of the sclerosing agent. The needle is introduced to the vein. The sclerosant is then diluted by the blood (Figure 7.8).[15] Foam sclerosants, however, displace the blood from the vein under treatment and completely fill it, making the treatment more effective. The needle is placed into the vein, the foam is injected and displaces the blood from the vein, and the vein then responds by developing a spasm (Figure 7.9).[15]

Advantages and Disadvantages of Foam Sclerotherapy

Foam sclerotherapy offers several advantages over traditional sclerotherapy. First, it allows increased contact between the sclerosant and the endothelium as the air within the foam pushes the material snugly against the vein wall. Foam sclerotherapy decreases the dilution of the sclerosant because the foam actually replaces the blood rather than mixing with it as in traditional sclerotherapy. Compared with traditional sclerosants, foam sclerosants are able to increase the duration of treatment, ie, the length of time the sclerosant stays in contact with the vein wall.[14] Variables in foam sclerosants include the type and concentration of sclerosant used, the type of gas used to create the foam, the ratio of liquid to gas in the solution, the method of sclerosant preparation, the time between processing and use of the sclerosant, and the bubble size of the foam.[14] Some new possible indications for foam sclerotherapy include interventional angioradiologic procedures, pelvic venous congestion syndrome, varicocele, hydrocele, angiodysplasia, metastatic lesions, vascular malignant tumors, and Baker's cysts.[16]

Adverse events can accompany injections of foamed sclerosant. These include dry cough, visual disturbance, panic attacks, chest pressure, paresthesias, and myoclonus.[17] Serious adverse events have been reported with foam sclerotherapy, including pulmonary embolism of less than 1%, DVT (less than 1%), visual disturbance (1%–4%), headaches (4.2%), thrombophlebitis (4.7%), matting and pigmentation (17.8%), pain at the injection site (25.6%), complete vein occlusion (87%), and vein recurrence (8.1%).[18]

Ultrasound-Guided Sclerosant Therapy

Indications for ultrasound-guided injections include incompetent small or great saphenous vein with associated saphenofemoral or saphenopopliteal incompetence, or obese individuals in whom it may be difficult to palpate the varicosities. It is useful to identify deeply seated perforating veins and also to map and diagnose complex pathologic processes.[14] Ultrasound-guided sclerotherapy offers several benefits. It allows the practitioner to place the needle accurately, to follow the infusion of the sclerosant and foam, and to monitor perforating veins. In addition, extravasation and intraatrial injections can be avoided.[14] Some precautions, however, are necessary when performing ultrasound-

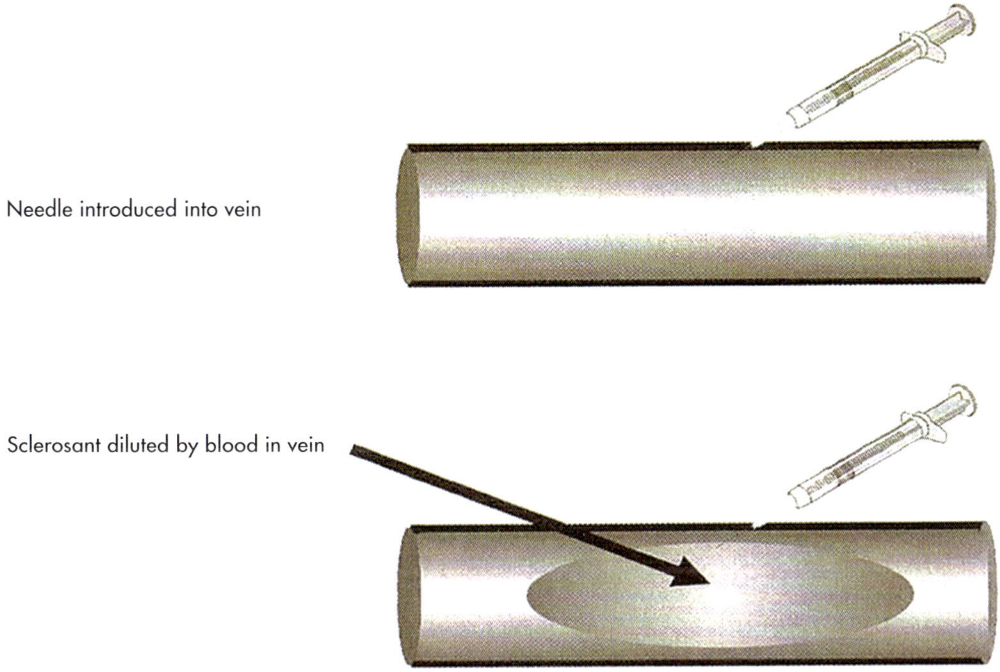

FIGURE 7.8 Liquid sclerosants mix with blood in the vein that is being treated, resulting in inactivation of the sclerosant. Reprinted from Smith PC. Saphenous ablation:sclerosant or sclerofoam. Semin Vasc Surg. 2005;18:19-2. With permission from Elsevier.

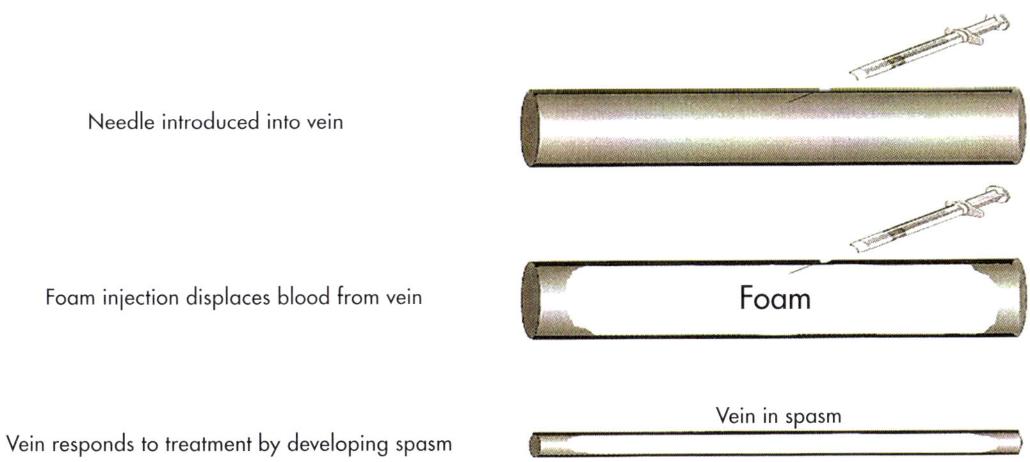

FIGURE 7.9 Foam sclerosants displace blood from the vein under treatment and completely fill it, making treatment more effective. Reprinted from Smith PC. Saphenous ablation:sclerosant or sclerofoam. Semin Vasc Surg. 2005;18:19-2. With permission from Elsevier.

guided sclerotherapy. First, the vessel to be injected should always be compressed prior to the injection. Veins should compress easily, while arteries will not compress easily without excessive pressure. This should help to prevent arterial injections. In addition, practitioners should aspirate and check for blood "flashback." They should never inject without seeing where the needle tip is; any practitioner who is not sure should simply not inject.

Intra-arterial injections can occur. Some tips to avoid this involve use of ultrasound guidance and compression of the vessel before injecting, always keeping the needle tip in view. An intra-arterial injection represents a true emergency. It can result in severe tissue destruction and loss of limb and thus requires immediate transport to the hospital for treatment.

The complications of foam sclerotherapy include "trapping," intravascular hematoma, hemosiderin staining, infection, pain, bruising, paresthesias, DVT, phlebitis, and skin burn (both chemical and thermal).

Polidocanol is currently in the process of obtaining FDA approval. Polidocanol foam sclerotherapy has been used widely in Europe. Table 7.5 presents the concentration of liquid in foam polidocanol and the appropriate vein sizes that have been studied.[19]

Primary and secondary outcomes with 1% and 3% polidocanol foam have been evaluated using duplex-guided sclerotherapy to treat the great saphenous vein and are listed in Table 7.6.[20]

Table 7.5 Concentrations of Polidocanol According to the Diameter of the Varices and Quantities Used per Injection

Diameter	Liquid	Foam
1.0–2.0 mm	1.00%	0.50%
2.1–3.0 mm	1.25%	0.65%
3.1–4.0 mm	1.50%	0.75%
4.1–5.0 mm	2.00%	1.00%
5.1–6.0 mm	2.50%	1.25%
Volume per injection	0.5 mL	2.00 mL
Quantity (polidocanol) per injection	0.5 mL	0.5 mL

From Alòs J, Carreño P, López JA, et al. Efficacy and safety of sclerotherapy using polidocanol foam: a controlled clinical trial. Eur J Vasc Endovasc Surg. 2006;31(1):101-7. With permission from Elsevier.

TABLE 7.6 **Primary and Secondary Outcomes of 1% and 3% Polidocanol Foam**

Outcome	Baseline		1 month			1 year		
	1%	3%	1%	3%	*P* Value	1%	3%	*P* Value
Occlusion			86.7%	91.5%		69.5%	80.1%	0.25
Cosmetic improvement			40.0%	52.5%	0.31	67.5%	77.5%	0.57
Venous complaints	66.7%	78.9%	6.7%	11.1%	0.51	29.7%	25.0%	0.45
Thrombophlebitis			32.1%	50.0%	0.16			
Hyperpigmentation			22.0%	28.2%	0.48	8.10%	17.5%	0.22
Fibrosis						5.40%	5.0%	0.94

From Ceulen RP, Bullens-Goessens YI, Pi-Van De Venne SJ, et al. Outcomes and side effects of duplex-guided sclerotherapy in the treatment of great saphenous veins with 1% versus 3% polidocanol foam: results of a randomized controlled trial with 1-year follow-up. Dermatol Surg. 2007;33(3):276-81 with permission.

Conclusion

The opportunities and use of sclerotherapy continue to grow. Ultrasound-guided sclerotherapy and foam will further expand the realm of possibilities for the use of sclerotherapy in the future. FDA-sanctioned studies aimed at increasing the number of agents approved for sclerotherapy, including foam, are currently underway.

References

1. Bergan JJ, Kumins NH, Owens EL, Sparks SR. Surgical and endovascular treatment of lower extremity venous insufficiency. J Vasc Interv Radiol. 2002;13(6):563-8.
2. Heyerdale WW, Stalker LK. Management of varicose veins of the lower extremities. Ann Surg. 1941;114(6):1042-9.
3. Duffey DM. In: Callen JP, Dahl MV, Golitz LE, et al, eds. Advances in Dermatology, Vol 3. Chicago: Year Book Publishers; 1988.
4. Goldman MP, Bergan JJ. Sclerotherapy: Treatment of Varicose and Telangiectatic Leg veins. 3rd ed. St. Louis: Mosby; 2001. p49.
5. Bartholomew JR, King T, Sahgal A, Vidimos AT. Varicose veins: newer, better treatments available. Clev Clin J Med. 2005;72(4):312-4, 319-21, 325-8.
6. TriHealth Inc. Venous mapping. lower extremities: great and small saphenous veins protocol. Good Samaritan Hospital John J. Cranley Vascular Laboratory; March 2007.
7. Wolff K, Goldsmith LA, Katz SI, et al. Fitzpatrick's Dermatology in General Medicine. 7th ed. New York: McGraw Hill Medical; 2008. p810.
8. Goldman MP, Bergan JJ. Sclerotherapy: Treatment of Varicose and Telangiectatic Leg Veins. 3rd ed. St. Louis: Mosby; 2001. p174.
9. Goldman MP, Bergan JJ. Sclerotherapy: Treatment of Varicose and Telangiectatic Leg Veins. 3rd ed. St. Louis: Mosby; 2001. p170.

10. Goldman MP, Bergan JJ. Sclerotherapy: Treatment of Varicose and Telangiectatic Leg Veins. 3rd ed. St. Louis: Mosby; 2001. p209.
11. Goldman MP, Bergan JJ. Sclerotherapy: Treatment of Varicose and Telangiectatic Leg Veins. 3rd ed. St. Louis: Mosby; 2001. p.231.
12. Scultetus AH, Villavicencio JL, Kao TC, Gillespie DL, Ketron GD, Iafrati MD, et al. Microthrombectomy reduces postsclerotherapy pigmentation: multicenter randomized trial. J Vasc Surg. 2003;38(5): 896-903.
13. Goldman MP, Bergan JJ. Sclerotherapy: Treatment of Varicose and Telangiectatic Leg Veins. 3rd ed. St. Louis: Mosby; 2001. p354.
14. Sadick NS. Advances in the treatment of varicose veins: ambulatory phlebectomy, foam sclerotherapy, endovascular laser, and radiofrequency closure. Adv Dermatol. 2006;22:139-56.
15. Coleridge Smith P. Saphenous ablation: sclerosant or sclerofoam? Semin Vasc Surg. 2005;18(1):19-24.
16. Breu FX, Guggenbichler S. European consensus meeting on foam sclerotherapy, April, 4-6, 2003, Tegernsee, Germany. Dermatol Surg. 2004;30(5):709-17.
17. Bergan J, Pascarella L, Mekenas L. Venous disorders: treatment with sclerosant foam. J Cardiovasc Surg (Torino). 2006;47(1):9-18.
18. Jia X, Mowatt G, Burr JM, Cassar K, Cook J, Fraser C. Systematic review of foam sclerotherapy for varicose veins. Br J Surg. 2007;94(8):925-36.
19. Alòs J, Carreño P, López JA, Estadella B, Serra-Prat M, Marinel-Lo J. Efficacy and safety of sclerotherapy using polidocanol foam: a controlled clinical trial. Eur J Vasc Endovasc Surg. 2006;31(1):101-7.
20. Ceulen RP, Bullens-Goessens YI, Pi-VAN DE Venne SJ, Nelemans PJ, Veraart JC, et al. Outcomes and side effects of duplex-guided sclerotherapy in the treatment of great saphenous veins with 1% versus 3% polidocanol foam: results of a randomized controlled trial with 1-year follow-up. Dermatol Surg. 2007;33(3):276-81.

CHAPTER 8

Foam Sclerotherapy for the Treatment of Chronic Venous Insufficiency

Javier E. Anaya-Ayala, Sofia Gonzalez-Morales, and Mark G. Davies

Sclerosants in foam form have been used for decades in phlebology. In 1944, Egmont James Orbach described his "air-block technique," in which a small amount of air was injected into the vein segment to be treated before the liquid sclerosing agent was injected in order to empty the vein of blood, making direct and undiluted contact of the agent with the endothelium possible.[1] Karl Sigg presented a sclerotherapeutic concept in which foam was added to the "air-block technique" in 1949.[2] The objective of sclerotherapy is the induction of irritation in the endothelial and subendothelial layers of the wall of the vein, collapse of the walls by compression, and obliteration of the lumen by inflammation and fibrosis.

Sclerotherapy gained a reputation for lack of efficacy in the latter part of the 20th century due to the works of Hobbs,[3] but subsequent advances in technology led to improvements in practice and techniques. The first sclerosing agents employed were 40% glucose solution (Varico-Calorose), sodium tetradecyl sulfate (STS; Sotradecol), monoethanolamine oleate (Varisyl), and iodine solution (Varigloban), and after 1966 the most commonly employed product licensed in Germany was Aethoxysklerol with the active ingredient polidocanol (POL; concentrations of 0.25%, 0.5%, 1.0%, 2.0%, 3.0%, and 4.0%).[4] The next significant advancement came in 1995, when Cabrera et al suggested using carbon dioxide mixed with polidocanol, a detergent sclerosant. Since the mid-1990s, sclerotherapy with foam has been widely discussed, especially for the treatment of larger varicose veins. In addition to Juan Cabrera Garrido (Spain), Alain Monfreux (France) and others,

Chronic Venous Insufficiency. Contemporary Endovascular Management series.
Cardiotext Publishing, ISBN 978-1-935395-09-6.

Lorenzo Tessari, and Alessandro Frullini (Italy) demonstrated therapeutic successes with sclerosing foam.[5-7]

Indications

Foam sclerotherapy (FST) is becoming established as a primary method of treating refluxing saphenous veins. Its popularity is related to its relatively low cost; feasibility as an anesthetic-free, outpatient procedure; minimal postprocedural pain; and easy repeatability. However, the correct indications, the best sclerosant, and the most effective technique are still unclear. Long-term data on quality of life (QOL) and symptomatic and cosmetic improvement are lacking. The results of a phase III European trial (surgery vs. sclerotherapy) and a phase II US study of Varisolve (polidocanol microfoam) are eagerly awaited.[8]

Suitability of a patient for foam sclerotherapy depends on the aims of treatment. The method can be performed successfully in almost any patient with clinical venous insufficiency, no matter how elderly, frail, obese, or ill they are. Varicosities with small and large diameters can be treated, but saphenous veins with diameters of 10 mm or more may require multiple treatments and large volumes of foam (up to 3 sessions and 15 mL of foam). It can be used in patients with severe chronic venous insufficiency (CVI) and may enhance ulcer healing. This technique is also used to treat perforator veins and congenital venous malformations.[9]

Contraindications

Some relative and absolute contraindications to treatment by foam sclerotherapy are as follows.[3]

Adverse Patient Factors (Relative Contraindications to Treatment)

- Morbid obesity (BMI >30)
- Extreme age or frailty
- Severe concomitant disease (malignancy, cardiovascular, respiratory); known thrombophilia or history of previous deep venous thrombosis (DVT)
- "Needle-phobic" patients or those preferring treatment under general anesthesia
- Very thin patients may be left with lumps where the veins were obliterated following sclerotherapy and are less suitable for treatment

Adverse Venous Anatomy (Relative Contraindications to Treatment)

- Severe postthrombotic damage in the deep veins (little advantage of treating varicose veins)
- Very large varices (more complications of skin pigmentation and lumps following treatment)
- The lesion is an arteriovenous malformation (more difficult to treat)

Absolute Contraindications to Treatment

- Severe allergy to sclerosants
- Severe systemic disease
- Deep venous thrombosis
- Obliteration of deep vein system (eg, following extensive previous DVT with no recanalization of the deep veins)
- Recurrent deep venous thrombosis
- Severe arterial disorders with critical limb ischemia
- Patent foramen ovale

Technique

In the definitive treatment of varicose veins, the aim is to abolish sources of venous reflux and remove long refluxing segments and varicose reservoirs; this can be achieved by conventional surgery or by endovenous ablation techniques.

Foam sclerotherapy treatment consists of the injection of a sclerosing agent into the vein, leading to its long-term occlusion. After the injection of the sclerosing agent, the endothelium is profoundly damaged, leading to a secondary thrombus adherent to the vessel wall and, in the long term, to a conversion of the treated vessel into a sclerosed connective tissue cord.[2]

Sclerosing foam is produced by mixing a sclerosing agent with surface activity with a gas. Sclerosing foams have different characteristics: type and concentration of the sclerosing agent, type of gas, ratio of liquid to gas, time between the foam production and use, and size of the bubbles.[2,3]

Liquids and gas have different densities: gases are less dense and can be compressed, whereas liquids cannot. This basic principle explains why use of a sclerosant in foam form enables the active agent to be in touch with the endothelium for a longer time and provide more intensive contact.

The most effective foam with regard to stability, viscosity, and displacement ability results from a mixture ratio of 1 part sclerosant with 3 parts (1:4) or 4 parts air (1:5).[2] The smaller bubble size, the higher the sclerosant concentration in the foam, the lesser its dilution with blood, and the greater the sclerosant activity.[10]

The technique consists in following pretreatment workup and informed consent. Digital photographs are taken of the patient's limbs for "before and after" comparisons. The varicosities are then marked with an indelible marker. Reticular veins and small surface varicosities can be accessed without ultrasound guidance; however, for larger varicose veins, the use of ultrasound-guided injection is preferred. The vein-accessing technique can be performed with the patient either standing or lying down.[8]

Branch veins can be accessed with an angiocatheter or a hypodermic or butterfly needle. Foam is created before accessing the vein using Tessari's technique (the liquid is then rapidly exchanged between the 2 syringes until thick white foam is produced; about 20 exchanges). No bubbles should be visible in the foam. The foam should be used immediately because it starts to separate within minutes. Stability of the foam depends on concentration (higher concentrations are more stable) and which solution is used. The concentration of the liquid sclerosant used depends on the size of the vessel to be treated (Table 8.1). The foam is injected and followed with ultrasonography to fill the desired vein. Volumes injected into side branches should be small (1–2 mL), and the distance of injection from the saphenofemoral or sapheno-

TABLE 8.1

Recommended Concentration of Solution for Creation of Foam

Vein Size	STS (%)	POL (%)
Telangiectasia	0.1	0.25–0.75
Reticular veins	0.2	0.5–1.0
Small varicose veins	0.3–1.0	1.0
Large varicose and saphenous veins	1.0–3.0	1.0–3.0

Modified table from Gibson KD, Ferris BL, Pepper D. Foam sclerotherapy for the treatment of superficial venous insufficiency. Surg Clin North Am. 2007 Oct;87(5):1285-95, xii-xiii. (Permission to reproduce granted by Elsevier.)

popliteal junction or major perforator veins should be noted to prevent inadvertent entry of large volumes of foam into deep veins. Gentle massage can help to work the foam farther along the vein. Further injections may be needed to fill all of the veins. On duplex ultrasonography imaging, the veins should be observed to go into intense vasospasm. When treating the greater saphenous vein (GSV), the saphenofemoral junction is compressed with digital or transducer pressure to prevent migration of foam into the common femoral vein. The pressure on the saphenofemoral junction (SFJ) is continued until spasm and lack of flow in the GSV is verified with ultrasonography. Following injection, compression pads are placed over the path of the vein and secured with tape. The patient is then placed in a compression stocking (Class II or III) that is worn constantly for at least 48 hours.[11] Immediate or early closure in medium to large veins was achieved in over 85% cases usually requiring more than one sitting; 80% to 90% of these remained occluded 3 years after foam sclerotherapy. High patient satisfaction and significant improvement in symptoms and QOL was noted at a mean follow-up of 2 years after foam sclerotherapy.[10]

Ultrasound-Guided Cannulation[3]

Both saphenous trunks and major tributaries are treated through an intravenous cannula or butterfly needle. Once foam is injected, it spreads rapidly to many superficial veins, which makes further ultrasound injection more difficult. Ultrasound guidance is not needed for superficial varices, which can be treated by direct needle injection without prejudicing safety and efficacy.

Primary GSV

An 18-gauge cannula is placed in the GSV in the lower third of the thigh. This treats the vein between the injection point and the SFJ. If the GSV lies more superficially in part of its track, this is strictly speaking an accessory vein and not the main saphenous trunk. It is better to inject sclerosant of a lesser strength into the trunk in these situations. A butterfly needle is then placed in the superficial accessory vein, usually in the distal third of the thigh. Any further accessory veins in the region of the GSV are treated by placing additional butterflies in them.

Next, any major tributaries of the GSV in the thigh are identified, especially those above the level of cannulation of the GSV. Larger tributaries (3-mm diameter and above) may supply enough venous flow to the GSV to keep it above the level of the junction of the GSV with its tributaries. They can be managed by direct needle injection with foam.

In the calf, a 23-gauge butterfly needle is used to cannulate the saphenous trunk and any varices, again inserting all cannulae and butterflies before any treatment is commenced. In patients with primary varicose veins, 2 or 3 cannulations are required to treat GSV reflux and associated varices.

Primary Small Saphenous Vein Varices

With the patient lying in the left lateral position, the small saphenous vein (SSV) is punctured in the midcalf region using an 18-gauge cannula. This avoids making an injection in the popliteal fossa and inserting foam close to the popliteal vein. A 23-gauge butterfly is used to treat the distal SSV. Varices can be managed using an additional butterfly or by direct needle injection; 2 or 3 cannulations are usually needed for the management of SSV varices.

Combined GSV and SSV Reflux

In patients in whom both the GSV and SSV are incompetent, both veins are cannulated in order to treat the 2 saphenous trunks in one session. More limited treatment of superficial varices may be required to minimize the number of cannulations and volume of foam injected during the first treatment session.

Incompetent Perforating Veins

In the calf, most incompetent perforating veins can be managed by cannulation of a superficial vein immediately fed from the perforators. Foam is used for proximal calf-perforating veins, popliteal fossa perforators, and perforating veins in the thigh. In the popliteal fossa, the cannula is positioned within the perforator so that its tip lies at or near the fascial opening. Medial thigh-perforating veins are cannulated with an 18-gauge cannula to ensure reliable injection.

Superficial varices are injected first with 1% sclerosants foam using a syringe and 30- or 25-gauge needle; 1 mL is given per injection, and the foam is distributed to varices near the point of injection by massaging the leg with the ultrasound probe or by hand. Next, all previously placed butterflies and cannulae are injected with foam, working from the calf toward the groin. The leg should be elevated well above the heart to minimize the diameter of the veins achieving the Fegan's empty vein, although this is not universally used by the sclerotherapist. No more than 2 mL of foam should be injected at time, even into the largest veins. In small veins the calf injection of 1 mL at a time may be adequate.

After injection, the patient is asked to perform a series of dorsiflexions to clear any foam that has reached the deep veins. Foam always reaches the deep veins within a few moments of injection. There is significant difference of opinion among vascular surgeons over this point; some recommend that the patient should be still after injection of foam. Further injections of 1 to 2 mL of foam into each needle and cannula reinforce the treatment already given. This strategy results in the veins being treated and then retreated. Retreatment has been suggested by French and Italian phlebologists as a way of achieving more effective sclerosis than a single injection. This first injection produces spasm of the treated vein and facilitates the passage of foam to more proximal veins with the subsequent injections. The last vein to be treated is the GSV in the thigh, for which 2 mL of 3% sodium tetradecyl sulfate (STS) foam is injected; this is repeated 2 more times, making sure the patient dorsiflexes between each one. The extent of spread of the foam is monitored using duplex ultrasonography and injection is discontinued at any site where extravasation of foam is seen. Butterflies work well but sometimes cut through the side of the vein. The development of spasm in treated veins is widely regarded as a measure of success following vein sclerotherapy. The total amount of foam required to treat the GSV in the thigh is usually 6 to 8 mL if it is a large vein. In the calf section of the GSV 2 to 4 mL of 1% STS foam is sufficient. In the SSV, 4 to 6 mL of 3% STS foam is required depending on the size of the vein. Additional foam is required for accessory veins and varices. In perforating veins other than the medial ankle (Cockett's) perforators, 2 to 4 mL of 3% foam is used. Robust treatment of perforators is required to achieve a permanent result. For medial calf perforators connecting directly to the posterior tibial vein, 1 mL of 3% liquid STS is needed.

Compression

Two days after the procedure, the patient is allowed to take off the stocking and remove the compression pads. It is recommended that the patient continue wearing compression stockings for 2 to 3 weeks. Injections are performed without the need for sedation, and the majority of patients are very comfortable during the follow-up interval.[12] Patients will occasionally complain of tenderness over the treated veins, and nonsteroidal anti-inflammatory medications are usually all that is required for relief. The extremity is bandaged for 7 to 10 days using a short-stretch cohesive bandage. A compression roll is placed between layers of the bandage to increase compression over the treated veins. The compression regimen is recommended after each treatment session. Using elastic compression stockings without bandaging may lead to excessive retained thrombus, thrombophlebitis, and skin pigmentation over treated veins. As with earlier practices in sclerotherapy, immediate ambulation and return to normal activity are encouraged. There is little need for time away from work. Patients can flex the knee sufficiently; it is acceptable for them to drive since the leg is not normally painful or weak following treatment.

Follow-up

Patients should be reviewed 2 weeks following their first treatment, as this is the optimum time for managing any adverse consequences, such as thrombophlebitis. Patients usually return having removed the bandages themselves. The treated leg may be checked using duplex ultrasonography, including visualization of the femoral and popliteal veins and saphenous trunks containing excessive amounts of thrombus. Any residual segment of vein can be managed by further foam sclerotherapy, as described previously. Rebandaging the leg in the region of further sclerotherapy is usually appropriate.

Safety

Endovenous injection of foam may cause local cutaneous side effects such as hyperpigmentation and, rarely, skin necrosis. Compared with classic liquid sclerotherapy, foam sclerotherapy is more likely to induce post-inflammatory hyperpigmentation but less likely to induce skin necrosis because it has much higher sclerosing power at 3- to 4-fold dilution. A few weeks following therapy, patients may experience a stringlike induration of the injected vein due to venous obstruction. Most adverse events are comparable to those after liquid sclerotherapy and include rare events such as migrainelike neurologic symptoms and scotomas, especially with people with an open foramen ovale. Although sclerosing foam enters to the systemic circulation and can be detected in the right ventricle of the heart seconds after the administration, very few deep vein thromboses and emboli have been reported.[11]

The likelihood of these serious side effects may depend on the volume of the injected foam.[13] Some authors recommend the use of low-molecular-weight heparins for 5 days to prevent DVTs, especially in patients with a higher risk for thromboembolic complications.[7,12]

Outcomes

With regard to the efficacy of foam sclerotherapy as compared with liquid sclerotherapy, foam sclerotherapy is 4 times more effective because of increased contact time with the venous wall, and increased agent contact surface area with the venous wall leading to increased venous spasm.[13] It has been reported that after 1 session, about two-thirds of the truncal varicosities were occluded and more than 90% of treatments were successful after 2 or 3 sessions.[14,15]

Cabrera, in his large clinical series of patients treated with foam sclerotherapy published in 2000,[23] reported that after 3 or more years, 81% of treated great saphenous trunks remained occluded and 97% of superficial varices had disappeared. This required 1 session of sclerotherapy in 86% of patients, 2 sessions in 11%, and 3 sessions in 3% of patients. No DVT or pulmonary embolism (PE) was reported. A number of authors have published based in this technique.

Published outcomes are summarized in Table 8.2. It should be noted that the efficacy reports vary depending on the number of injection sessions needed and the defined endpoint.

Comparisons of FST compared with liquid sclerosants have demonstrated significantly better efficacy of FST in ablating GSV reflux. Efficacy of closure or elimination of reflux of saphenous veins ranges from 63% to 97% in a time range of 3 to 22 months. In many studies, however, a substantial percentage of patients required more than one session of treatment to adequately treat the saphenous veins.[8]

Complications

Complications include skin hyperpigmentation and necrosis, phlebitis, transient lymphoedema, allergic reaction, transient scotoma, or confusional states. Five cases of DVT following foam sclerotherapy to the SSV have been reported. None of these led to pulmonary embolism.[10]

In experienced hands, foam sclerotherapy is a safe procedure, and serious complications are rare. Superficial thrombophlebitis is the most common complication but is usually minor and self-limited. Patients who have trapped coagulum in a closed vein segment often have decreased tenderness over the veins after expression of the coagulum. This can be readily accomplished during a follow-up visit using a small wheal of local anesthetic, and then puncture and drainage of the coagulum with an 18-gauge needle or the tip of an 11 blade. Skin pigmentation following FST is also common, and patients should be counseled regarding the possibility before treatment. In most cases, the pigmentation will gradually fade over a period of months.

Other less common complications include skin necrosis causing ulceration or blistering, and telangectasia matting. Dry cough, transient scotoma, migraine, chest discomfort, and other self-limited visual and neurologic disturbances have been noted.

More serious complications such as deep venous thrombosis have been reported. Rates of DVT have ranged from 0% to 1.8%.[12] The most common sites noted for DVT are gastrocnemius and calf veins. In most of these cases, these clots do not require anticoagulation and may be followed with serial duplex scans.

One of the most severe complications reported is neurological deficit following foam sclerotherapy; this event occurred in a patient later found to have a patent foramen ovale (PFO). Although this is an isolated report, it does demonstrate the embolic potential of foam sclerosant and the need to use caution in volumes injected.[8,11]

Conclusion

There are no defined standards for treatment of venous diseases, but there is sufficient evidence that ultrasonography foam sclerotherapy is a surgical technique with promise of great efficacy.[16] Foam sclerotherapy is an effective and well-tolerated treatment for nonsaphenous varicose veins and recurrent or residual veins after surgery without evidence of venous reflux. This treatment is suitable for the management of primary uncomplicated varices, recurrent varicose

TABLE 8.2 **Summary of Published Data**

Author	Year	N	Study Summary
Cabrera et al[17]	2000	500	Retrospective trial including GSV, SFV treatment.
Hamel-Desnos et al[18]	2003	88	Prospective randomized trial comparing FST vs. liquid sclerotherapy of GSV. Endpoint elimination of reflux in treated veins.
Barrett et al[19]	2004	100	Retrospective review of GSV or SSV treatment. Endpoint elimination of reflux and quality of life (QOL) questionnaire.
Kakkos et al[20]	2006	38	Treated recurrent varicose veins in 45 limbs. Endpoint elimination of reflux in treated veins.
Bergan et al[21]	2006	56	77 limbs, CEAP 4–6 treated. Comparison groups compression only, and crossovers that failed compression. Endpoints relief of pain and inflammation, and ulcer healing.
Bergan et al[21]	2006	261	328 limbs, CEAP 2 and 3. Endpoint "abolishment of reflux and obliteration of varicose clusters."
Wright et al[22]	2006	710	Randomized trial comparing FST with "alternative" treatment (sclerotherapy or surgery) in phlebologist and vascular surgeon groups. Endpoint occlusion of trunk veins and elimination of reflux.
Bountouroglou et al[23]	2006	60	Randomized trial comparing GSV ligation and stripping with SFJ ligation plus FST. Endpoint elimination of reflux.
Darke et al[24]	2006	181	220 limbs treated, GSV, SSV, or side branches. Endpoint closure of saphenous vein or closure of 85% of varicosities.

Modified table from Gibson KD, Ferris BL, Pepper D. Foam sclerotherapy for the treatment of superficial venous insufficiency. Surg Clin North Am. 2007 Oct;87(5):1285-95, xii-xiii. (Permission to reproduce granted by Elsevier.)

veins, and patients with lipodermatosclerosis and pain.

Foam has been used successfully for an ever-expanding list of other indications, including male varicocele and pelvic congestion.[15] With increasing awareness and continued international research and discussion, it will be important for the entire vascular specialist community to further characterize the efficacy profile of this tool and establish a treatment guideline.

TABLE 8.2 **Summary of Published Data (*continued*)**

Results
After 3 or more years, 81% of treated great saphenous trunks remained occluded and 97% of superficial varices had disappeared. This required 1 session of sclerotherapy in 86% of patients, 2 sessions in 11%, and 3 sessions in 3% of patients. No DVT or PE was reported.
3 weeks and 6 months: 84% and 80% of FST group showed elimination of reflux compared with 40% and 26% treated with liquid sclerotherapy.
Mean follow-up of 22.5 months, 97% complete saphenous occlusion or fibrosis with "minimal flow," 94% of patients reported improved QOL.
Endpoint reached in 87% limbs: 58% required 1 session only; 11% needed >3 sessions.
10/22 ulcers in compression group healed at 6 weeks. All FST and crossovers healed at 6 weeks. VCSS improvement greatest in FST group (*P* <0.041).
Endpoint reached in 79.8% of limbs.
Success of FST at 3 months and 12 months was 93.0% and 89.6%, respectively, in the phlebology group and 68.2% and 63.1% in the vascular surgeon group.
Short-term success with FST 87%. Decreased operative time and return to work with FST.
Endpoints reached after 1 treatment in 163 limbs, 2 in 32 limbs, and 3 in 1 limb (91% success)

References

1. Orbach EJ. Sclerotherapy of varicose veins. Utilization of an intravenous air block. Am J Surg. 1944;LXVI:362-6.
2. Sigg K. Newer aspects of the technique of treating varicosities. Therapeutishce Umschau. 1949;6:127-134. Translated into English.
3. Coleridge Smith P. Foam and liquid sclerotherapy for varicose veins. Phlebology. 2009;24 (Suppl) 1:62-72.
4. Wildenhues B. Rediscovered one foam sclerotherapy in the treatment of varicose veins therapy. Vasomed. 2006;18:106-8.
5. Cabrera J, Cabrera J Jr. Nuevo método de

esclerosis en las varices tronculares. Patologia Vascular. 1995;4:55-73.

6. Monfreux A. Traitement sclérosant des troncs saphéniens et leurs collaterals de gros calibre par la méthode mus. Phlébologie. 1997;50: 351-3.
7. Tessari L, Cavezzi A, Frullini A. Preliminary experience with a new sclerosing foam in the treatment of varicose veins. Dermatol Surg. 2001;27:58-60.
8. Gibson KD, Ferris BL, Pepper D. Foam sclerotherapy for the treatment of superficial venous insufficiency. Surg Clin N Am. 2007;87:1285-95.
9. Nijsten T, van den Bos RR, Goldman MP, Kockaert MA, Proebstle TM, et al. Minimally invasive techniques in the treatment of saphenous varicose veins. J Am Acad Dermatol. 2009;60:110-9.
10. Subramonia S, Lees TA. The treatment of varicose veins. Ann R Coll Surg Engl. 2007;89:96-100.
11. Guex JJ, Allaert FA, Gullet JL, Chleir F. Immediate and midterm complications of sclerotherapy; report of prospective multicenter registry of 12,173 sclerotherapy sessions. Dermatol Surg. 2005;31:123-8.
12. Smith PC. Chronic venous disease treated by ultrasound guided foam sclerotherapy. Eur J Vasc Endovasc Surg. 2006;32: 577-83.
13. Yamaki T, Nozaki M, Iwasaka S. Comparative study of duplex-guided foam sclerotherapy and duplex-guided liquid sclerotherapy for the treatment of superficial venous insuffiency. Dermatol Surg. 2004;30:718-22.
14. Ceulen RP, Bullens-Goessens YI, Pi-Van De Venne SJ, Nelemans PJ, Veraart JC, Sommer A. Outcomes and side effects of duplex-guided sclerotherapy in the treatment of great saphenous veins with 1% versus 3% polidocanol foam: results of a randomized controlled trial with 1-year follow up. Dermatol Surg. 2007;33:276-81.
15. Frullini A, Cavezzi A. Sclerosing foam in the treatment of varicose veins and teleangiectases: history and analysis of safety and complications. Dermatol Surg. 2002;28:11-5.
16. Belcaro G, Cesarone MR, Di Renzo A, et al. Foam-sclerotherapy, surgery, sclerotherapy, and combined treatment for varicose veins: a 10 year, prospective, randomized, controlled tiral (VEDICO trial). Angiology. 2003;54: 307-15.
17. Cabrera J, Cabrera J Jr, Garcia-Olmedo MA. Treatment of varicose long saphenous veins with sclerosant in microfoam form: long-term outcomes. Phlebology. 2000; 15:19-23.
18. Hamel-Desnos C, Desnos P, Wollmann JC, Ouvry P, Mako S, Allaert FA. Evaluation of the efficacy of polidicanol in the form of foam compared with liquid form in sclerotherapy of the greater saphenous vein: initial results. Dermatol Surg. 2003;30:6-12.
19. Barrett JM, Allen B, Ockerford A, Goldman MP. Microfoam ultrasound-guided sclerotherapy of variocose veins in 100 legs. Dermatol Surg. 2004;30:6-12.
20. Kakkos SK, Bountouroglou DG, Azzam M. Effectiveness and safety of ultrasound-guided foam sclerotherapy for recurrent varicose veins: immediate results. J Endovasc Ther. 2006;13:357-64.
21. Bergan J, Pascarella L, Mekenas L. Venous disorders: treatment with sclerosant foam. J Card Surg. 2006;47:115-24.
22. Wright D, Gobin JP, Bradbury AW, Coleridge-Smith P, Spoelstra H, Berridge D, et al, and the Varisolve European Phase III Investigators Group. Varisolve polidocanol microfoam compared with surgery or sclerotherapy in the management of varicose veins in the presence of trunk

vein incompetence: European randomized controlled trial. Phlebology. 2006;21(4): 180-90.

23. Bountouroglou DG, Azzam M, Kakkos SK, Pathmarajah M, Young P, Geroulakos G. Ultrasound-guided foam sclerotherapy combined with sapheno-femoral ligation compared to surgical treatment of varicose veins: early results of a randomized controlled trial. Eur J Vasc Endovasc Surg. 2006;31: 93-100.
24. Darke SG, Baker SJA. Ultrasound-guided foam sclerotherapy for the treatment of varicose veins. Br J Surg. 2006;93(8):969-74.

CHAPTER 9

Perforator Veins
Indications, Techniques, and Outcomes

Nyla Ismail and Eric K. Peden

The treatment options for chronic venous insufficiency have changed dramatically over the last 10 years. Current procedures are clinic-based with local aesthesia compared to previous surgery in a hospital operating room requiring general anesthesia. Contemporary methods utilize ablation of the vein with endoluminal techniques rather than physical removal of the diseased veins. The endoluminal vein treatments can be performed for both the superficial venous system of greater and small saphenous veins as well as for perforator veins. Perforator veins serve as connectors between the superficial and deep veins in the feet, calves, and thighs. Most treatment options have been focused on superficial veins; however, perforator veins may play a fundamental role in some patients with venous disease.

Treatment of perforator veins has fluctuated considerably over time, both in popularity and technique. Generally, patients with chronic venous insufficiency consider and choose surgery. Still, approximately 4% of these patients develop ulcers in their lower extremities, at which point durable healing becomes increasingly challenging.[1] A multisystem approach may be the best solution, at least initially, to determine the right options for each patient.[2,3]

Perforator vein treatment in the algorithm for chronic venous disease has been the subject of multiple debates and significant controversy.[4,5] It is generally agreed that perforator veins do play a significant role in advanced venous disease, but benefits from their treatment are poorly studied. In addition, the appeal of perforator vein treatment has fluctuated considerably over time. Initial description of the perforator veins and the

Chronic Venous Insufficiency. Contemporary Endovascular Management series. © 2011 Mark G. Davies MD and Alan B. Lumsden MD, eds. Cardiotext Publishing, ISBN 978-1-935395-09-6.

Linton procedure led to early enthusiasm but was later tempered by high wound-complication rates.[4] Later endoscopic techniques led to operative procedures but that too faded with poor results in postthrombotic limbs. Currently, the use of percutaneous techniques has caused resurgence in the popularity of treating perforator veins.[6]

The most current procedure, termed PAPS—percutaneous ablation perforator surgery—shows some promising results. In this trial by Bergan et al, treatment resulted in improved venous clinical severity scores and ulcer healing.[7] Also, recurrence of ulcers and perforator veins was shown to occur simultaneously, establishing a link between the 2 symptoms.[4] Taken together, the results from these trials suggest a role for the treatment of perforator veins in patients with advanced venous disease.[8]

Techniques: Perforator Veins

Depending on the use of radiofrequency, laser, or sclerotherapy, perforator treatment techniques vary. All the treatments, however, do involve the use of ultrasound guidance to accurately visualize access to the perforator veins and to validate treatment effect. Certain commonalities exist: (1) ultrasound-guided percutaneous intraluminal access; (2) application of some energy source within the lumen leading to vein wall contraction or occlusion; (3) local anesthesia with possibly some form of sedation (oral or intravenous); (4) an outpatient office location and no incisions; and (5) simple retreatment, if needed.

For radiofrequency and laser techniques, the perforator vein is accessed directly at or preferably below the level of the fascia. For the radiofrequency perforator probe, 2 techniques of work are described: an over-the-wire technique and direct puncture and treatment. Preferably, a length of the vein is treated, or if not possible, then treatment at 2 focal areas. In the clinic setting, infusion of local anesthetic around the area of the ablation catheter prevents pain, and use of external pressure ensures good contact between the probe and the vessel wall. The laser fiber can then be passed directly through a 21-gauge needle, similarly allowing for treatment along a length of vein or 2 to 3 focal treatments for 5 seconds each. Just as with radiofrequency, it is important to infuse local anesthetic around the catheter tip and hold external pressure. The manufacturer for radiofrequency ablation suggests a 4-minute treatment, toggling the probe to contact each of the 4 walls for 1 minute each. During treatment, the impedance reading on the machine can be helpful to confirm intravascular treatment. Following treatment, the vein is tested for flow with duplex imaging, although the presence of the anesthetic can limit visualization. Generally, the perforator vein should appear shrunken and more echogenic with no color flow visualized (Figures 9.1 and 9.2). After completion of the procedure, the area is compressed for a few minutes, and a compression bandage or stockings are applied.

Both foam and liquid sclerotherapy have also been utilized to treat perforator veins. Direct perforator access is not mandatory and commonly a nearby varix can be accessed. Ultrasonography is used to visualize passage of the sclerosant into the perforator vein. Elevation of the leg is recommended, and anesthetic is not required. As with radiofrequency and laser ablation, digital compression for a brief time followed by application of compressive bandaging is common.

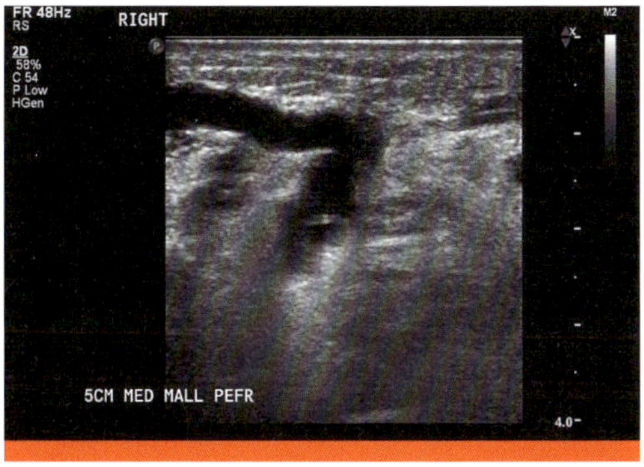

FIGURE 9.1 Duplex ultrasound showing the perforator vein prior to ablation.

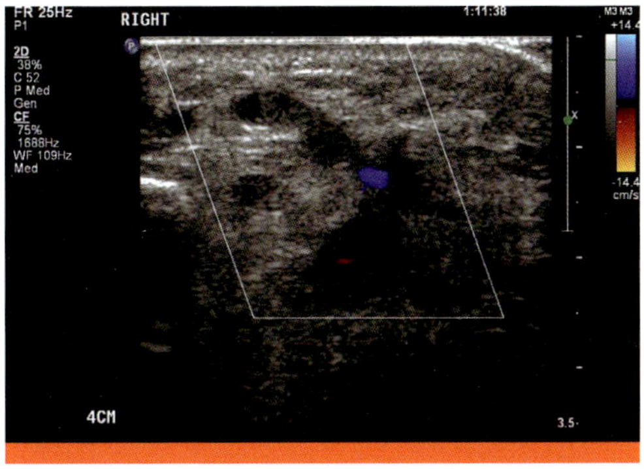

FIGURE 9.2 Duplex ultrasound showing successful perforator vein ablation.

Perforator Vein Treatment Results

Although sclerotherapy was reported for perforator vein treatment more than 4 decades ago,[9] results from perforator treatment are few and most of the information available is in the form of abstracts from national conferences. In general, the results do report high occlusion rates and few complications.[6] Occlusion rates of 75% to 98% were reported with few complications; however, repeat intervention may be necessary.[6]

Similarly, a report of percutaneous ablation of perforator veins with a saphenous style radiofrequency probe has been achieved successfully.[10] In fact, 81% of the veins shown in this study had successful ablation in a 5-year follow-up, including just under half of the original patients. A recent review indicated that 90% of perforator veins that were treated with radiofrequency were occluded in short-term follow-up.[6]

Success using laser ablation of perforators is equally promising. An 85% to 100% early closure rate with few complications using laser ablation for perforator veins has been reported.[11] In addition, no deep venous thromboses, rare paresthesias, and few blisters have been reported.[6]

Overall, perhaps the biggest advantage of the PAPS technique is that it is repeatable. Clearly, perforator veins have been documented to recur, and previous, more invasive techniques of direct or endoscopic perforator ligation are very difficult to repeat. Patients with advanced chronic venous disease often have recurrence; therefore, repeatability of the treatments becomes increasingly more important.

Conclusion

Endoluminal treatment of venous insufficiency has rapidly gained widespread acceptance and has entered into mainstream practice. The advancement of minimally invasive techniques has enabled ambulatory clinic treatment in the majority of patients with varicose veins, getting patients back to normal activity and work more rapidly than traditional open-surgical methods. In addition, a more comprehensive view of the venous system, including both superficial and perforator veins, has achieved better results for patients with chronic venous disease. Increasing numbers of reports are being published in the literature with good results and low complication rates. As techniques continue to evolve, patients will clearly benefit from these advances in technology.

References

1. Nitecki S, Kantarovsky A, Portnot I, Bass A. The contemporary treatment of varicose veins (strangle, strip, grill or poison). Isr Med Assoc J. 2006;8:411-5.
2. Hanrahan LM, Kechejian GJ, Cordts PR, Rodriguez AA, Araki CA, LaMorte WW, et al. Patterns of venous insufficiency in patients with varicose veins. Arch Surg. 1991;126(6):687-90; discussion 690-1.
3. Hanrahan LM, Araki CT, Rodriguez AA, Kechejian GJ, LaMorte WW, Menzoian JO. Distribution of valvular incompetence in patients with venous stasis ulceration. J Vasc Surg. 1991;13(6):805-11; discussion 811-2.
4. O'Donnell TF Jr. The present status of surgery of the superficial venous system in the management of venous ulcer and the evidence for the role of perforator interruption. J Vasc Surg. 2008;48(4):1044-52.
5. Meissner MH. "I enjoyed your talk, but . . .": evidence-based medicine and the scientific foundation of the American Venous Forum. J Vasc Surg. 2009; 49(1):244-8.
6. Elias S, Peden E. Ultrasound-guided percutaneous ablation for the treatment of perforating vein incompetence. Vascular. 2007;15(5):281-9.
7. Bergan JJ. Perforating Veins. In: Bergan JJ, Goldman MP, eds. Varicose Veins and Telengiectasias: Diagnosis and Treatment. St. Louis: Quality Medical Publishing; 1993.
8. Masuda EM, Kessler DM, Lurie F, Puggioni A, Kistner RL, Eklof B. The effect of ultrasound-guided sclerotherapy of incompetent perforator veins on venous clinical severity and disability scores. J Vasc Surg. 2006;43(3):551-6; discussion 556-7.
9. Hobbs JT. Surgery and sclerotherapy in the treatment of varicose veins, a random trial. Arch Surg. 1974;109:793-6.
10. Bacon JL, Dinneen AJ, Marsh P, Holdstock JM, Price BA, Whiteley MS. Five-year results of incompetent perforator vein closure using trans-luminal occlusion of perforator. Phlebology. 2009;24(2):74-8.
11. Fegan WG. Continuous compression technique of injection varicose veins. Lancet. 1963;2:109-12.

PART

2

Chronic Venous Reconstructions

In contrast to superficial venous incompetence, the understanding of and interventions for chronic venous occlusive disease have progressed at a slower pace with a lower penetration of new technologies. Many ideas and therapies have been borrowed from the equivalent obstructive scenarios in arterial disease, although the pathophysiology is markedly different since obstruction alone causes symptoms in about one-third of postthrombotic limbs, while the remainder have a combination of reflux and obstruction. This transfer of techniques and knowledge may have underserved the development of therapy in the field. The increasing use of CTV/MRV and the resurgence of venography have increased the awareness of iliofemoral obstruction in patients with chronic venous disease. Introduction of intravascular ultrasonography has further enhanced the three-dimensional understanding of occlusive and nonocclusive iliac venous obstructive disease. The adoption of both recannulization and stenting techniques is altering perceptions of therapy in these conditions. May-Thurner syndrome is now considered a treatable condition.

The increasing use of endoluminal techniques has decreased the utilization of venous bypasses, but these techniques remain a viable alternative in the appropriately selected patient. Expansion of the evidence from a few select centers and development of better evidence-based protocols are necessary for this field to advance further. However, while these modalities can change the outlook for occlusive disease and lessen the clinical impact of the combination of reflux and obstruction, treatment of deep venous reflux will require both refinements in autologous valve transfers and the development of a viable artificial venous valve. This is the next frontier in chronic venous disease.

CHAPTER 10

Stenting of Chronic Obstruction

Indications, Techniques, and Outcomes

Peter Neglén

Chronic venous disease (CVD) is still among many physicians equated with venous valve incompetence, and diagnosis and therapy have been focused on venous reflux. The main reason for this is poor understanding of the importance of venous outflow obstruction in the pathophysiology of primary and secondary chronic venous disease. The lack of accurate tests and the sole treatment being invasive surgery also explain the lack of previous enthusiasm. However, it has been well known for some time that obstruction alone causes the symptoms in more than one-third of postthrombotic limbs, that the most symptomatic limbs have a combination of reflux and obstruction,[1,2] and that persistent obstruction of proximal veins is associated with progressive distal vein incompetence.[3] It has also been pointed out that the obstruction of the iliofemoral vein, that is, the final pathway for the venous outflow above the confluence of the profunda and femoral veins, more frequently results in leg complaints, especially venous claudication and leg ulcers. Studies have also shown that cumulative incidence of the postthrombotic syndrome is more common than previously realized (all symptoms 27% and ulcer rate 4% at 20 years following acute deep vein thrombosis [DVT]).[4] Even without thrombosis, the existence of iliac vein compressions with or without intraluminal lesions are in themselves more pathogenic than previously thought, although they have been considered a common finding of little clinical importance.

Percutaneous endovenous stenting was introduced more than a decade ago and has emerged as the method of choice for the treatment of chronic obstruction of the femoro-ilio-caval venous outflow. It has replaced

Chronic Venous Insufficiency. Contemporary Endovascular Management series. © 2011 Mark G. Davies MD and Alan B. Lumsden MD, eds. Cardiotext Publishing, ISBN 978-1-935395-09-6.

bypass surgery as the primary treatment. Stenting is a relatively simple and effective endovenous treatment with low morbidity and mortality. Venous stenting has been slow to be widely adopted despite these advantages. The key is to increase awareness among treating physicians of the possible presence of iliofemoral obstruction in patients with CVD, and, consequently, the need for more extensive evaluation of the pelvic venous outflow and less reliance on infrainguinal duplex Doppler investigation alone. Patients complaining of significant symptoms of chronic venous insufficiency should make the physician think obstruction rather than reflux.

Chronic Postthrombotic Obstruction

Poor recanalization following acute deep vein thrombosis is presently thought to be the most common cause of chronic venous blockage.[1] Most symptomatic outflow obstruction occurs following deep vein thrombosis involving the iliac segment. It may be limited to the iliofemoral segment or contiguous from the calf to the iliac veins. Only approximately 20% of these iliac veins will completely recanalize on anticoagulation treatment, while the remaining veins recanalize only partially and develop varying degrees of obstruction and collateral formation.[5,6] In the 1960s, Cockett and his associates performed groundbreaking studies and published numerous "classic" reports on venous outflow obstruction, compression of the iliac veins, and its relationship to thrombosis.[7-11] They observed that the obstructive lesion that precipitated the thrombosis impeded its resolution, and the postthrombotic perivenous fibrosis appeared to develop excessively at the site of the initiating lesion. Recently, this observation has been confirmed by serial spiral computed tomography venography (CTV) studies, which showed inhibited and incomplete recanalization in the presence of an external compression, eg, left iliac vein compression.[12] This finding is of great importance, as it has been reported that 80% of limbs with iliofemoral DVT have underlying extrinsic iliac compression-type lesions revealed by the same technique (67% and 84%, right and left iliofemoral veins, respectively).[13]

The typical postthrombotic iliofemoral lesion often involves both common and external iliac veins with irregular stenosis or occlusions and axial, transpelvic, and ascending lumbar collaterals are present (Figure 10.1). Infrequently, a diffusely narrowed long segment of the iliac vein with no collateral formation is found. We have designated this entity a "Rokitansky" stenosis, from the 19th-century pathologist who described the phenomenon. As the severe inflammation of the wall (phlebitis) subsides, a fibrotic cylinder is formed, which impedes any collateral development and expansion of the vein. Thus, significant outflow obstruction cannot be excluded because of lack of collaterals.

Nonthrombotic Iliac Vein Lesion

Even without previous thrombosis, studies have shown frequent findings of intraluminal lesions and varying degrees of external compression of the iliac vein in the general population (22%–33%[14-16] and 66%–88%,[9,11,17] respectively). They have often been considered a common finding of little clinical importance. Symptomatic nonthrombotic iliac vein lesions (NIVL) have previously been described as May-Thurner syndrome[14] or Cockett's or "iliac vein com-

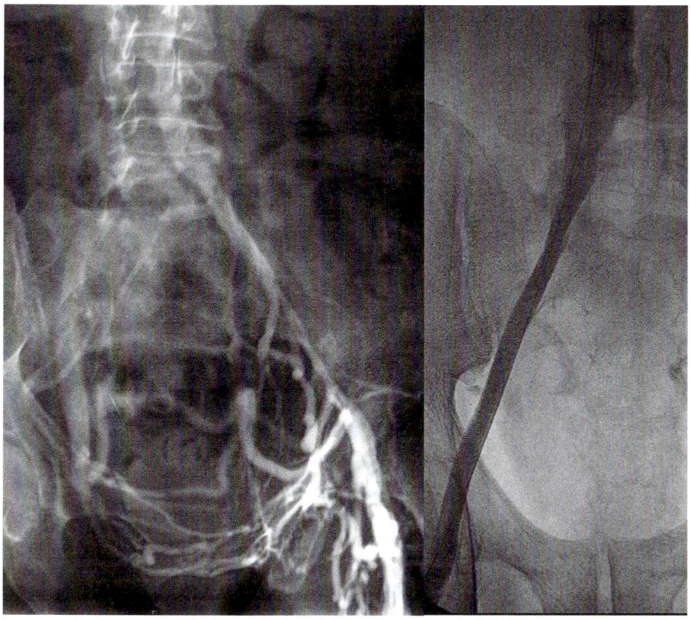

FIGURE 10.1 Transfemoral venogram showing typical postthrombotic iliofemoral vein segments. Obstructed iliac vein with marked collateralization **(left)**; and **(right)** long uniform noncollateralizing stenosis ("Rokitansky" stenosis).

pression" syndrome.[11] Why a silent lesion should suddenly become significant in the pathophysiology is not fully understood. It has been suggested that the NIVL is a so-called permissive lesion, which does not become clinically significant until other components of the venous circulation of the lower limb fail. Correction of a permissive lesion alone often results in cure, which may explain the surprisingly good results of venous stenting in CVD even in the presence of untreated reflux. Compression of the common iliac vein was seen in 36%, external iliac vein in 18%, and both sites in 46% of symptomatic limbs.[18]

Typically, a stenosis of the left proximal common iliac vein is caused by compression by the right common iliac artery with secondary band or web formation, but may involve both the common and the external iliac veins.[8,18] The prevailing concept is that iliac vein compression syndrome is clinically expressed only in the lower left extremity of predominantly young women of childbearing age. This limitation is not true, since compression lesions are not uncommon in males and in elderly patients and may involve the right limb (Figure 10.2). In our experience in the treatment of iliofemoral obstruction in 938 limbs in 879 patients, 53% of limbs had nonthrombotic compression lesions (defined as absent history of DVT, no venographic or ultrasonography findings indicating previous DVT); 40% had postthrombotic obstruction; and 7% had a combined etiology. The ages of the patients with nonthrombotic blockage ranged from 18 to 90 years (median: 54 years), 20% of patients were men, and 25% of the symptomatic lower limbs were on the right side.[18]

Typical Symptoms of Obstruction

Symptoms of obstruction may be any of those associated with chronic venous disease, ranging from moderate swelling and pain to discoloration and stasis ulcer. Venous outflow obstruction plays an important role in the clinical expression of chronic venous disease, especially of pain.[19] The iliac vein is the common outflow tract of the lower extremity, and chronic obstruction of this segment appears to result in more severe

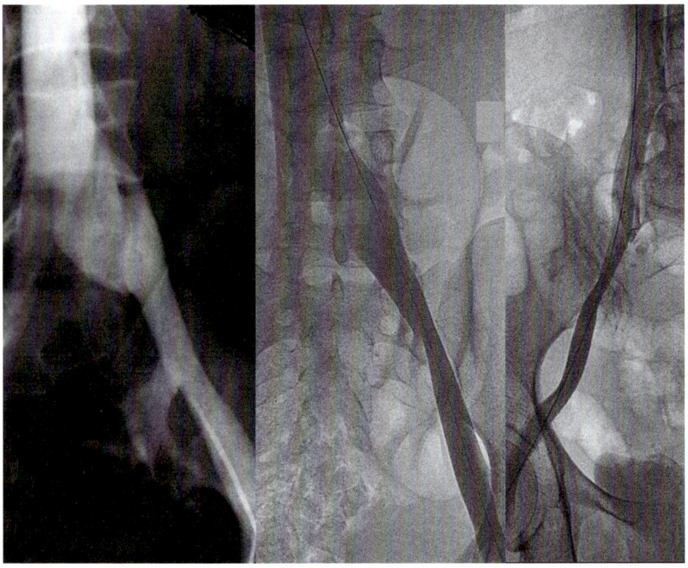

FIGURE 10.2 Venographic changes suggest a nonthrombotic iliac lesion (NIVL) such as **(left)** "pancaking" with collaterals due to common left iliac vein compression; **(center)** translucency and widening of the common iliac vein and stenosis of the proximal external iliac vein; and **(right)** multiple smooth stenoses of the left iliac vein.

symptoms than does lower segmental blockage. Femoro-popliteal venous obstruction appears to be better compensated for by collateral formation than obstruction of the iliac and common femoral veins.[20] The clinical expression is influenced by any concomitant deep or superficial reflux. Negus et al suggested that limb swelling and pain were related to the obstructive component, whereas limb ulceration resulted from valve reflux.[8] It has been shown that ulcers occur rarely in the presence of isolated iliofemoral obstruction (4%), but occur more often when obstruction is associated with reflux (30%).[19] A substantial number of patients with chronic venous disease complain of disabling pain and swelling of the lower limbs without skin changes. Clinical outcomes after stenting suggest that these symptoms are mainly attributable to obstruction rather than to reflux. Five years after iliofemoral DVT treated conservatively with anticoagulation, 90% of patients suffer symptoms of CVD. Debilitating "venous claudication" is found in 15% to 44% of patients and venous ulcer has developed in 15% of limbs.[5,21] "Venous claudication" is a dramatic condition described as an exercise-induced "bursting" pain, which requires several minutes of rest and sometimes leg elevation to achieve relief. Certainly, patients with significant outflow obstruction may also have less distinct lower extremity pain and discomfort with decreased quality of life and less extreme disability.

What Is the Definition of a Significant Hemodynamic Obstruction?

The degree of hemodynamic venous obstruction depends on multiple factors, such as the number, location, degree of narrowing, and length of the lesions; development of collaterals; and the volume flow varying at rest and during exercise. Any test to measure venous outflow obstruction must be identified as to whether it evaluates anatomic or functional aspects. The concept of a hemodynamically significant vessel obstruction being a stenosis of more than 70% to 80% is derived from observations on the arterial system. An arterial stenosis does not become significant until it supersedes the high peripheral resistance. Contrarily to the high-pressure, high-velocity, small-volume, and high-resistance diverging arterial system ("water supply system"), the venous circulation is a low-pressure, low-velocity, large-volume converging vascular system ("sewage draining system") with a very low central resistance.[22] Logically, a significant stenosis in the venous system would occur at a much lesser degree. However, it is presently not known at what degree a venous stenosis is hemodynamically significant. Consequently, there is no accurate hemodynamic test ("gold standard") available to properly assess venous outflow obstruction and its improvement after stenting in individual limbs. Plethysmographic outflow fraction determination and pressure tests (hand-foot pressure differential, hyperemia-induced dorsal foot venous pressure increase) are global hemodynamic tests and may suggest obstruction to the venous outflow at any anatomic site and level, but significant blockage may exist in the presence of a normal result.[23-25] Positive tests may support further investigation and intervention, but a negative test does not exclude clinically significant venous outflow obstruction.

Femoral venous pressure is a test for focal outflow obstruction. A pull-through pressure differential over a lesion or a pressure increase peripherally to the lesion with augmentation of venous inflow may be indicative of a significant stenosis.[7,26] The venous pressure is not only a function of resistance to the flow but is also highly dependent on the flow velocity and magnitude of volume flow. It is not known to what degree the resting venous flow must be increased to detect a functionally significant stenosis, nor a method to reproduce this flow rate consistently. Pressure gradients recorded in the venous system are much lower than in the arterial system, and only small pressure differentials may indicate significant obstruction. Studies suggest that a prestenotic pressure rise in the supine position greater than 2 to 4 mm Hg on provocation, a slow return to base level (>30s), or a gradient compared to the contralateral femoral pressure exceeding 2 to 5 mm Hg indicates a hemodynamically significant obstruction.[7,26] It has been suggested that a pressure differential on exercise should be at least 5 mm Hg to warrant intervention, but none of these pressure limitations have been validated. Good clinical results have been obtained treating morphologic obstruction with normal pressure findings.[27]

The accuracy of these tests is insufficient to detect borderline obstructions. Thus, they play only a limited role in the management of obstructive disease, as a positive hemodynamic test may indicate hemodynamic significance but a normal test does not necessarily exclude it.

Investigations for Morphological Venous Obstruction

In lieu of an adequate hemodynamic test, morphological tests must be utilized. Ascending venography after injection of contrast dye in a foot vein or an antegrade transfemoral venography reveals the distribution and nature of the morphologic changes, including occlusion, stenosis, and the presence of collateral circulation, but is unable to show any hemodynamic impact of visualized lesions. Ascending venography usually insufficiently visualizes the iliac vein to permit assessment of any obstruction of that segment. It is mainly used today as a preoperative mapping tool to delineate the inflow to a postthrombotic iliac vein segment considered for stenting. To increase accuracy, all antegrade transfemoral venograms should be performed using arterial angiographic techniques with subtraction imaging, multiple oblique projections, and pressure injectors (Figure 10.3). With this technique, the quality of the images improves and the contrast medium load is minimal. A single-plane venogram was actually considered "normal" in 25% to 45% of patients, despite the fact that intravascular ultrasonography (IVUS) showed >50% obstruction.[28] Interestingly, Cockett and colleagues made similar observations. Venography was diagnostic in only 65% of obstructed limbs in their experience and collaterals were visualized in only 63%. It was noted that in 54% of symptomatic patients, transfemoral venography appeared "normal," with smooth contours of contrast in the iliac vein and without collaterals. The authors noted that absence of collateral formation should not negate consideration of the pathology.[8,9,11]

Although the formation of collaterals is classically regarded as a compensatory mechanism to bypass and thus alleviate an obstruction, the precise mechanism and

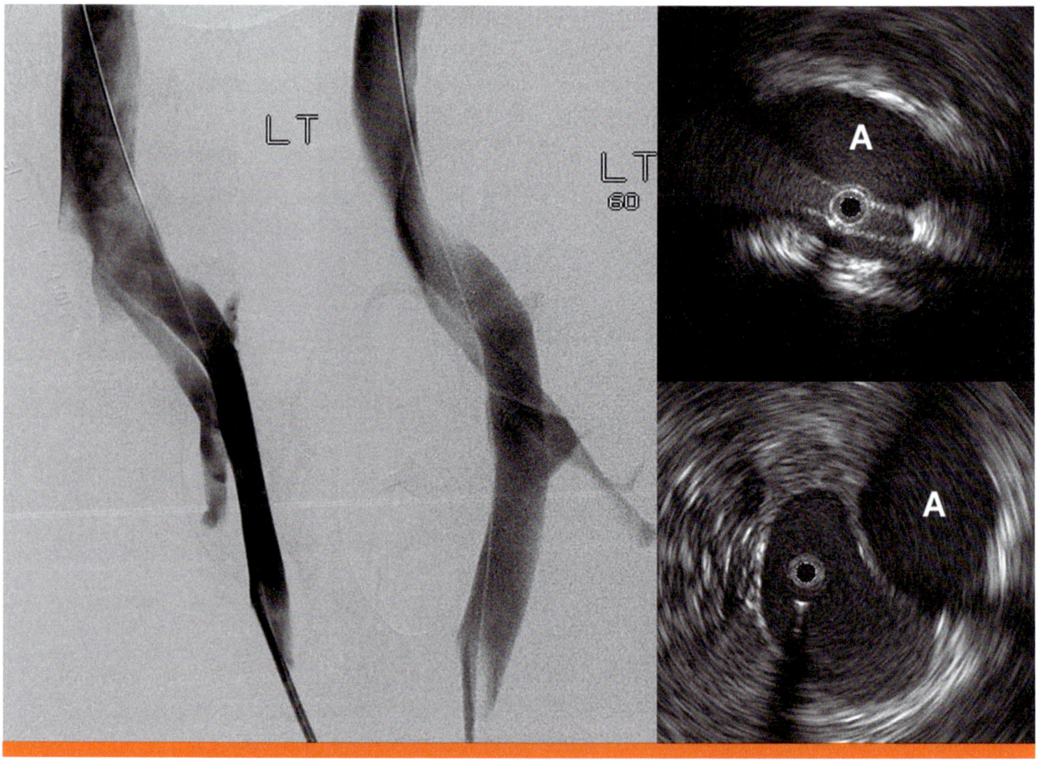

FIGURE 10.3 **Left.** Left transfemoral venogram with multiple projections in a patient with nonthrombotic iliac vein obstruction. The oblique view (60° rotation) reveals stenosis, which is not visualized on the anter-posterior projection (0°). **Right.** Corresponding images by intravascular ultrasonography (IVUS). The compression of the left proximal common iliac vein is clearly shown as it is crossed by the right common iliac artery A **(top)** and the artery still impinging on the vein in the middle part of the common iliac vein **(bottom)**. The black circle inside the vein represents the inserted IVUS catheter.

inducement of collateral formation are unknown. Collateral circulation shown prior to stenting is often not visualized following stenting of a venous stenosis. The flow through the stent is obviously favored. Limbs with collateral formation have been shown to have a significantly tighter stenosis than limbs with no collaterals, as measured by IVUS.[29] The rate of limbs with femoral pressure increase on intra-arterial injection of papaverine was 3 times more common in patients with collaterals. These observations support the concept of pelvic collateralization as an indicator of obstruction and that collaterals poorly compensate for the blockage in symptomatic patients.

Ultrasonography of the iliac vein is under development but still lacks the adequate accuracy to detect partial or complete chronic obstruction and to separate axial collaterals from main stem veins. It can be used to evaluate patency of inserted stents. Spiral CT imaging and magnetic resonance venography (MRV) are under evaluation and may replace transfemoral venogram for screening in the future. Like ultrasonography, none of these tests have been validated.

Intravascular ultrasonography is superior to single- and multi-plane venography in detection of the extent and type of morphologic lesion of the vein.[29-33] It is the most accurate test in this aspect and should be used to validate findings of other morphological imaging methods. IVUS has proven superior in showing intraluminal details (eg, trabeculations and webs), which may be hidden in the contrast medium. Venous wall thickness, in-stent restenosis, and movement can be adequately assessed. An external compression with the resulting deformity of the venous lumen or postthrombotic remodeling can be directly visualized (Figure 10.3). The degree of stenosis can be precisely calculated by measurement of the cross-cut areas and diameters of the normal and compressed or diseased veins using the software built into the IVUS apparatus. In addition to being a diagnostic tool, it is also a crucial aid to guide stent insertion. Morphologic obstruction >50% as measured by IVUS has arbitrarily been chosen for stenting based on clinical outcome.

Which Patient Should Have Pelvic Outflow Studies?

As pointed out previously, there is no accurate hemodynamic test to select patients for venous outflow stenting. The key for the physician is to be aware of the importance and possibility of venous blockage combined with increased suspicion in patients with history and clinical signs and symptoms suggestive of outflow obstruction. Patients with previous DVT; patients with limb symptoms, especially pain out of proportion to detectable pathology; patients not improving on conservative treatment or following reflux intervention; and patients with no other detectable pathology to explain their symptoms are specifically targeted. Although a positive noninvasive or invasive test may support further studies, a negative test should not exclude it. The diagnosis and treatment must presently be based on morphological investigations of the iliac venous outflow, although hemodynamic criteria would be preferred. IVUS investigation is the ultimate test and should be generously utilized in symptomatic patients with a suspicion of outflow obstruction. Other morphological tests, eg, MRV or CTV, need to be validated by comparison to IVUS. Limiting workup of patients with significant chronic venous disease to only duplex ultrasonography will not suffice, especially not when restricted to the infrainguinal vein segments.

Stenting Technique

Although venous stenting may appear a simple procedure, attention to details is important to ensure an optimal outcome. The following is a list of important technical points that are vital to achieve patency rates and clinical outcome as reported; attention to details cannot be overemphasized:

- Consider venous balloon angioplasty and stenting a different procedure from that employed in the arterial system.
- Balloon venoplasty alone is insufficient in the venous system. Stent placement is mandatory.
- The "kissing" balloon technique utilized at the aortic bifurcation is unnecessary at the confluence of the common iliac veins, and bilateral stents are not needed to treat unilateral obstruction at this location.
- Ultrasonography to guide cannulation of the femoral vein is an absolute essential to prevent access complications.
- IVUS is essential, both as a diagnostic tool and as an intraoperative aid in directing placement of the stent. The degree of obstruction and the extent of the lesion are often greater than visualized on venogram.
- Cover the entire disease venous segment as outlined by the IVUS. The most common cause of early occlusion is inadequate stenting of the entire lesion.
- Stenting of a stenosis adjacent to the confluence of the common iliac veins by braided stents requires the stent to be placed well into the IVC to avoid early restenosis (distal migration).
- Venoplasty should be performed with large-diameter balloons (14–18 mm) followed by insertion of a large-diameter stent (14–18 mm wide). Unlike the artery, the vein accepts extensive dilation without clinical rupture. Oversize the balloon and stent with diameters at least 2 mm over normal size.
- It is important to redilate the stent after insertion to avoid its possible movement.
- Avoid skip areas between 2 stents because they are prone to develop secondary stenosis.

It is crucial for the clinical outcome that the stent procedure is guided by IVUS imaging. Venous balloon angioplasty and stenting is a different procedure from that employed in the arterial system. Experience acquired from arterial dilation and stenting may not necessarily be extrapolated to the venous system, mainly because of the different nature of the lesions. Balloon angioplasty alone is insufficient in the venous system due to the severe fibrosis encapsulating the lesion or unyielding external compression. Severe recoil of the vein is observed intraoperatively in the majority of limbs, and simple balloon dilation leads to early restenosis.[34-37] Stent insertion is mandatory. The procedure may be performed under local infiltration analgesia in combination with monitored sedation or general anesthesia. Since the balloon dilation may be quite painful, the latter is recommended when tight stenoses or occlusions are stented. Attempts to recanalize occluded veins are also often time-consuming. The procedure should be performed in a fully equipped endovascular or angiographic suite, and availability of intravascular ultrasonography (IVUS) and external ultrasonography for cannulation guidance is essential.

Accessing the Vein

Ultrasound-assisted guidance of the cannulation is mandatory and has largely eliminated access complications. Access to the iliac segment can be achieved retrogradely through the jugular or contralateral femoral vein, but an antegrade approach through an ultrasound-guided access distal to the obstruction in the thigh portion of the femoral vein or through the popliteal vein is preferred. In our hands, popliteal vein access is rarely used and often not possible because of segmental occlusion of the distal femoral vein. We prefer the mid-thigh access, which facilitates recanalization of occlusions from below (shorter distance and better "pushability"), evaluation of the inflow, and precise placement of the stent in relationship to distal tributaries when necessary. Ultrasound guidance is necessary in this situation to avoid inadvertent arterial puncture, as the femoral vein occupies a variable postero-lateral or postero-medial location in reference to the femoral artery. In contrast to arterial access at the thigh level, control of the venopuncture site is not a problem because of the low venous pressure and the routine use of tamponade devices (VasoSeal).

Crossing the Obstructive Lesion in Nonocclusive Obstruction

A hydrophilic guidewire (0.035 in.) is inserted and the cannula replaced by a 9 to 11 Fr sheath, which accommodates the appropriate balloon and stent sizes. A stiff guidewire and predilation with serial dilators may be necessary to facilitate sheath placement in case of perivenous fibrosis of the postthrombotic femoral vein. Except in the event of complete obstructions (occlusions), the guidewire can usually be passed through the stenosis and into the inferior vena cava (IVC) with ease. An initial contrast venogram is then performed. Multiplane venograms (antero-posterior, 45° and 60° oblique projections) are helpful to delineate a stenosis that may not be revealed in the antero-posterior projection, especially if IVUS is not available (Figures 10.3 and 10.4). IVUS is superior to venography in delineating any obstructive lesion and is recommended for diagnosis of the extent and degree of obstruction.

Crossing the Obstructive Lesion in Occlusion

When an occlusion is present, the initial venogram may suggest the direction of manipulation of the guidewire beyond the point of occlusion. Recanalization is a challenging procedure and can be quite time-consuming (Figure 10.5). Success or failure in recanalization of occlusions cannot be predicted by age of occlusion, the extent of the lesion, or its venographic appearance. The initial venogram may appear discouraging, but more often than not, a guidewire can be passed through the occlusion by sight and feel (Figure 10.5a–b). Patience is the key. In the event of initial failure, one or more additional attempts at reopening the occlusion are warranted in all cases. A 0.035-in. soft or stiff Glidewire (Terumo Medical Corporation, Somerset, NJ) is inserted up to the occlusion. Further progress into the

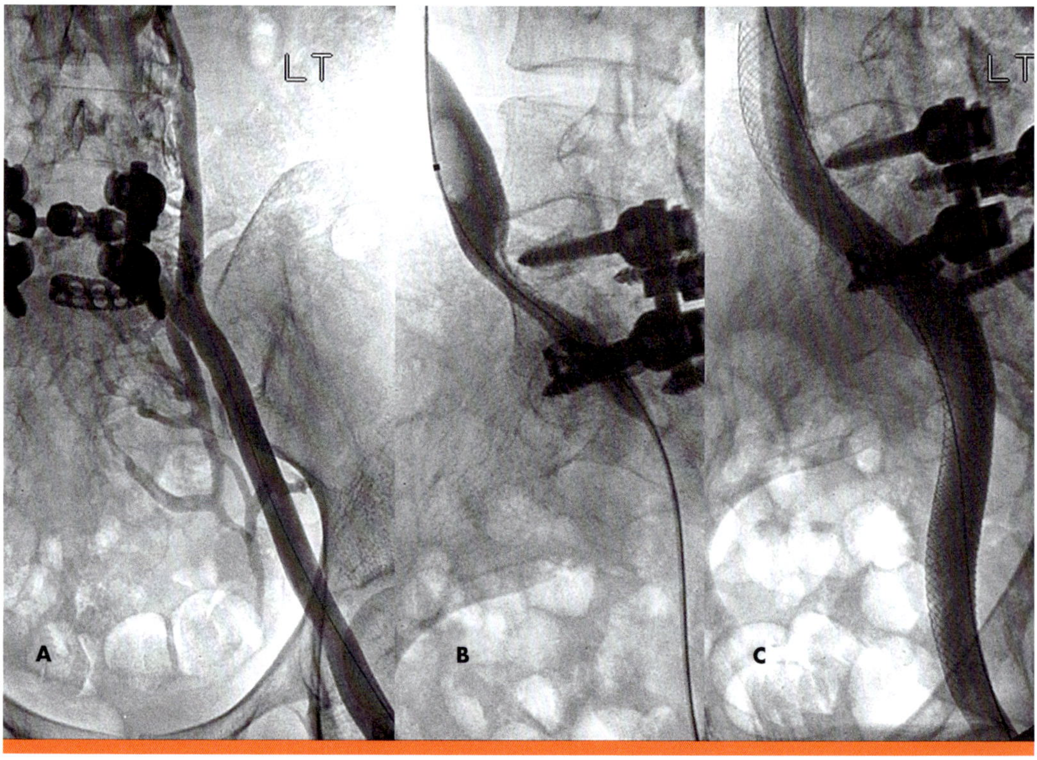

FIGURE 10.4 Balloon dilation and stenting of a left nonthrombotic iliac vein obstruction. **A.** Transfemoral venogram showing occlusion of the common iliac vein and filling of transpelvic collaterals and the ascending lumbar vein. **B.** In a 60° oblique view, it is obvious that the fixation plate and screws are placed posteriorly. A severe obstruction is dilated. **C.** Poststent venogram in the same oblique view reveals no remaining stenosis and good venous outflow. No collaterals are visualized, and the stent is placed well into the IVC.

occlusion is made with the tip of the Glidewire with straight or angled catheter support. Unlike in arterial occlusions, a leading loop is not helpful at this stage. After presumably gaining access to the occluded vein, rapid progress can usually be achieved without perforation by developing a loop or extended "J" at the end of a stiff guidewire or catheter-supported soft wire during manipulation. Usually a combination of soft and stiff Glidewires with straight, angled, and "J" tips of different sizes (0.018–0.035 in) and supporting catheters (straight or angled) are required to advance. The Glidewire tracks through the occluded vein, probably through small vascular channels present in the organizing fibrous tissue within the thrombus, which can frequently be seen on IVUS imaging. Multiple small-volume contrast injections and multiple oblique projections are performed to ensure that the guidewire stays in the vessel and progresses in the correct anatomical direction in the pelvis (Figure 10.5c). Limited extravasations of contrast can be safely ignored, and the procedure continued. Larger dye extravasation calls for cessation of the procedure, which can be reattempted a few weeks later. Once the guidewire has traversed the occluded common iliac vein, passage through the iliocaval junction usually meets with additional resistance, again requiring extended manipulation in the

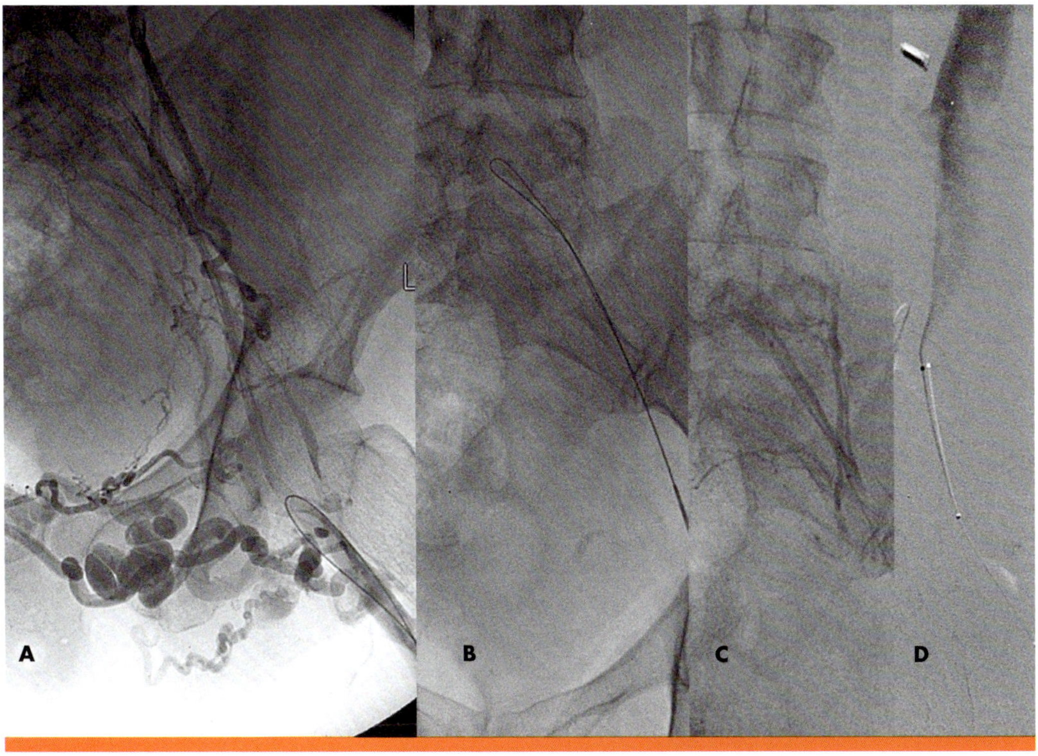

FIGURE 10.5 **A–D.** Recanalization of an occluded vein. **A.** Transfemoral venogram performed through a sheath inserted after ultrasound-guided cannulation of the left femoral vein. A postthrombotic chronic occlusion of the left common iliac vein and cephaled iliac vein with collateral formation is shown. **B.** The obstruction is being traversed by manipulation with soft and stiff hydrophilic guidewires supported by guiding catheters. **C.** Intermittent injection of contrast dye shows that catheter is in a vessel. **D.** A cavogram obtained by contrast dye injection through a catheter ensures that the IVC has been penetrated.

area with coaxial catheter support. Specialized techniques such as those described to cross the occluded aorto-iliac junction are usually not of value. Successful vena cava entry is indicated by further easy passage of the guidewire into the right atrium and is confirmed by contrast injection through an angiography catheter (5 Fr) exchanged for the guidewire (Figure 10.5d).

Iliofemoral Venoplasty and Stent Placement

As pointed out, the IVUS is used to diagnose a significant obstruction. IVUS is also essential during the stenting procedure to determine the size of the balloon, the appropriate diameter of the stent, and the extent of the lesion requiring stent cover, since the diseased vein segment is frequently more extensive in reality than indicated by venography.[29,30] Overdilatation and oversizing of the stent diameter by 2 to 4 mm for the anatomic location are recommended to allow for the inevitable variable recoil of the recanalized channel. An obstruction is always predilated by an appropriately sized balloon, usually 16 to 18 mm for the distal cava and common iliac veins, 14 to 16 mm for the external iliac vein, and 12 to 14 mm for the common femoral vein. Predilation of

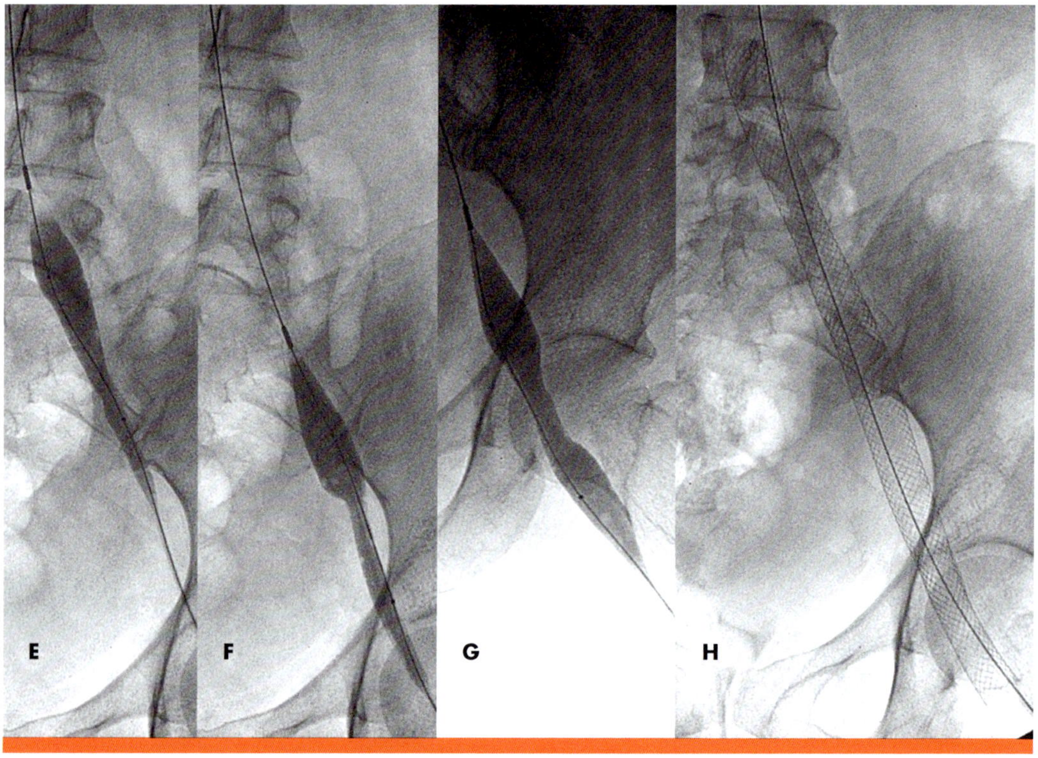

FIGURE 10.5 (*continued*) **E–H.** The intravascular ultrasonography (IVUS) catheter is inserted to assess the extent of the lesion. If necessary, the vessel is recanalized by a smaller balloon to allow passage of the IVUS catheter. **E–G.** Sequential ballooning of the entire iliofemoral venous segment to final diameter size (in this case 14-mm width) is performed then followed by stent placement. **H.** This plain image shows the entire stent system comprising 3 stents, proximally placed well into the IVC and then telescoped over each other to cover the entire iliofemoral vein.

the tract over the wire with 4- to 6-mm balloons is usually required when an occlusion has been recanalized to allow the passage of the IVUS catheter and larger balloons.

The entire tract is ultimately dilated with 12- to 18-mm balloons (Figure 10.5 e-h). There may be hesitation to dilate the obstructive vein because of fear of rupture. There has been no clinically apparent, procedure-related hemorrhage with the recommended balloon sizes in more than 1500 patients in our experience (one case of contained hematoma requiring transfusion occurred in 2008). If rupture should indeed occur, bleeding would probably be contained owing to the comparatively low prevailing venous pressure and the constraining influence of perivenous fascia, surrounding fibrosis, and retroperitoneal cover. CT-scanning performed because of postoperative back pain, which occurs infrequently (10%–15%), has failed to show rupture as causative. Limiting dilation and stenting to 8 to 12 mm diameter in the iliac vein are likely to result in residual stenosis in the stented segment and subsequent stent malfunction or thrombosis.

We exclusively use self-expanding woven braided stainless stents (WALLSTENT, Boston Scientific, Natick, MA) if necessary in series with 3 to 5 cm overlap to minimize shelving along the complex course

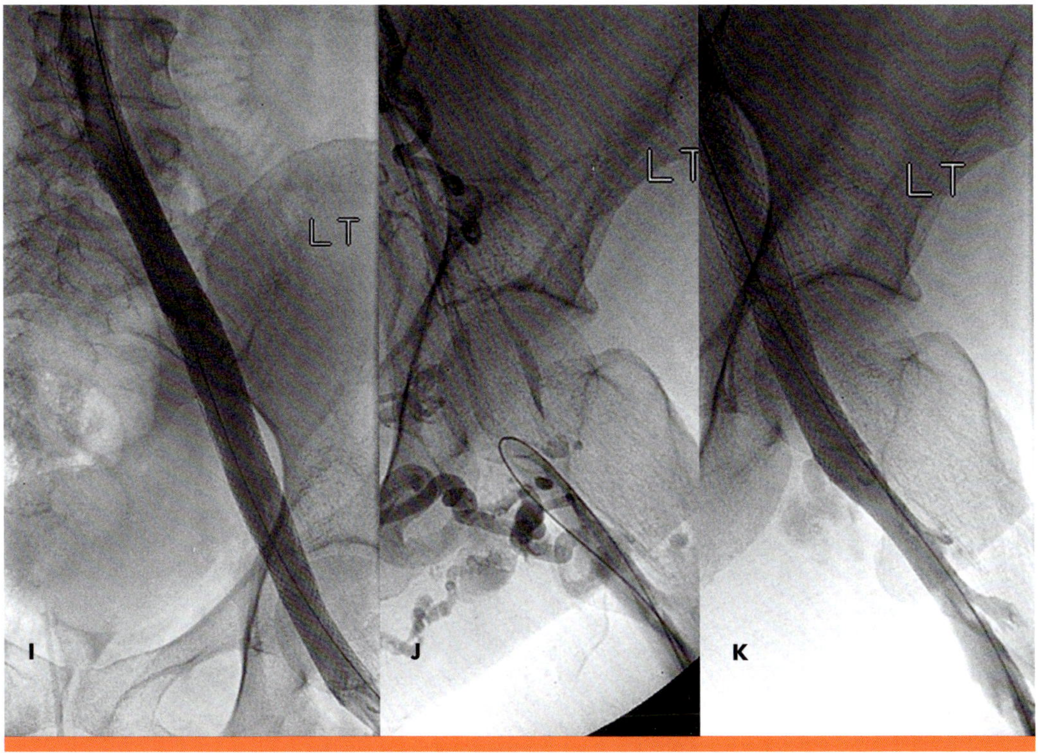

FIGURE 10.5 (*continued*) **I–K.** Final transfemoral venogram, which shows uninterrupted venous outflow and no visualization of any collaterals. **J–K.** It is vital to cover the entire postthrombotic obstruction, even when it requires placement of the stent underneath the inguinal ligament into the common femoral vein, to ensure sufficient inflow.

of the iliac vein (Figure 10.5h). Insertion of one or several large-diameter stents corresponding to the size of the dilating balloon is recommended. It is important to redilate the stent after insertion to ensure a good apposition to the vessel wall and to avoid possible migration. A completion IVUS examination and venogram terminate the procedure after noted defects are corrected by repeat dilation (Figure 10.5i).

To ensure a sufficient venous inflow, it is vital to cover the entire obstruction. Initially, we chose to minimize the length of stented area to avoid stent occlusion, fearing that the stent in itself was a risk factor for stent occlusion. If too short a stent is used, it might migrate proximally into the atrium during the stenting procedure.[38] Stents were inserted covering only the common iliac vein, with its lower end placed just proximal to the internal-external iliac vein confluence in early cases of left iliac vein compression syndrome. This site is usually the lowest point of the iliac vein in the pelvis, where the vein turns anteriorly on its course toward the groin. In more than half of limbs with compression lesion (primary disease), this site is involved due to compression of the external iliac vein by the internal iliac artery "diving" into the pelvis.[18] Secondary stenting procedures for distal recurrent stenosis were either due to a primarily overlooked compression lesion at this site or a predilection of this site for de novo stenosis. The iliac vein confluence should be carefully assessed by IVUS at the time of stenting and the stenting commonly extended "around the curve" well into the external iliac vein. Short (<5-cm) skip areas between 2 stents should be avoided. When multiple stents are placed, they should be sufficiently overlapped to prevent separation. It appears that the occlusion rate and frequency of in-stent recurrent stenosis are not related to stent length or metal load per se; on the contrary, failure to support the entire diseased vein segment with a stent commonly results in early in-stent recurrent stenosis or occlusion of the stent system.

As emphasized previously, adequate inflow into the stent system is essential for future patency. In extensive lesions, especially when recanalization of an occluded vein is obtained, it may be necessary to extend the stent below the level of the inguinal ligament (Figure 10.5j–k). The great saphenous, circumflex, and profunda veins are easily identified by IVUS, and the stent can be extended caudad to the inguinal ligament into the common femoral vein just above the inflow from these and other tributaries. Blood flow, especially from a healthy profunda vein, appears to provide sufficient inflow into the newly recanalized segment, even when the femoral vein is severely diseased or occluded. Contrary to arterial stenting, it has been shown that braided stainless stents (WALLSTENT) can be safely placed in the venous system across the inguinal crease with no risk of stent fractures, narrowing due to external compression, or focal development of severe in-stent restenosis, and no effect on long-term patency.[39]

Most often self-expanding stents (braided stainless steel or nitinol mesh stents) are inserted, but sometimes balloon-expanded stainless steel stents with strong radial force must be used. Stenting of a focal obstruction adjacent to the confluence of the common iliac veins requires that the stent be placed well into the IVC to avoid early recurrence of the stenosis. This is especially important when a braided stent is used. Owing to its inherent property, this stent may be "squeezed" (migrate) caudally when placed slightly beyond the stenosis to avoid extension of the stent into the inferior vena cava. A cephaled recurrent stenosis has been shown to develop in 40% of such limbs.[31] The placement of the stent into the IVC does not appear to significantly impair the flow from the contralateral limb so as to result in thrombosis. Cases of contralateral limb thrombosis have been observed (<1%) and raised concern.[40] This should be compared to the approximately 40% rate of proximal restenosis when a braided stent (WALLSTENT) was not extended into the IVC. The "kissing" balloon technique utilized at the aortic bifurcation is unnecessary at the confluence of the common iliac veins, and bilateral stents are not inserted at this location in the treatment of unilateral lesions.

Stenting of the IVC and Its Confluence

Segmental obstruction of the supra- or infrarenal IVC rarely causes symptoms due to excellent collateral development and function. Only when associated with thrombosis of hepatic veins (Budd-Chiari syndrome), the segmental IVC obstructions may result in liver failure and portal hypertension. Contrarily, when the infrarenal IVC obstruction is combined with chronic iliac vein obstruction, or when acute thrombosis of this segment and ascending collaterals occur, the patient develops limb symptoms.[41]

Essentially the same technique for access, transversing of the obstruction with the guidewire, venoplasty, and stenting are used in the IVC as described for the iliofemoral vein obstruction. Both self-expandable and balloon-expandable stents have been placed with success in the IVC, since flexibility in this straight vessel is not of importance. As in all instances, all diseased segments should be covered by the stent to ensure adequate inflow and outflow of the stent. Even extensive stenting of the occluded IVC from the atrium to the confluence of the iliac veins does not appear to have any adverse effect on the splanchnic outflow.

When both limbs are symptomatic with bilateral iliac vein disease, stenting may have to include the caval confluence. Several techniques have been described. A "double-barrel" stent placement into the IVC may be used when simultaneous bilateral stenting is performed. This is only possible when the caval lesion is limited to the distal infrarenal IVC or when cephaled bilateral lesions of the iliac veins require stent extension into the IVC. The healthy IVC must be wide enough to accommodate 2 parallel stents. The caval confluence is dilated with balloons inserted from both sides and inflated simultaneously, similar to the "kissing balloon" technique used at the aortic bifurcation. Two braided stainless steel stents (9 cm long and 14 mm wide) are then placed and released concurrently starting at the same level in the IVC.

The "double-barrel" technique cannot be used when iliocaval stenting has previously been performed or when bilateral iliac vein stenting is necessary in the presence of extensive cephaled caval obstruction. In those situations, a "Y fenestration" must be performed, which configures the stents in the form of an inverted "Y."[42] The IVC stents are initially placed and extended into one of the iliac veins. The guidewire is introduced through the contralateral side and manipulated through the mesh of the side of the stent. Inflation of a low-profile balloon creates a fenestrum (window) in the side of the stent. A stent is then inserted over the wire through the window. The inflow of the contralateral iliac vein will be covered with this technique. An alternative technique is to place a wide IVC stent down to the confluence and then place bilateral "double-barrel" stents into the IVC stent.

If all other techniques fail, a contralateral stent may be placed as close to the primary stent as possible (appositioned). This always creates a skip area between the stents and may be performed only if the cephaled common iliac vein is relatively healthy. This alternative technique is poor and often results in later restenosis in the uncovered area, which necessitates placement of a bridge stent.

Perioperative Anticoagulation

The perioperative thrombosis prophylaxis may vary but is fairly standardized in our hands. The perioperative anticoagulation management is important, especially when postthrombotic complete occlusions are recanalized, balloon dilated, and stented. The management outlined next has been successful in our experience. Patients on warfarin preoperatively owing to prior deep vein thrombosis, those with thrombophilia discovered during workup and history of previous thrombosis, and those who are recanalized and stented for occlusion are anticoagulated postoperatively. Other patients are discharged on oral aspirin 81 mg daily.

The preoperatively anticoagulated patients are instructed to discontinue the warfarin 3 days prior to the intervention and to self-inject daltaparin sodium 5000 units daily subcutaneously. A slight increase of preoperative prothrombin time (INR ≤1.7) is not a contraindication to proceeding with the procedure. On the day of intervention, all patients are given 2500 units of daltaparin sodium subcutaneously before and after surgery. Patients on warfarin resume taking the medication the same day of the intervention. Daltaparin sodium 5000 units is self-injected subcutaneously daily combined with the warfarin treatment for 5 postoperative days, at which time the INR level is usually found to be therapeutic. Patients treated for occlusion are fully anticoagulated with daltaparin, usually for 14 days before Coumadin is started. All patients receive 3000 to 5000 units of intravenous unfractionated heparin after placement of the sheath in the femoral vein, followed by an intravenous ketorolac tromethamine injection of 30 mg at the time of stenting. The ketorolac and 5000 units of daltaparin sodium injections are repeated the next morning before discharge. Generally, the patients are hospitalized less than 23 hours.

Complications and Thrombotic Events

Venous stenting is performed with low morbidity and no mortality.[28,38,40] The nonthrombotic complication rate related to the endovascular intervention is minimal and usually related to the cannulation site, although a few cases of retroperitoneal hematoma requiring blood transfusions have been described.[28,38] After introduction of ultrasound-guided access of the femoral vein, the morbidity is virtually nil.

Early thrombotic events (<30 days) after iliofemoral stenting for chronic venous disease is low (1.5%). All thrombi involving iliac veins were found in limbs stented for chronic thrombotic obstruction (mainly occlusions). The overall poststent rate of thrombotic events was found to be 4% to 5%.[38,40] The late thrombosis rate in our report of 982 stented iliac veins occurred in 3% of limbs 2 to 77 months after stenting, and only in limbs treated for thrombotic obstruction. Stenting of primary iliac compression lesions (NIVL) with the technique presented has very favorable long-term results with no thrombotic occlusions in that report (we have later experienced thrombosis in 2 patients with NIVL, not included in that study).

Stent Outcome

Although there are numerous small-case reports in the literature, only a few larger series with acceptable short- to mid-term follow-up have been published. The majority of these reports mix limbs stented for chronic obstruction with those stented following clot removal. Knipp et al reported in 2007 an update with a retrospective analysis of 50 stented patients. Nearly half the patients had lysis before stenting and more than 90% had thrombotic obstruction.[43] Cumulative primary, assisted-primary, and secondary patency rates at 48 months were 58%, 71%, and 83%, respectively. Hartung et al reported results of iliocaval stenting in 44 patients with chronic obstruction of primary, secondary, and congenital etiologies in 32, 10, and 2 limbs, respectively.[38] Stenting was not preceded by thrombolysis. Overall cumulative primary, assisted-primary, and secondary patency rates at 36 to 60 months were 73%, 88%, and 90%, respectively, with intention to treat.

We have reported 982 limbs stented under IVUS guidance for chronic nonmalignant obstructive lesions of the femoro-ilio-caval vein.[40] The overall cumulative primary, assisted-primary, and secondary patency rates found in this study at 72 months were 67%, 89%, and 93%, respectively. The stent-related outcome in this study was related mainly to presence and severity of thrombotic disease. Primary and secondary patency rates dropped markedly from NIVL limbs to thrombotic limbs with obstruction, and to thrombotic limbs with occlusion (79% and 100%, 57% and 86%, and 54% and 74%, respectively). Despite the fact that the thrombotic state was such a high-risk factor and thrombophilia was more frequent in limbs with thrombotic disease, the presence of thrombophilia in itself was not significantly associated with occlusion. The operation side and gender did not influence stent outcome in this study, but younger age appeared to do so. Knipp et al found that gender, recent trauma, and age under 40 years were predictive of decreased primary patency.[43] This different finding may be explained by selection of patients, since half of the patients were enrolled with acute DVT in that study. Only 10% of the limbs presented without current or previous DVT, possibly too few to detect the thrombotic state as being predictive.

In our study, the cumulative severe (>50%) in-stent recurrent stenosis (ISR) rate was assessed in 464 limbs and remained low in the long term, 5% at 72 months.[44] The cumulative rate of ISR was higher in thrombotic limbs than in nonthrombotic limbs (10% and 1%, respectively). Despite this observation, it has not been conclusively proven that progressive ISR results in occlusion. Hartung et al reported a 13% restenosis rate, but these authors appear to have included stenosis at the lower stent-vein border area, which is not considered true ISR.[38] The nature and mechanism of development of ISR is not yet known.

Clinical Outcome

Patients with chronic venous disease are younger, will live longer, and have a better prognosis than patients with arterial atherosclerotic disease. Chronic venous disease rarely threatens the survival of limb or patient, so the goal is to improve symptoms and the quality of life. Hurst et al showed resolution or substantial improvement in 72% of limbs, and Hartung et al reported a marked improvement of Venous Clinical Severity and Venous Disability Scores (VCSS and VDS; median score decreased from 8.5 to 2.0, and from 2 to 0, respectively).[25,38] Postinterventional clinical follow-up in our report on 982 stented limbs ranged up to 8¾ years (mean: 24 months; range: 1–107).[40] Information was available in 918 of 982 limbs (93%). The incidence of ulcer healing after stent placement in 148 limbs with active ulcer was 68%, and the cumulative ulcer recurrence-free rate at 5 years was 58%. Ulcers recurred in only 8 limbs of 101 healed ulcers during the follow-up period. Thus, if healing of the ulcer was achieved after this intervention, ulcer recurrence was rare within the study period. The pre- and postoperative mean pain and swelling scores improved substantially (3.7 [range: 0–9] and 0.8 [range: 0–10] [Visual Analogue Pain Scale], and 1.7 [range: 0–3] and 0.8 [range: 0–3] [degree of swelling 0–3], respectively [P <0.0001]). This improvement was sustained with cumulatively 62% and 32%, respectively, remained completely free of pain and swelling (grade 0 swelling and 0 level of pain), and 74% and 62%, respectively, substantially improved.

It has previously been shown that both primary CVD with "simple" varicose veins and secondary CVD with development of postthrombotic stigmata significantly reduce quality of life. Specifically, previous iliofemoral DVT may cause clinically pertinent iliac outflow obstruction, resulting in a marked compromise of quality-of-life (QOL).[21] A validated health-related quality of life questionnaire (CIVIQ)[45] assessing subjective leg pain, sleep disturbance due to leg problems, work-related leg problems, and the effect of leg symptoms on morale and social activities was filled out by stented patients prospectively before and after intervention (mean follow-up 5 months, range: 1–79 months, n = 381).[40] There was significant improvement in all 5 problem categories after stenting of both NIVL and thrombotic outflow obstructions. Chronic venous disease regardless of etiology affects QOL adversely, and stenting in patients with chronic venous outflow obstruction frequently markedly improved it. Stenting is a minimally invasive outpatient procedure with low morbidity, which results in marked clinical improvement of pain and swelling with sustained ulcer healing and measurable improvement of VCSS, VDS, and QOL.

Follow-up

Patients having had iliocaval stenting should be followed on a regular basis. Transfemoral venogram, ascending venogram, or iliocaval duplex ultrasonography should be performed before the patient is discharged, 6 weeks to 3 months later, 6 months after intervention, and then annually. Patients with high risk of developing early thrombosis, mainly in limbs with recanalization of postthrombotic occlusion, may be seen more often. Adequate anticoagulation is vital for stent patency in this group of patients. When a recurrent in-stent stenosis >50% is found on routine surveillance, balloon angioplasty should be performed to maintain stent patency whether or not the patient is symptomatic. On emergence of significant interval symptoms, even with normal venography or ultrasonography findings, IVUS should be performed generously to ensure that an in-stent restenosis or extra stent de novo stenosis does not go undetected and untreated.

References

1. Johnson BF, Manzo RA, Bergelin RO, Strandness DE Jr. Relationship between changes in the deep venous system and the development of the postthrombotic syndrome after an acute episode of lower limb deep vein thrombosis: a one- to six-year follow-up. J Vasc Surg. 1995;21:307-12; discussion 313.
2. Nicolaides AN, Hussein MK, Szendro G, Christopoulos D, Vasdekis S, Clarke H. The relation of venous ulceration with ambulatory venous pressure measurements. J Vasc Surg. 1993;17:414-9.
3. Caps MT, Manzo RA, Bergelin RO, Meissner MH, Strandness DE Jr. Venous valvular reflux in veins not involved at the time of acute deep vein thrombosis. J Vasc Surg. 1995;22:524-31.
4. Kahn SR. Frequency and determinants of the postthrombotic syndrome after venous thromboembolism. Curr Opin Pulm Med. 2006;12:299-303.
5. Akesson H, Brudin L, Dahlstrom JA, Eklof B, Ohlin P, Plate G. Venous function assessed during a 5 year period after acute ilio-femoral venous thrombosis treated with anticoagulation. Eur J Vasc Surg. 1990;4:43-8.
6. Plate G, Akesson H, Einarsson E, Ohlin P, Eklof B. Long-term results of venous thrombectomy combined with a temporary arterio-venous fistula. Eur J Vasc Surg. 1990;4:483-9.
7. Negus D, Cockett FB. Femoral vein pressures in post-phlebitic iliac vein obstruction. Br J Surg. 1967;54:522-5.
8. Negus D, Fletcher EW, Cockett FB, Thomas ML. Compression and band formation at the mouth of the left common iliac vein. Br J Surg. 1968;55:369-74.

9. Cockett FB, Thomas ML, Negus D. Iliac vein compression—its relation to iliofemoral thrombosis and the post-thrombotic syndrome. Br Med J. 1967;2:14-9.
10. Cockett FB. The iliac compression syndrome alias 'iliofemoral thrombosis' or 'white leg.' Proc R Soc Med. 1966;59:360-1.
11. Cockett FB, Thomas ML. The iliac compression syndrome. Br J Surg. 1965;52: 816-21.
12. Fraser DG, Moody AR, Morgan PS, Martel A. Iliac compression syndrome and recanalization of femoropopliteal and iliac venous thrombosis: a prospective study with magnetic resonance venography. J Vasc Surg. 2004;40:612-9.
13. Chung JW, Yoon CJ, Jung SI, Kim HC, Lee W, Kim YI, et al. Acute iliofemoral deep vein thrombosis: evaluation of underlying anatomic abnormalities by spiral CT venography. J Vasc Interv Radiol. 2004;15:249-56.
14. May R, Thurner J. The cause of the predominantly sinistral occurrence of thrombosis of the pelvic veins. Angiology. 1957;8:419-27.
15. Ehrich WE, Krumbhaar EB. A frequent obstructive anomaly of the mouth of the left common iliac vein. Am Heart J. 1943;26: 737-50.
16. McMurrich JP. The occurrence of congenital adhesions in the common iliac veins, and their relation to thrombosis of the femoral and iliac veins. Am J Med Sci. 1943;135:342-6.
17. Kibbe MR, Ujiki M, Goodwin AL, Eskandari M, Yao J, Matsumura J. Iliac vein compression in an asymptomatic patient population. J Vasc Surg. 2004;39:937-43.
18. Raju S, Neglén P. High prevalence of nonthrombotic iliac vein lesions in chronic venous disease: a permissive role in pathogenicity. J Vasc Surg. 2006;44:136-43; discussion 144.
19. Neglén P, Thrasher TL, Raju S. Venous outflow obstruction: an underestimated contributor to chronic venous disease. J Vasc Surg. 2003;38:879-85.
20. Mavor GE, Galloway JM. Collaterals of the deep venous circulation of the lower limb. Surg Gynecol Obstet. 1967;125:561-71.
21. Delis KT, Bountouroglou D, Mansfield AO. Venous claudication in iliofemoral thrombosis: long-term effects on venous hemodynamics, clinical status, and quality of life. Ann Surg. 2004;239:118-26.
22. Strandness DE Jr, Sumner DS. The Effect of Geometry on Arterial Blood Flow. Hemodynamics for Surgeons. New York: Grune & Stratton, 1975. p96-119.
23. Neglén P, Raju S. Detection of outflow obstruction in chronic venous insufficiency. J Vasc Surg. 1993;17:583-9.
24. Labropoulos N, Volteas N, Leon M, Sowade O, Rulo A, Giannoukas AD, Nicolaides AN. The role of venous outflow obstruction in patients with chronic venous dysfunction. Arch Surg. 1997;132:46-51.
25. Hurst DR, Forauer AR, Bloom JR, Greenfield LJ, Wakefield TW, Williams DM. Diagnosis and endovascular treatment of iliocaval compression syndrome. J Vasc Surg. 2001;34:106-13.
26. Albrechtsson U, Einarsson E, Eklof B. Femoral vein pressure measurements for evaluation of venous function in patients with postthrombotic iliac veins. Cardiovasc Intervent Radiol. 1981;4:43-50.
27. Raju S, Owen S Jr, Neglén P. The clinical impact of iliac venous stents in the management of chronic venous insufficiency. J Vasc Surg. 2002;35:8-15.
28. Neglén P, Berry MA, Raju S. Endovascular surgery in the treatment of chronic primary and post-thrombotic iliac vein obstruction. Eur J Vasc Endovasc Surg. 2000;20: 560-71.
29. Neglén P, Raju S. Intravascular ultrasound scan evaluation of the obstructed vein. J Vasc Surg. 2002;35:694-700.

30. Forauer AR, Gemmete JJ, Dasika NL, Cho KJ, Williams DM. Intravascular ultrasound in the diagnosis and treatment of iliac vein compression (May-Thurner) syndrome. J Vasc Interv Radiol. 2002;13:523-7.
31. Neglén P, Raju S. Balloon dilation and stenting of chronic iliac vein obstruction: technical aspects and early clinical outcome. J Endovasc Ther. 2000;7:79-91.
32. Ahmed HK, Hagspiel KD. Intravascular ultrasonographic findings in May-Thurner syndrome (iliac vein compression syndrome). J Ultrasound Med. 2001;20:251-6.
33. Satokawa H, Hoshino S, Iwaya F, Igari T, Midorikawa H, Ogawa T. Intravascular imaging methods for venous disorders. Int J Angiol. 2000;9:117-21.
34. Marzo KP, Schwartz R, Glanz S. Early restenosis following percutaneous transluminal balloon angioplasty for the treatment of the superior vena caval syndrome due to pacemaker-induced stenosis. Catheter Cardio Diag. 1995;36:128-31.
35. Neglén P, al-Hassan HK, Endrys J, Nazzal MM, Christenson JT, Eklof B. Iliofemoral venous thrombectomy followed by percutaneous closure of the temporary arteriovenous fistula. Surgery. 1991;110:493-9.
36. Wisselink W, Money SR, Becker MO, Rice KL, Ramee SR, White CJ, et al. Comparison of operative reconstruction and percutaneous balloon dilatation for central venous obstruction. Am J Surg. 1993;166:200-4; discussion 204-5.
37. Walpole HT Jr, Lovett KE, Chuang VP, West R, Clements SD Jr. Superior vena cava syndrome treated by percutaneous transluminal balloon angioplasty. Am Heart J. 1988;115:1303-4.
38. Hartung O, Otero A, Boufi M, Decaridi G, Barthelemy P, Juhan C, et al. Mid-term results of endovascular treatment for symptomatic chronic nonmalignant iliocaval venous occlusive disease. J Vasc Surg. 2005;42:1138-44; discussion 1144.
39. Neglén P, Tackett TP Jr, Raju S. Venous stenting across the inguinal ligament. J Vasc Surg. 2008;48:1255-61.
40. Neglén P, Hollis KC, Olivier J, Raju S. Stenting of the venous outflow in chronic venous disease: long-term stent-related outcome, clinical, and hemodynamic result. J Vasc Surg. 2007;46:979-90.
41. Raju S, McAllister S, Neglén P. Recanalization of totally occluded iliac and adjacent venous segments. J Vasc Surg. 2002;36:903-11.
42. Raju S, Hollis K, Neglén P. Obstructive lesions of the inferior vena cava: clinical features and endovenous treatment. J Vasc Surg. 2006;44:820-7.
43. Knipp BS, Ferguson E, Williams DM, Dasika NJ, Cwikiel W, Henke PK, et al. Factors associated with outcome after interventional treatment of symptomatic iliac vein compression syndrome. J Vasc Surg. 2007;46:743-9.
44. Neglén P, Raju S. In-stent recurrent stenosis in stents placed in the lower extremity venous outflow tract. J Vasc Surg. 2004;39:181-7.
45. Launois R, Reboul-Marty J, Henry B. Construction and validation of a quality of life questionnaire in chronic lower limb venous insufficiency (CIVIQ). Qual Life Res. 1996;5:539-54.

CHAPTER 11

Venous Bypass

Indications, Techniques, and Outcomes

Joseph J. Ricotta II and Peter Gloviczki

Reconstruction of the occluded iliofemoral vein or the inferior vena cava (IVC) may be required in patients with chronic venous insufficiency (CVI). Iliofemoral venous occlusion is responsible for CVI in at least 10% of the patients afflicted by this disease. Endovascular treatment for iliocaval obstruction has progressed rapidly, and today venous stenting is the primary choice for treatment of benign iliac vein or iliocaval venous occlusions in patients who failed conservative compression therapy. Venous stenting is used for patients with malignancy only in those cases when excision of the tumor is not possible and the goal of therapy is palliation. In the last 2 decades, results of open surgical reconstructions have also improved, and symptomatic patients who are not candidates for, or who have failed, endovascular reconstructions can be treated with venous bypasses to relieve venous outflow obstruction. Venous reconstruction is also performed in those patients who undergo excision of malignant tumors invading large veins such as the IVC or the iliac veins. Patient selection for surgical treatment of postthrombotic syndrome (PTS) can be challenging, since proximal occlusion is frequently combined with infrainguinal venous valvular incompetence. Thorough preoperative evaluation to identify significant venous outflow obstruction in these patients is essential.

Chronic Venous Insufficiency. Contemporary Endovascular Management series. © 2011 Mark G. Davies MD and Alan B. Lumsden MD, eds. Cardiotext Publishing, ISBN 978-1-9353950-9-6.

An Open Surgical Treatment

Patients who are not candidates for, or who have failed endovascular reconstruction for, chronic venous insufficiency can be treated with venous bypasses to relieve symptomatic venous outflow obstruction. Venous reconstruction is also performed in those patients who undergo excision of malignant tumors invading the vena cava or iliac veins. In the infrainguinal location, autologous grafts have the best chance of long-term success. If available, the ipsilateral or contralateral great saphenous vein (GSV) is the preferred conduit, followed by arm vein. Harvesting the contralateral femoral vein (FV) in the post-thrombotic leg is best avoided unless absolutely necessary because of the potential for significant morbidity. Externally supported ePTFE is currently the best choice for prosthetic replacement of large veins when an autologous vein is not available.

Factors responsible for poor patency in venous grafts include low flow and pressure, external compression, and hypercoagulability. Some surgeons consider thrombophilia to be a contraindication to venous bypass surgery. All procedures are performed under the cover of intra- and postoperative anticoagulation and intermittent pneumatic compression. Many authors have confirmed that a distal arteriovenous fistula (AVF), first suggested by Kunlin in 1953, improves the patency of grafts placed in the venous system. However, elevated cardiac output secondary to a large fistula may potentially accentuate the venous outflow obstruction and cause worsening of symptoms until the fistula is taken down. A femoral arteriovenous fistula is recommended for prosthetic grafts anastomosed to the femoral vein and iliocaval grafts longer than 10 cm. The fistula is closed surgically or by endovascular embolization 3 to 6 months after the operation, although fistulas that cause no symptoms can be left indefinitely. A small silastic sheet wrapped around the fistula facilitates its localization at time of subsequent surgical closure. Palma procedures can be performed without a fistula in patients with a high pressure gradient (10–20 mm Hg), but those with a lower pressure gradient and those with low initial flow (<100 mL/min) benefit from temporary fistula formation.

Saphenopopliteal Bypass

First advocated by Warren and Thayer in 1954 and reintroduced by Husni[1] and by May,[2] saphenopopliteal bypass (May-Husni operation) is indicated for patients with occlusion of the superficial femoral or proximal popliteal veins. In the original operation, the ipsilateral saphenous vein was used for conduit. A single distal anastomosis is performed, usually end-to-side, between the mobilized and divided saphenous vein and the distal popliteal vein, using running 6/0 or 7/0 prolene sutures. An end-to-side arteriovenous fistula can be constructed at the ankle between the posterior tibial artery and one of the paired posterior tibial veins or the saphenous vein. Alternatively, a bypass graft may be performed with free contralateral saphenous or arm vein.

Cross-Pelvic Venous Bypass (Palma-Dale Procedure)

Initially described by Palma in Uruguay and popularized by Dale in the United States, the Palma-Dale procedure has remained a useful technique for venous reconstruction in patients with chronic unilateral iliac vein obstruction of any etiology.[3,4] A prerequisite for the procedure is a normal contralateral iliofemoral venous system to ensure adequate venous drainage. Absence of distal deep venous obstruction or reflux is associated with superior results.

Patients with unilateral iliac vein obstruction and minimal, if any, infrainguinal disease are the best candidates for saphenous vein transposition (Palma procedure) (Figure 11.1). Unfortunately, many patients with postthrombotic syndrome have extensive femoral venous obstruction, and patients with poor inflow to the groin have less chance of a durable result. The contralateral saphenous vein is mapped with duplex ultrasonography and marked on the skin preoperatively for bypass. The vein should be 5 to 6 mm in size for a good conduit. The common femoral vein on the affected side is exposed first through a 5- to 7-cm-long longitudinal groin incision. The collateral veins are preserved if possible. If an arteriovenous fistula is planned, the proximal superficial femoral artery is also dissected. The GSV of the contralateral leg is dissected through a 3- to 4-cm-long longitudinal or oblique incision in the groin crease, starting just medial to the femoral artery pulse. Tributaries of the saphenous vein are ligated and divided, and adequate saphenous vein is mobilized. A short, second, upper-thigh incision is made to dissect a total of 20 to 25 cm GSV. After heparinization, the saphenous vein is ligated and divided distally and pulled up to the groin incision.

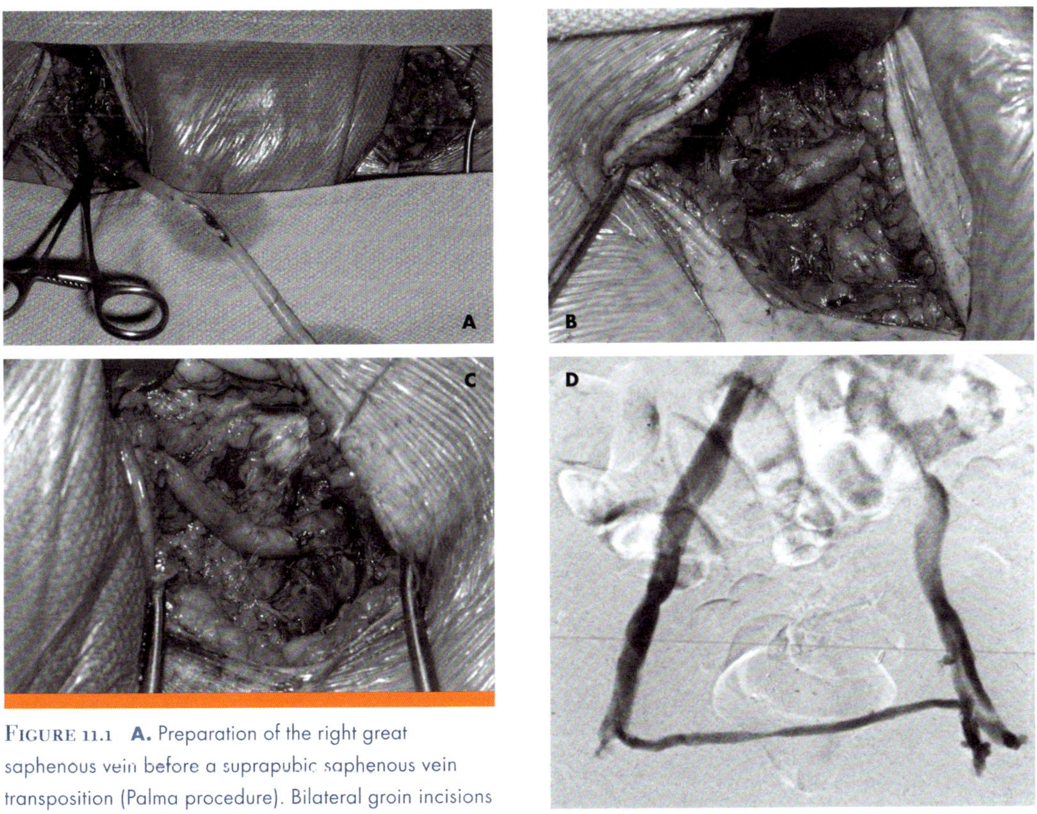

FIGURE 11.1 **A.** Preparation of the right great saphenous vein before a suprapubic saphenous vein transposition (Palma procedure). Bilateral groin incisions are performed to expose the left common femoral vein and the right saphenofemoral junction. The right saphenous vein is harvested through short incisions in the thigh, and a clamp is placed to occlude the saphenous vein and partially the common femoral vein as well. The vein is distended with heparinized papaverine solution before tunneled to the left side for anastomosis with the femoral vein. **B.** The right saphenofemoral junction after tunneling the vein to the left side in the suprapubic space. Note excellent inflow without kink in the saphenous vein. **C.** Anastomosis of the saphenous vein with the left common femoral vein. **D.** Postoperative CTV confirms patent saphenous vein graft.

Alternatively, the GSV can be harvested endoscopically. The saphenofemoral junction is dissected, but the vein is not divided proximally. Before tunneling, a small side-biting vascular clamp is placed on the common femoral vein, and the saphenous vein distended with heparinized papaverine solution (Figure 11.1a). This is an important part of the procedure, since the saphenous vein is usually in spasm and distention increases the size of the conduit. The suprapubic tunnel has to be wide to avoid external constriction of the vein graft and is made proximal to the external opening of the inguinal canal to avoid any injury to the spermatic cord structures in men. If there is a kink in the vein at the saphenofemoral junction after tunneling, sometimes it is necessary to disconnect the GSV with a 2-mm cuff from the common femoral vein and reanastomose it with a running 6/0 polypropylene suture, after turning it upwards through 180°. The common femoral vein of the affected limb is then cross-clamped with soft vascular clamps and opened longitudinally over about 2 cm. The anastomosis between the GSV and the femoral vein is performed with running 6/0 or 7/0 polypropylene sutures. If the vein is small, interrupted sutures can be employed. If the vein is less than 5 mm in diameter, or the pressure difference between the 2 femoral veins is less than 3 mm Hg, femoral arteriovenous fistula is indicated. This is performed between the superficial femoral vein and the hood of the saphenous vein using a separate reversed segment of the right GSV. An alternative is to use a segment of 4- by 7-mm tapered PTFE graft to create 4- or 5-mm-diameter fistula. The Palma procedure, however, should not be performed with veins 4 mm or smaller.

Although few large series have been reported, overall patency of Palma grafts in 9 series including 412 operations ranged between 70% and 83% at 3 to 5 years.[4-7] Results were better in patients who had none, or minimal infrainguinal venous disease and in those with May-Thurner syndrome without previous deep vein thrombosis.

Crossover Femoral Venous Prosthetic Bypass

When the saphenous vein is small or not available, crossover femoral venous prosthetic bypass with an 8-mm or 10-mm externally supported ePTFE is a good alternative (Figure 11.2). The femoral veins are exposed bilaterally, the ePTFE graft is positioned in the subcutaneous suprapubic tunnel, and an end-to-side anastomosis performed to the common femoral veins on each side. It is not unusual to require endophlebectomy of the partially recanalized femoral vein, to optimize inflow into the graft (Figure 11.2a). A distal AVF on the affected side is routinely added to the procedure using a 4- to 5-mm PTFE graft between the PTFE graft and the superficial femoral artery (Figure 11.2b). Sottiurai recommends cutting out a small window rather the just making a longitudinal cut in the cross-femoral graft at the hood of the femoral anastomosis to optimize inflow and decrease intimal hyperplasia.[8] A small silastic sheath is placed around the fistula and marked with metal clips and a large prolene stitch positioned under the skin (Figure 11.2c). When surgery is undertaken to close the fistula after 3 to 6 months, it is easy to find by following the thread and the silastic sheath that prevents tissue in-growth into the PTFE graft.

The patency rates of ePTFE grafts in this location are extremely variable, ranging between 0% and 100%. At the Mayo Clinic, long-term patency is about 50%, and preference is given to saphenous crossover grafts, where possible.[9]

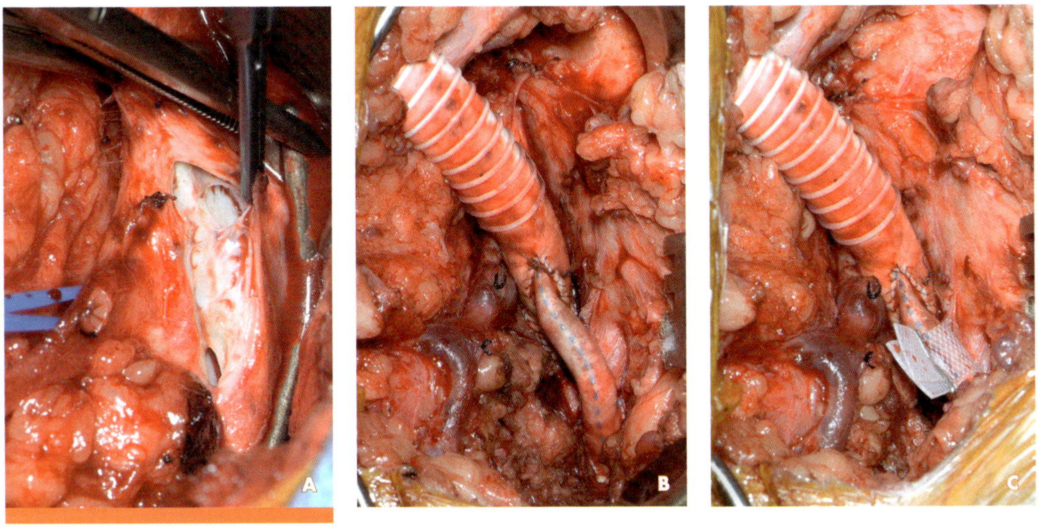

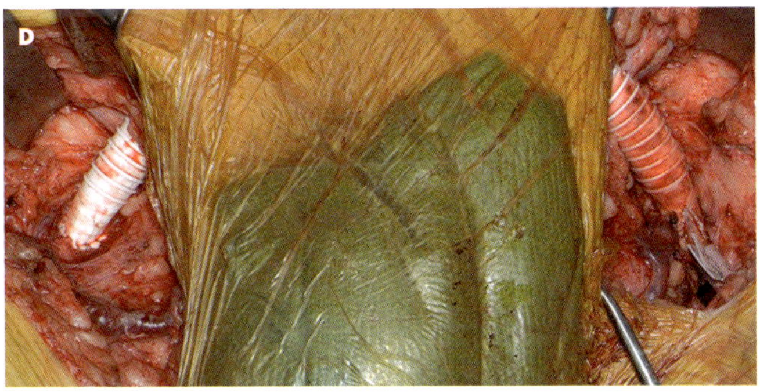

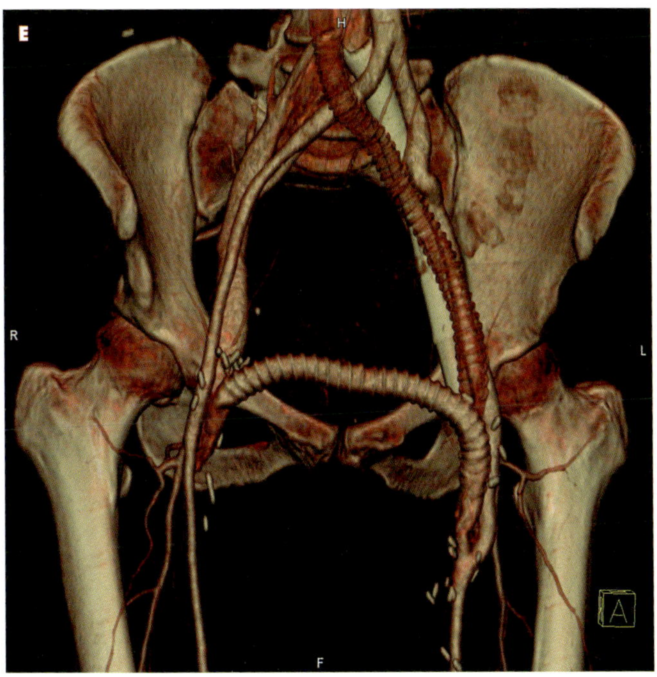

FIGURE 11.2 **A.** Partially recanalized femoral vein found after venotomy. Endophlebectomy was performed to remove the organized thrombus and improve inflow into a femoro-femoral crossover venous PTFE bypass. **B.** A PTFE arteriovenous fistula was performed between the superficial femoral artery and the hood of the cross-femoral PTFE graft. **C.** A small silastic sheath is placed around the fistula and marked with metal clips for easy identification at reoperation when the fistula is closed. **D.** Completed left-to-right femoral crossover PTFE graft with an arteriovenous fistula. **E.** Computed tomographic venography of the cross-femoral PTFE graft with a patent arteriovenous fistula 8 months after surgery.

Iliocaval and Femorocaval Bypass

Low-risk patients with bilateral iliac obstructions or with iliocaval obstruction that cannot be treated with stents should be considered for an in-line femorocaval (Figure 11.3) or iliocaval (Figure 11.4) bypass. For in-line reconstruction of iliocaval or caval occlusions, ePTFE graft with external support is the preferred conduit. Short, large-

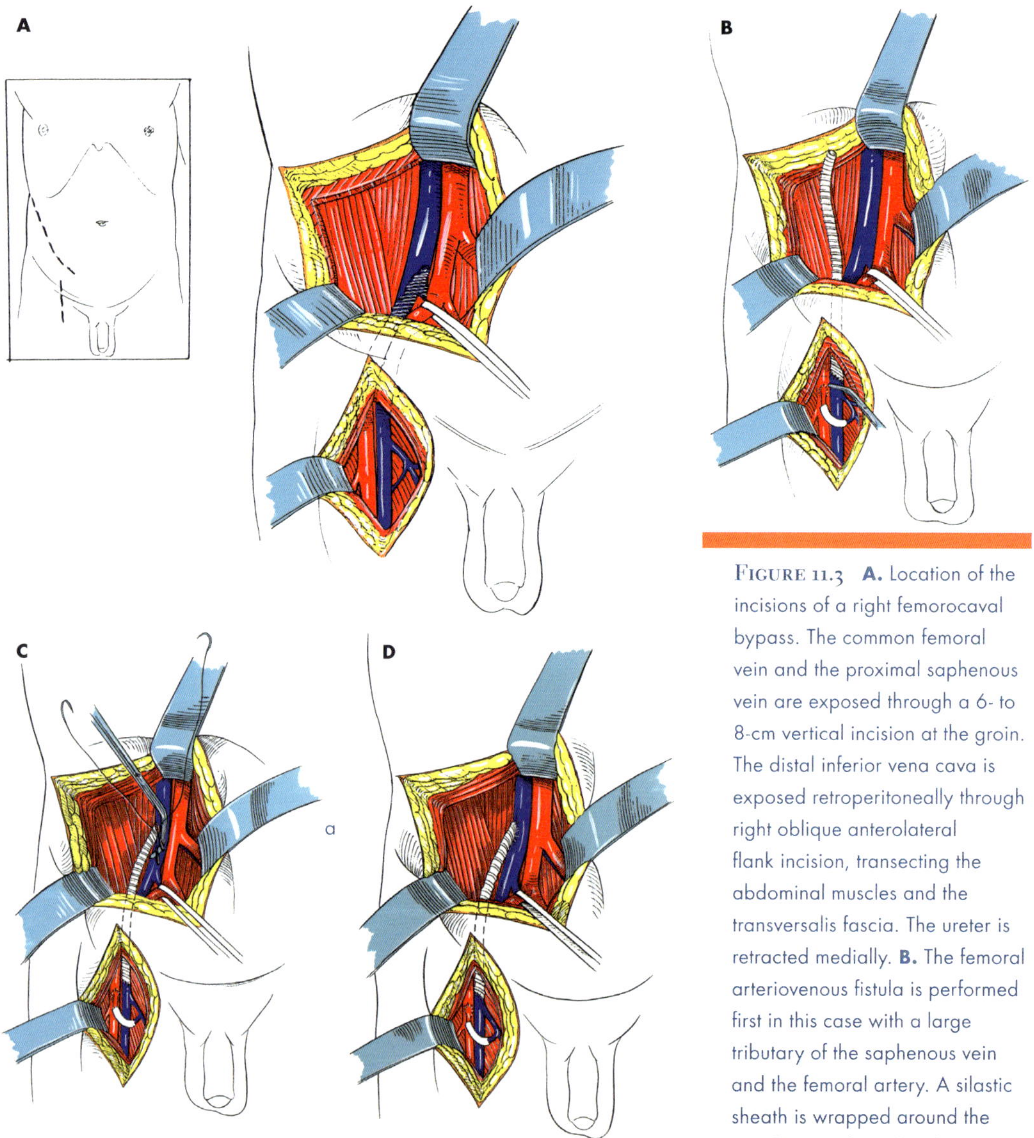

FIGURE 11.3 **A.** Location of the incisions of a right femorocaval bypass. The common femoral vein and the proximal saphenous vein are exposed through a 6- to 8-cm vertical incision at the groin. The distal inferior vena cava is exposed retroperitoneally through right oblique anterolateral flank incision, transecting the abdominal muscles and the transversalis fascia. The ureter is retracted medially. **B.** The femoral arteriovenous fistula is performed first in this case with a large tributary of the saphenous vein and the femoral artery. A silastic sheath is wrapped around the vein for easy late identification. The distal anastomosis is then performed in an end-to-end fashion between the common femoral vein and the 10-mm externally supported PTFE graft. **C.** The anastomosis between the graft and the inferior vena cava is performed in an end-to-end fashion using 5/0 polypropylene suture. Air is carefully flushed from the graft before removing the clamp from the inferior vena cava. **D.** Completed femorocaval bypass with a saphenofemoral arteriovenous fistula. Reprinted with permission from the Mayo Foundation.

diameter (≥12-mm) grafts are used most frequently. We recommend a diameter of 12 to 14 mm for iliocaval bypasses and at least 10 mm for femorocaval bypass. The superior portion of the infrarenal IVC, at and immediately distal to the renal veins, is best approached transperitoneally, through a midline incision, reflecting the ascending colon medially and mobilizing the duodenum using the Kocher maneuver. The inferior portion of the IVC, just above the iliac bifurcation, is best approached retroperitoneally, through a right flank incision (Figure 11.3a). If the occlusion is limited to the right common iliac vein, the same incision is used to expose the external iliac vein for the distal anastomosis and the graft is tunneled under the ureter.

If a femorocaval graft is required, a separate 8-cm-long vertical groin incision is made on the affected side, and the graft is tunneled under the inguinal ligament (Figure 11.3a). For all grafts originating from the femoral vein and for most long iliocaval grafts, an arteriovenous fistula is added at the groin (Figure 11.3b). Local heparin therapy (500 units per hour) is initiated via a 20-gauge catheter, which is introduced through a tributary of the saphenous vein (Figure 11.4), and advanced to the distal anastomosis. This catheter can be used for completion venography 24 to 48 hours after reconstruction and removed on the third postoperative day, when full anticoagulation is started. Early clinical improvement can be expected in the majority of patients, but the presence of coexisting femoropopliteal reflux can still be the cause of significant disability.

The use of autologous vein for femoroiliac or femorocaval reconstruction is also an option. However, because of its relatively small size, saphenous vein in this location can only rarely be used. If a short segment of the common femoral or iliac vein has to be reconstructed, a better size match is a spiral saphenous vein graft, prepared using the contralateral saphenous vein (Figure 11.5). The excised vein is opened longitudinally, the valves are excised, and the graft is wrapped around a 28-mm or 32-mm argyle chest tube. The edges are approximated with running 6/0 polypropylene sutures or with stainless steel nonpenetrating vascular clips. The internal or external jugular veins are alternative conduits that can be considered for venous reconstruction. Femoral vein is also an alternative for reconstruction of

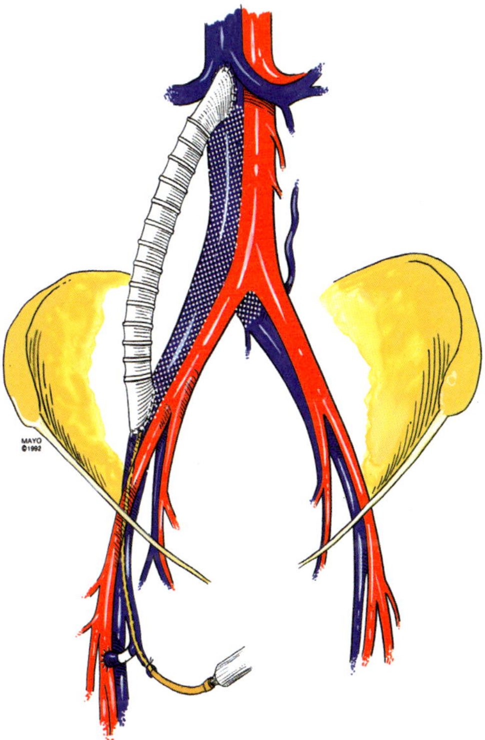

FIGURE 11.4 Iliocaval PTFE bypass between the right external iliac vein and the infrarenal inferior vena cava. Note saphenofemoral arteriovenous fistula and placement of a 20-gauge pediatric central line into the saphenous vein and advanced up to the graft to perfuse heparin to prevent early thrombus formation on the graft surface. Reprinted with permission from the Mayo Foundation.

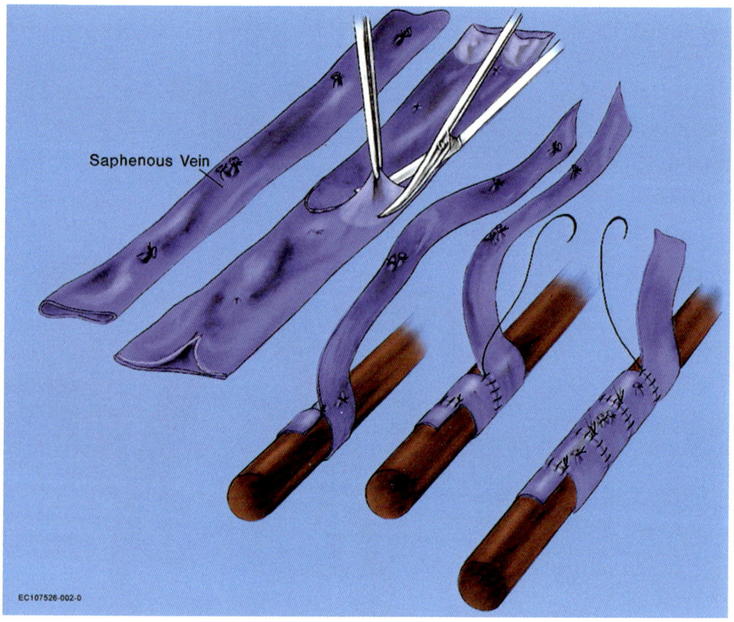

FIGURE 11.5 Technique to prepare a spiral saphenous vein graft. The vein is cut open longitudinally, valves are excised, and the vein is wrapped around a 28- or 32-gauge argyle chest tube. The edges are approximated with running 6/0 polypropylene sutures, making interrupted stitches after each circle to minimize purse stringing. Alternatively, nonpenetrating vascular clips can be used for this purpose. Reprinted with permission from the Mayo Foundation.

abdominal veins, although the morbidity of removing this vein in many of these patients with underlying thrombophilia or postthrombotic syndrome is high, and other options are recommended. Cryopreserved saphenous or femoral vein has also been reported for venous reconstruction; however, long-term patency of these grafts for venous replacement in our experience has been poor.

Results of Deep Venous Bypass

Although the first successful venous reconstruction was reported more than 40 years ago by Warren and Thayer, results of surgical treatment for venous obstruction have been less than satisfactory for many years. There has been some improvement in diagnosis, patient selection, and surgical technique over the last 2 decades. The original May-Husni transposition is rarely performed and popliteofemoral bypasses are also infrequent. In 9 series that included 218 operations, functional improvement was reported in 77%.[4,5,10] In an earlier review of 59 operations, Smith and Trimble[11] reported clinical success in 76% of the patients. Crude patency rates at variable follow-up ranged from 5% to 100%, but only 4 of 9 studies reported on late imaging of the grafts to ascertain patency.[5,6,10,11]

Patency rates of 412 Palma operations, published in 9 series, were somewhat better, with clinical improvement in 63% to 89% and patency rates between 70% and 85% (Table 11.1). However, follow-up was variable and objective graft assessment with imaging was rarely employed. Husni reported patency of 47 of 67 grafts, followed from 6 months to 15 years.[1] Four-year patency of the 18 Palma grafts performed at the Mayo Clinic was 83%.[9] ePTFE grafts in this location are not so good, with early occlusion of all 3 grafts implanted at the Mayo Clinic and 5 of 6 grafts performed by Eklof.[12] However, Comerota et al[13] reported patency in 2 of 3 grafts at 40 and 63 months. The best results with PTFE were reported by Sottiurai and associates, who observed 100% patency (26/26) at a follow-up ranging from 11 to 139 months.[14] Gruss et al have the most experience with ePTFE graft in this position. These authors

TABLE 11.1 **Results of Femoro-femoral Crossover Bypass**

Author, Year	No. of Limbs	Follow-up (years)	Post-operative Imaging (%)	Patency Rate (%)	Clinical Improve-ment (%)	Graft Material
Palma et al,[3] 1960	8	Up to 3	13	N/A	88	vein
May,[2] 1981	66	N/A	N/A	73	N/A	vein
Dale,[19] 1979	56	N/A	N/A	N/A	80	vein
Husni,[1] 1983	85	0.5 ~ 15.0	N/A	70	74	vein (n = 83) PTFE (n = 2)
Halliday et al,[20] 1993	47	Up to 18	72	75 (cumulative)	89	vein
Danza et al,[6] 1991	27	N/A	N/A	N/A	81	vein
AbuRahmaet al,[5] 1991	24	5.5	100	75	63	vein
Gruss et al,[4] 1977	19 32	N/A N/A	N/A N/A	71 85	82 overall	vein PTFE
Jost et al,[7] 2001	21	3.5	100	75	67 overall*	18 vein, 3 ePTFE

*Includes outcome for all deep venous bypasses.

reported an 85% (27/32) patency rate in a long-term follow-up study.[4] Based on his results and those of others, Gruss now recommends using externally supported ePTFE grafts with AVF for all cross pubic venous bypasses

An alternative is in-line femorocaval bypass for patients without suitable saphenous vein for a Palma procedure. Secondary patency of 13 ilio-femoro-caval ePTFE bypasses was, however, only 54% (Table 11.2). Sottiurai et al reported patency in 9 of 13 femorocaval ePTFE bypass grafts at 1 year.[14] Overall, open venous reconstruction for iliofemoral or inferior venacaval obstruction offers 3-year patency rates of 62%.

Cavoatrial Bypass

Patients with symptomatic short membranous occlusion of the IVC, or longer congenital or acquired narrowing (caval coarctation) without or with hepatic venous outflow obstruction (Budd-Chiari syndrome) can be treated by cavoatrial bypass when attempts at percutaneous angioplasty or stenting have failed, or if transcardiac membranotomy is not feasible.

The suprahepatic inferior vena cava or right atrium is approached through an anterolateral right thoracotomy (Figure 11.6). The pericardium is opened anterior to the phrenic nerve. If the membranous occlusion is short and is confined to this area, a short ePTFE interposition graft can be performed from this exposure. If the occlusion extends distal to the hepatic veins, the abdomen is entered through the same thoracotomy, transecting the diaphragm circumferentially and mobilizing the liver forward and medially. Division of the triangular and the right coronary ligament will help with

TABLE 11.2 **Results of Femorocaval/Iliocaval Bypass**

Author, Year	No. of Limbs	Follow-up (months)	Imaging (%)	Patency Rate (%)	Clinical Improvement (%)	Graft Material
Husfeldt et al,[21] 1979	4	4–30	100	100	100	ePTFE
Dale et al,[22] 1984	3	1–30	100	100	100	ePTFE
Alimi et al,[23] 1997	8	Mean: 19.5	100	88	88	ePTFE
Sottiurai et al,[14] 1997	45	11–139	100[a]	93[b]	89[c]	ePTFE
Jost et al,[7] 2001	18	42	100	56	67	13 ePTFE, 5 spiral vein

[a] Postoperative duplex scan, followed by annual air plethysmography and selective venography.

[b] Includes 6 femoroiliac, 26 femoro-femoral, 8 femorocaval, and 5 femoro-femoral-caval grafts.

[c] An additional 8 patients (18%) developed recurrent ulcers during follow-up.

mobilization of the liver. The adrenal gland and the kidney are left in their anatomical positions, and dissection is performed more medially. Excellent exposure of the suprarenal IVC can be achieved through this approach. If the distal anastomosis must be made more distally, a separate right subcostal or midline incision can be performed as previously described.

For a cavoatrial bypass an end-to-side anastomosis to the IVC is performed and the graft is routed under the liver parallel to the IVC. The graft is then anastomosed end-to-side to the suprarenal IVC or the lower portion of the right atrium. Partially occluding clamps are used to perform the anastomoses, and cardiopulmonary bypass is not needed. Traumatic or iatrogenic occlusions can also be managed by this technique. The use of a 16-mm to 20-mm externally supported ePTFE graft is recommended.

Reported clinical success rate with cavoatrial grafts is about 77%, with a perioperative mortality of 3% and 2-, 5-, and 10-year patency rates of 86%, 78%, and 57%, respectively.[15,16]

Inferior Vena Cava Reconstruction Following Excision of Malignant Tumors

Primary venous leiomyosarcoma or secondary tumors invading the inferior vena cava, such as hepatic tumors, retroperitoneal sarcomas, or adrenal tumors are the most frequent indications for IVC reconstruction. Most renal carcinomas that extend into the vena cava do not invade the wall of the vessel, and the tumor thrombus can frequently be removed from the IVC without the need for venous reconstruction. Attention must be paid to avoid tumor embolization into the pulmonary arteries. Patients with extension of the tumor thrombus into the right atrium need cardiopulmonary bypass to permit safe removal of the tumor.

The incision for resection of primary IVC tumors is transperitoneal, usually midline or right subcostal. Hepatic tumor resection may require a right thoracolaparotomy (Figure 11.7). The IVC is exposed by mobilizing the ascending colon and performing

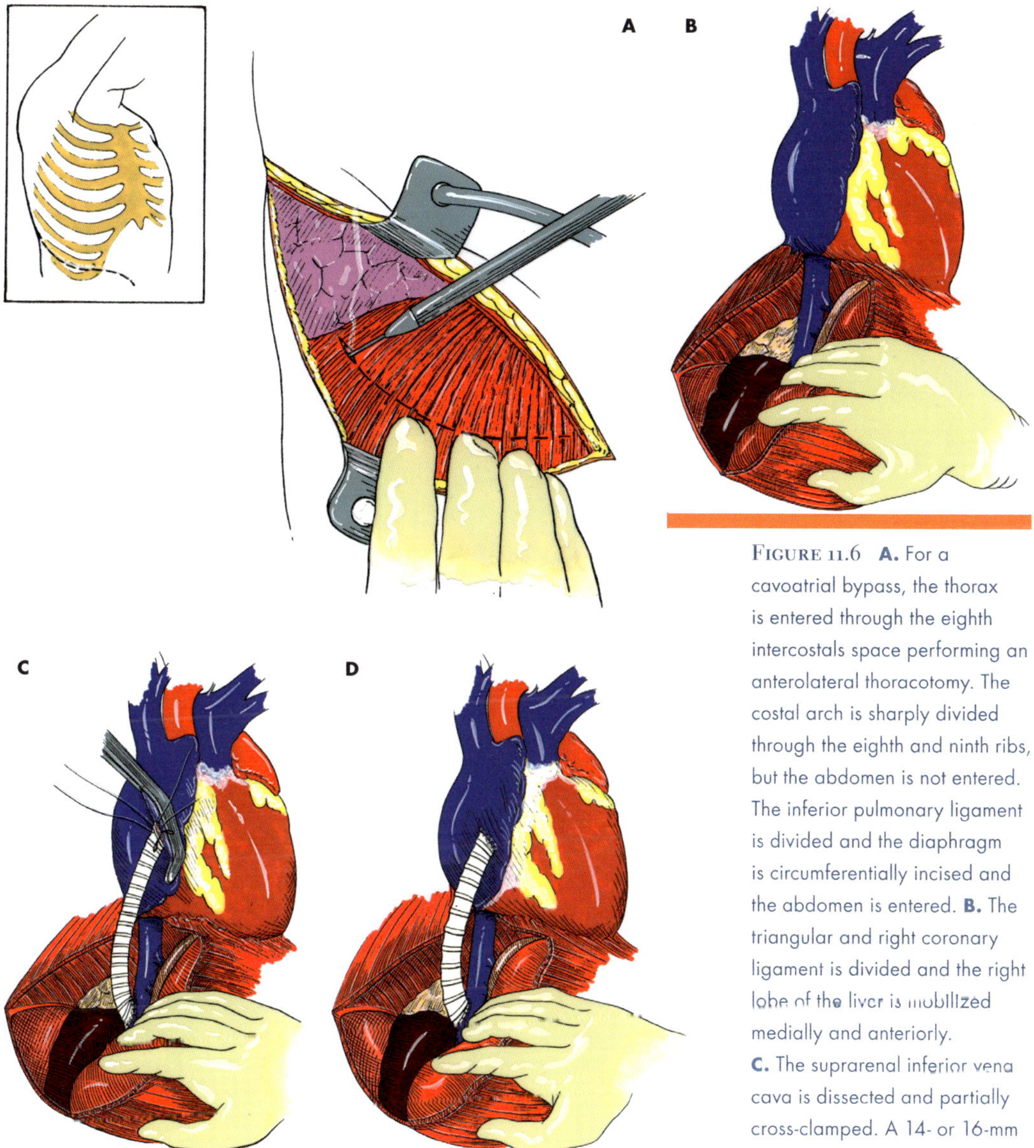

FIGURE 11.6 **A.** For a cavoatrial bypass, the thorax is entered through the eighth intercostals space performing an anterolateral thoracotomy. The costal arch is sharply divided through the eighth and ninth ribs, but the abdomen is not entered. The inferior pulmonary ligament is divided and the diaphragm is circumferentially incised and the abdomen is entered. **B.** The triangular and right coronary ligament is divided and the right lobe of the liver is mobilized medially and anteriorly. **C.** The suprarenal inferior vena cava is dissected and partially cross-clamped. A 14- or 16-mm externally supported PTFE graft is anastomosed first to the cava then to the right atrium. Air is carefully flushed before opening up flow in the graft. **D.** Completed cavoatrial PTFE bypass. Reprinted with permission from the Mayo Foundation.

the Kocher maneuver to mobilize the second portion of the duodenum medially, as described previously. ePTFE grafts (14–20 mm) with external support provide excellent patency of the reconstructed suprarenal or infrarenal inferior vena cava, since inflow is usually robust and there is no associated iliac vein thrombosis. Short, 8- or 10-mm-wide, externally supported ePTFE grafts can also be used to reconstruct the renal veins if nephrectomy for treatment of the tumor is not required. For partial invasion of the IVC, wide excision of the wall and direct suture or patch venoplasty using ePTFE or bovine pericardial patch are options for reconstruction.

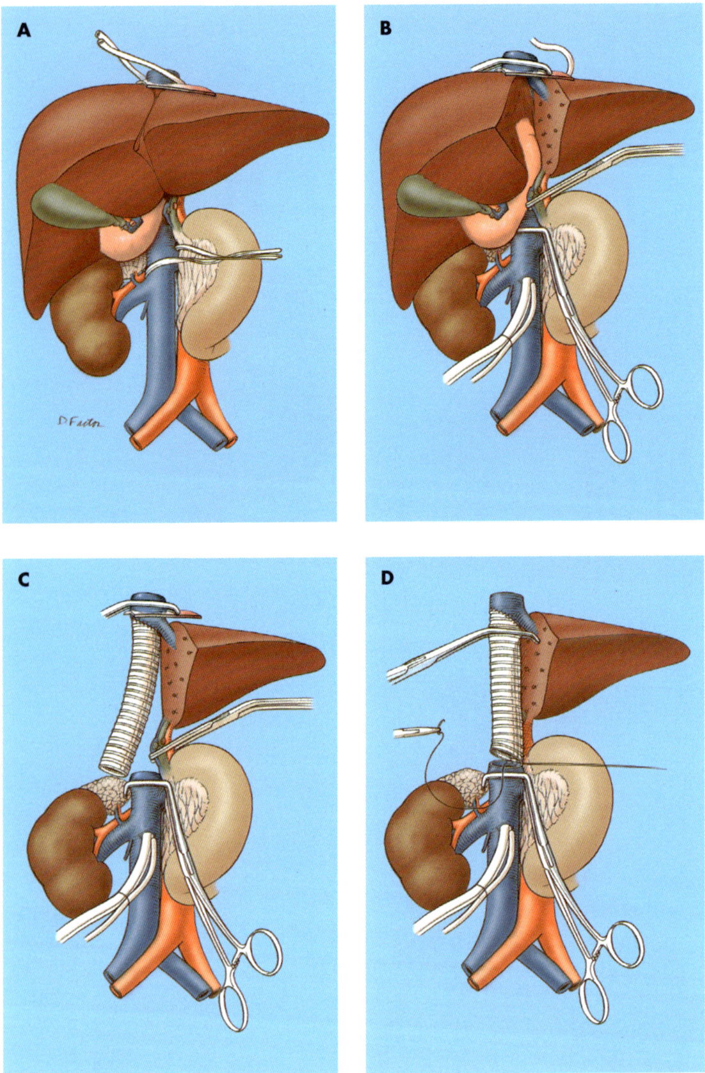

FIGURE 11.7 Technique for PTFE graft replacement of the suprarenal inferior vena cava following right hepatic lobectomy for a malignant tumor with caval invasion. **A.** Isolation of the suprahepatic and suprarenal segments of the vena cava and division of the right hepatic artery and portal vein branches. **B.** Hepatic vascular exclusion used to complete resection of the liver, tumor, and retrohepatic vena cava. If necessary, venovenous bypass via an infrarenal cannula is used. **C.** The upper caval anastomosis is performed first to minimize hepatic ischemia. **D.** The suprahepatic caval clamp is transferred across the graft after acid metabolytes have been flushed from the liver. The lower caval anastomosis is completed. From Bower TC, Nagorney DM, Toomey BJ, Gloviczki P, Pairolero PC, Hallett JW Jr, Cherry KJ Jr. Vena cava replacement for malignant disease: is there a role? Ann Vasc Surg. 1993;7:51-62. With permission from Elsevier.

A venovenous bypass between the IVC or iliac vein and the axillary or internal jugular vein, using a mechanical (Bio-Medicus) pump, is needed only in those patients with poor cardiac function who cannot maintain a systolic blood pressure above 100 mmHg when both the IVC and the hepatic veins are occluded for creation of the anastomoses. When resection of the retrohepatic suprarenal inferior vena cava must be performed, the proximal anastomosis is fashioned first to allow early restoration of hepatic venous outflow (Figure 11.7c–d.). A femoral AVF is usually not required because of the excellent venous inflow.

Perioperative complications are frequent (43%) and operative mortality because of the associated liver resection can be as high as 7%. Graft patency is 93% at 3 years.[17] Early patency of caval reconstruction for malignant disease is excellent, but survival in many patients is limited due to recurrent local tumor or distant metastases. Nevertheless, aggressive surgical management may offer the only chance for cure or palliation of symptoms for patients with primary or secondary IVC tumors. Caval reconstruction may result in significant improvement in the quality of life in these patients even if their survival is limited because of the underlying malignant disease.

Special Considerations

Endophlebectomy

Postthrombotic femoral veins frequently have multiple lumens due to partial recanalization of the thrombus. Excision of the organized and usually fibrotic thrombus will enlarge the lumen, although the exposed collagen in the media of the vein wall is more thrombogenic than the intact venous wall. Still, careful endophlebectomy will improve inflow substantially; however, attention must be paid to avoid injury to the thin residual venous wall. This procedure has long been performed combined with deep venous valve transplantation in patients with PTS, but it has become evident recently that it can be equally effective for treatment of venous obstruction as well. In patients who have localized high-grade stenosis of the common femoral vein, this operation alone is sufficient to improve venous outflow. The defect is closed with a patch using a segment of the saphenous vein or bovine pericardium. The endophlebectomized segment can also be used to improve inflow for iliocaval stenting or for a cross-femoral or femorocaval bypass. In a series of 10 patients who underwent endophlebectomy alone, early results showed 77% patency of the operated segments at 8 months.[18] Results of a larger number of patients to assess long-term patency with this technique have not yet been reported.

Adjunctive Procedures

With the exception of caval reconstructions or short iliocaval grafts, prosthetic bypasses used for venous outflow obstruction of the legs need an adjunctive temporary arteriovenous fistula to maintain patency. The optimal conduit is a 4- to 5-mm ePTFE graft that is about 2 cm long and is placed between the superficial femoral artery and the lower portion of the PTFE venous graft. We prefer to use a tapered 4- by 7-mm ePTFE graft to obtain a segment suitable for AVF. Both anastomoses are performed with 6/0 polypropylene sutures. A small silastic sheet is wrapped around the bypass to avoid healing and to permit easy identification later when the fistula is closed. A 2/0 polypropylene suture is tied to the silastic sheath and positioned under the skin incision for easy identification. Patients who have saphenous Palma grafts undergo takedown of the fistula at 3 months. Patients who have PTFE grafts will keep the arteriovenous fistula longer, if possible. The AVF increases flow through the graft, decreases platelet and fibrin deposition, and contributes to improved patency. It also provides time for pannus formation over the anastomoses during the initial period when the graft surface is most thrombogenic. Potential side effects of the temporary AVF are high cardiac output, functional outflow obstruction resulting in high distal venous pressures, and accelerated intimal hyperplasia.

Prevention of Complications

In general, large vein reconstructions for benign disease are performed in good surgical candidates only, with a low risk of systemic complications. Of the local, nonvascular complications, wound infection and lymphatic leaks (fistula, lymphocele) are the most frequent. Atraumatic surgical technique, antibiotic prophylaxis, and standard surgical principles are helpful in prevention.

Intraoperative air embolism, especially during caval reconstruction, is a potentially fatal complication and may be prevented by meticulous flushing of the grafts before reestablishment of the circulation, by performing a passive Valsalva's maneuver (30 mm Hg), and by placing the patient in Trendelenburg position before release of the proximal clamp.

Deep venous thrombosis and pulmonary embolism are also serious systemic vascular complications. Perioperative anticoagulation with heparin and warfarin, the use of elastic stockings, intermittent pneumatic compression pumps, and early ambulation help prevent thromboembolic complications, which are fortunately rare occurrences. Local vascular complications are specific to venous reconstructions and include graft stenosis or thrombosis, perioperative bleeding, graft infection, and injury to the surrounding vascular and nonvascular structures.

Anticoagulation

Grafts placed in the venous system have a higher rate of thrombosis than arterial grafts due to low venous flow. Infrainguinal venous obstruction and valvular incompetence further decrease inflow to the graft and are significant contributors to postoperative failure. Thrombophilia is prevalent among patients undergoing venous reconstructions. Many patients have absent circulating anticoagulants such as protein factor C, protein factor S, or antithrombin III, or they may have Factor V Leiden mutation. The thrombogenic surface of any prosthetic graft also increases the risk of graft failure. For these reasons, perioperative anticoagulation is indicated in patients undergoing reconstructive venous surgery for deep venous obstruction.

The patient is fully heparinized during reconstruction and protamine is avoided at the completion of the procedure. Heparin in a dose of 500 units per hour is started in the operating room through a 20-gauge pediatric central line that is placed through the saphenous vein of the affected limb and advanced to the distal anastomosis of the prosthetic graft. Complete postoperative systemic heparinization is achieved by 48 hours, and full-dose low-molecular-weight heparin is continued subcutaneously for another 3 to 5 days, given simultaneously with warfarin. The incidence of postoperative bleeding has been reported to be between 5% and 10%, mainly as a result of anticoagulation. Warfarin is continued indefinitely in most patients with prosthetic grafts and in all with a known underlying coagulation abnormality.

Follow-up and Reinterventions

Duplex scan on the first postoperative day or contrast venography is performed to confirm graft patency. Stenosis or thrombosis is corrected immediately after recognition. If thrombosis occurred in a graft without fistula, thrombectomy is done with addition of a fistula. Grafts stenosis discovered during surveillance in the late postoperative period is treated first with angioplasty or venous stenting. Late graft thrombosis is treated with thrombolysis, most commonly in conjunction with angioplasty and stenting to correct the underlying etiology of the graft thrombosis (graft stenosis). Surgical revision is usually limited to patch angioplasty of the stenotic portion of the graft, although occasionally aneurysmal dilation of the saphenous crossover graft may also need surgical correction.

References

1. Husni EA. Reconstruction of veins: the need for objectivity. J Cardiovasc Surg. 1983;24: 525-8.
2. May R. The Palma operation with Gottlob's endothelium preserving suture. In: May R, Weber J, eds. Pelvic and Abdominal Veins: Progress in Diagnosis and Therapy. Amsterdam: Excerpta Medica; 1981. p192-7.
3. Palma EC, Esperon R. Vein transplants and grafts in the surgical treatment of the postphlebitic syndrome. J Cardiovasc Surg. 1960;1:94-107.
4. Gruss JD, Hiemer W. Bypass procedures for venous obstruction: Palma and May-Husni bypasses, Raju perforator bypass, prosthetic bypasses, and primary and adjunctive arteriovenous fistulae. In: Raju S, Villavicencio, eds. Surgical Management of Venous Disease. Baltimore: William & Wilkins; 1977. p289-305.
5. AbuRahma AF, Robinson PA, Boland JP. Clinical, hemodynamic, and anatomic predictors of long-term outcome of lower extremity venovenous bypasses. J Vasc Surg. 1991;14:635-44.
6. Danza R, Navarro T, Baldizan J. Reconstructive surgery in chronic venous obstruction of the lower limbs. J Cardiovasc Surg. 1991;32:98-103.
7. Jost CJ, Gloviczki P, Cherry KJ Jr, McKusick MA, Harmsen WS, Jenkins GD, et al. Surgical reconstruction of iliofemoral veins and the inferior vena cava for nonmalignant occlusive disease. J Vasc Surg. 2001;33:320-7.
8. Sottiurai VS. Venous bypass and valve reconstruction: indication, technique and results. Phlebology. 1997;25:183-8.
9. Gloviczki P, Cho JS. Surgical treatment of chronic occlusions of the iliocaval veins. In: Rutherford RB, ed. Rutherford's Vascular Surgery. 6th ed. Philadelphia: Elsevier; 2005. p2303-2320.
10. Lalka SG, Lash JM, Unthank JL, Lalka VK, Ckirit DF, Sawchuk AP, et al. Inadequacy of saphenous vein grafts for cross-femoral venous bypass. J Vasc Surg. 1991;13:622-30.
11. Smith DE, Trimble C. Surgical management of obstructive venous disease of the lower extremity. In: Rutherford RB, ed. Rutherford's Vascular Surgery. Philadelphia: WB Saunders; 1977. p1247-68.
12. Eklof BG, Kistner RL, Masuda EM. Venous bypass and valve reconstruction: long-term efficacy. Vasc Med. 1998;3:157-64.
13. Comerota AJ, Aldridge SC, Cohen G, Ball DS, Pliskin M, White JV. A strategy of aggressive regional therapy for acute iliofemoral venous thrombosis with contemporary venous thrombectomy or catheter-directed thrombolysis. J Vasc Surg. 1994;20:244-54.
14. Sottiurai VS. Results of deep vein reconstruction. Vasc Surg. 1997:31:276-78.
15. Gloviczki P, Pairolero PC, Toomey BJ, Bower TC, Rooke TW, Stanson AW, et al. Reconstruction of large veins for nonmalignant venous occlusive disease. J Vasc Surg. 1992;16:750-61.
16. Ricotta JJ II, Gloviczki P. Surgical treatment of chronic venous insufficiency. In: Hallett J, Mills J, Earnshaw J, Reekers J, eds. Comprehensive Vascular and Endovascular Surgery. 2nd ed. Philadelphia: Elsevier; 2009. p783-806.
17. Bower TC, Nagorney DM, Cherry KJ Jr, Toomey BJ, Hallett JW, Panneton JM, et al. Replacement of the inferior vena cava for malignancy: an update. J Vasc Surg. 2000;31:270-81.
18. Puggioni A, Kistner RL, Eklof B, Lurie F. Surgical disobliteration of postthrombotic deep veins—endophlebectomy—is feasible. J Vasc Surg. 2004;39:1048-52.

19. Dale WA. Reconstructive venous surgery. Arch Surg. 1979; 114(11):1312-8.
20. Halliday AW, Mansfield AO. Congenital arteriovenous malformations. Br J Surg. 1993;80(1):2-3.
21. Husfeldt KJ, Gall FP, Schulz HP, Zirngibl H. Vein substitution using PTFE prosthesis—results of animal experiments and initial clinical experiences. German. Chir Forum Exp Klin Forsch. 1979:11-5.
22. Dale WA, Harris J, Terry RB. Polytetrafluoroethylene reconstruction of the inferior vena cava. Surgery. 1984 ;95:625-30.
23. Alimi YS, DiMauro P, Fabre D, Juhan C. Iliac vein reconstructions to treat acute and chronic venous occlusive disease. J Vasc Surg. 1997; 25:673-81.

CHAPTER 12

Valve Disease

Is It Really Important?

Kevin G. Burnand

Valves are present in the superficial and deep veins of the lower limb. Only two-thirds of the population have valves above the common femoral vein, and there are no valves in the inferior vena cava. Valves may be primarily absent or abnormal, or secondarily damaged by vein wall dilatation or thrombosis. Vein valves were originally discovered by Gian Bittista Canano in 1547 (as stated by Falopius in 1562). Amatus Lusitanus in 1551 also reported that veins contained valves. Precedence for their discovery has been disputed. Franklin and Friden thought it was possible that Lusitanus may have shown vein valves to Canano, following dissections carried out in Ferraro by both of the anatomists in 1547.

Chronic Venous Insufficiency. Contemporary Endovascular Management series. © 2011 Mark G. Davies MD and Alan B. Lumsden MD, eds. Cardiotext Publishing, ISBN 978-1-935395-09-6.

Versalius was told of their discovery by Canano in 1546 but failed to find any venous valves in his dissections and denied that they existed. It was left to Hieronymous Fabricius, a pupil of Versalius and Falopius, to confirm their existence when he redescribed them in his work *De Venarum Ostiolis* in 1579. He suggested that vein valves participated in the "ebb and flow" of blood, which had been proposed by Galen in AD 130 to 200.

William Harvey, an Englishman, went to Italy to study under Fabricius. The knowledge that valves existed in veins allowed him to conduct the "physiological experiments" illustrated in *De Motu Cordis*. He found that blood passed in only one direction through the superficial veins of the forearm. He stated that "blood moves in the veins from parts below to those above, and the heart, and not in the opposite way." This led to the concept of "circulation."

Brodie in 1896 showed that blood refluxed down the long saphenous vein of patients with varicose veins and that this reflux could be prevented by digital compression over the saphenofemoral junction. In 1866, John Gay performed cadaveric dissections on ulcerated limbs and noted the presence of "matter" within the lumens of the deep veins in some patients, though he did not recognize that "thrombosis" was responsible for the "matter" he described. In 1916, John Homans coined the term "post-thrombotic limb," recognizing that a previous deep vein thrombosis was the main cause of deep vein damage. Edwards and Edwards were the first to demonstrate that valves could be destroyed by thrombus. They reported that the vein lumen could be partially or completely restored by a process of recanalization. In the 1960s, Lindvall and Lodin described a small series of patients with total agenesis of the valves of the deep veins, and Kistner in 1980 reported the presence of floppy incompetent valves in the deep veins of a larger cohort of patients in Hawaii.

Physiology of the Vein Valves of the Lower Limb

The calf muscle pump permanently compresses the larger venous sinuses within the gastrocnemius and soleus muscles during walking or running. The presence of valves prevents "reflux" of blood that has been squeezed out of the calf veins in a caudal direction. This allows the venous pressure to fall from 200 mm Hg during muscular contraction to around 30 to 40 mm Hg on relaxation after a number of contractions. This fall in pressure draws blood from the superficial compartment into the deep compartment during diastole through competent communicating (perforating) veins. This process in turn lowers the superficial venous pressure. The relative venous hypotension caused by exercise does not occur when there is valvular incompetence in the saphenous or perforating veins. An incompetent long saphenous vein allows blood that has been pumped out of the calf and into the femoral veins to reflux back down to the calf again, rapidly returning the venous pressure to pre-exercise levels. Valvular damage in the deep veins also prevents any reduction in the exercising venous pressure, and venous obstruction causes severe ambulatory venous hypertension.

Measurements of Vavular Function

Foot vein pressure measurements during exercise provide an indication of calf pump function, and thigh and calf tourniquets can be applied to overcome the effects of long and short saphenous incompetence. Deep vein incompetence or obstruction is suspected when there is no venous pressure fall during exercise, which cannot be improved by application of tourniquets to prevent saphenous reflux.

Foot volumetry is a less invasive method of assessing calf pump function. Reduced emptying of the superficial veins during exercise is indicative of a raised venous pressure, and rapid recovery to pre-exercise levels is indicative of valvular incompetence. Tourniquets can again be used to overcome the effects of saphenous incompetence. Light reflection rheography (photoplethysmography) can also be used to measure capillary emptying in response to exercise. This provides an indirect measurement of calf pump function.

The development of the duplex scanner by Gene Strandness and his associates allowed the direction of flow in individual vein segments to be assessed. Prograde flow stimulated by compression is usually followed by a minute amount of retrograde flow as the valve leaflets fill to prevent venous reflux. An incompetent valve is associated with prolonged retrograde flow (0.5–1.0 second or more). The saphenous veins, perforating veins, and deep axial veins can all be assessed, and the presence of prolonged reflux noted.

There is, however, no really good test of venous obstruction, which is often a relative or functional obstruction. Recanalized veins, or those with large amounts of external fibrosis, are unable to dilate to allow more blood to leave the limb during periods of increased flow (eg, exercise). Venous obstruction is probably a much worse condition than pure venous reflux with valvular agenesis. Nevertheless, valvular incompetence can be corrected, whereas obstruction often cannot. Efforts are still being made to discover a good test for assessing venous obstruction.

Outcomes

Most patients with superficial venous incompetence do not have much in the way of symptoms, although the reflux through the valves of the superficial veins reduces the effectiveness of the calf muscle pump and increases the capillary pressure in the ulcer-bearing skin of the gaiter region. Patients with saphenous reflux rarely develop lipodermatosclerosis or ulceration. Some do, however, and it would be valuable to be able to identify this group of patients in order to treat them early and avoid future ulceration.

Many have suggested that the presence of coincidental incompetence of the calf perforating veins is essential for ulcers to develop. This does not seem to be the case, however, as some patients without any perforator incompetence later develop venous ulcers. Perhaps it is dependent on having a good calf pump that can overcome superficial venous incompetence. This is an important question that still needs an answer.

Many are now treating saphenous incompetence without bothering to treat perforator valve incompetence in patients with venous ulceration and normal deep veins in an effort to prevent ulcer recurrence. It is not known whether these patients would gain additional benefit from interrupting incompetent calf perforating veins. The trials of perforating vein ligation have failed to show that subfascial endoscopic perforator surgery (SEPS) has added anything to saphenous surgery in reducing ulcer recurrence. Many procedures on the superficial veins are often performed in tandem (eg, saphenous ablation and perforator ablation), and patients are also provided with elastic hosiery. The effect of perforator interruption on calf pump function has been shown to be very small and is much less marked than ablating an incompetent saphenous system.

Primary deep vein incompetence is still a relatively rare condition. It is interesting that patients with polymorphisms in the FOX2 gene have lymphatic valvular agenesis with associated abnormalities in the valves of the deep and superficial veins. This implies that the proteins encoded by these genes are important for the development of valves in both veins and lymphatics.

Valve repairs have consisted of external compression by tendons and plastic loops (the Psthakis valve), plastic collars (Lane Venocuff), reefing external sutures (Kistner, Sotterai), endovascular repair, transposition operations, and transplantation of a segment of the axillary vein into the leg (Taheri).

None of these procedures is regularly performed, and none to date have any level 1 data to support their use. There are no trials that compare valve repair with the intermittent wearing of elastic hosiery.

When it comes to venous obstruction, the results are even less clear. Lysis of acute iliac thrombus followed by stenting of a May-Thurner syndrome has been shown to reduce the symptoms of venous claudication. Raju and Neglén are stenting "venous obstructions" that can be detected only with an IVUS scan. A Palma bypass procedure using the contralateral long saphenous vein to bypass an occluded ililac vein and other vein bypass procedures primarily relieve obstructive symptoms. The avalvular section that is left as a consequence does not appear to cause problems. Most patients subsequently continue to wear elastic stockings.

Individual valves have been created using biological or prosthetic materials, but as yet there is no convincing evidence to support their insertion, and they can cause a deep vein thrombosis.

Venous valves clearly are important, but how many are required to function within which segment of the venous system of the lower limb to prevent future ulceration remains to be established.

CHAPTER 13

Valve Replacement Therapy

Indications, Techniques, and Outcomes

Dušan Pavčnik

Chronic deep venous insufficiency (CDVI) of the lower extremities is a common medical problem. Primary valve incompetence often involves valves in all 3 venous leg systems: superficial, deep, and perforator veins.[1-3] Secondary valve incompetence develops after deep venous thrombosis involves valves of the deep venous system. As venous thrombi organize, there is damage or complete destruction of the venous valves, leaving them incompetent and leading to CDVI. Recently, nonthrombotic iliac vein lesions were reported.[4] Clinical symptoms of CDVI depend on the degree of valve incompetence and the extent of venous involvement. Symptoms can range from minor cosmetic changes to disabling, ulcerating skin conditions.[2,5] The management of CDVI, however, still remains a problem. Selected patients can benefit from surgical valve repair, femoral vein transposition, venous segment transplantation, or neovalve construction.[6-8] The majority of patients with CDVI, particularly patients with secondary valve insufficiency, are not candidates for these procedures. The need for a percutaneous artificial venous valve becomes evident when no other options exist or have been successful in managing the venous reflux associated with CDVI.[9]

In the last 17 years, attempts have been made to develop an artificial valve based on an expandable stent that could be placed percutaneously into the femoral vein to replace the diseased or absent natural valve. In experimental work in 1993, Uflacker explored an artificial monocusp valve consisting of a thin polyether-urethane membrane in a single-body Z stent.[10] Thorpe et al in 2000 tested a bicuspid venous valve made of the porcine small intestinal submucosa

Chronic Venous Insufficiency. Contemporary Endovascular Management series. © 2011 Mark G. Davies MD and Alan B. Lumsden MD, eds. Cardiotext Publishing, ISBN 978-1-935395-09-6.

(SIS) mounted in a double-body Z stent.[11] A trimmed segment of a glutaraldehyde-fixed bovine external jugular vein sutured inside a nitinol stent was examined in animals in 2000 by Gomez-Jorge et al.[12] These valves were placed through 10 Fr to 24 Fr diameter sheaths and some valves remained patent for up to 2 weeks. The fixed bovine valve was also placed in a few patients with CDVI, but most of them thrombosed despite adequate anticoagulation.[13-15]

We have developed 3 types of bioprosthetic venous valves (BVV 1–3) and have tested them in animals (Figure 13.1). These bioprosthetic venous valves consisted of a small leaflet of SIS (Cook Biotech, West Lafayette, IN) attached to different types of square stent frames. SIS is a relatively acellular, nonimmunogenic, biodegradable, xenogenic, collagen-based biomaterial derived from the submucosal layer of porcine small intestine. After implantation, the SIS is remodeled by host tissue responses and reabsorbs over time.[16] Following successful testing of the BVVs in animals,[17-19] we used them clinically, using BVV1 in 3 and BVV3 in 15 patients with advanced CDVI, respectively.[20,21] We also investigated percutaneous autologous venous valve transplantation.[22] For our experimental work, we used an ovine jugular vein (JV) due to its anatomical and functional similarities to the human femoral vein.[17-19]

Valve Implantation—Experimental Work

First Generation of Bioprosthetic Venous Valve

Our original valve design, the bioprosthetic venous valve (BVV1), was developed in 1999. Its frame was formed by a single self-expandable stainless steel square stent with 4 barbs at its corners (Cook Inc., Bloomington, IN).[17] The valve leaflets were made of 120- to 180-µm-thick SIS sheets (Cook Biotech) and were sutured to the stent frame with 7/0 Prolene monofilament (Figure 13.1a). An 11 Fr sheath was used for the valve placement. Of 26 BVV1s placed bilaterally into JVs of 12 sheep, 22 valves self-expanded completely and were well centered in the JVs. Three valves were tilted and did not expand evenly, and one valve migrated and eventually occluded a branch of the pulmonary artery.[17] Immediate venograms showed uninterrupted flow in all valves. At 1-, 3-, and 6-month follow-up venograms, one of the 3 tilted valves thrombosed, and the other 2 were incompetent, exhibiting reflux, and thus were clinical failures. The other 22 valves were competent but demonstrated limited cusp flexibility due to leaflet thickening. Gross and microscopic examination of the valve and vein specimens at 1 month revealed partial remodeling of SIS leaflets with host cells including fibroblasts, lymphocytes, plasma cells, smooth muscle cells, and histiocytes. Endothelial cells were also present on both sides of the leaflets. On 3- and 6-month specimens, the completely remodeled SIS matrix was covered with neointima consisting of fibroblasts with collagen deposits that caused leaflet thickening, which was most prominent at the leaflet base. The leaflet bases were incorporated into the vein wall with some foreign-body giant cell reaction around the sutures and wires attached to the vein.[17]

Second Generation of Bioprosthetic Venous Valve

We explored several stent frame modifications to improve valve positioning during placement and to ensure its centering in the vein without tilting. The second generation

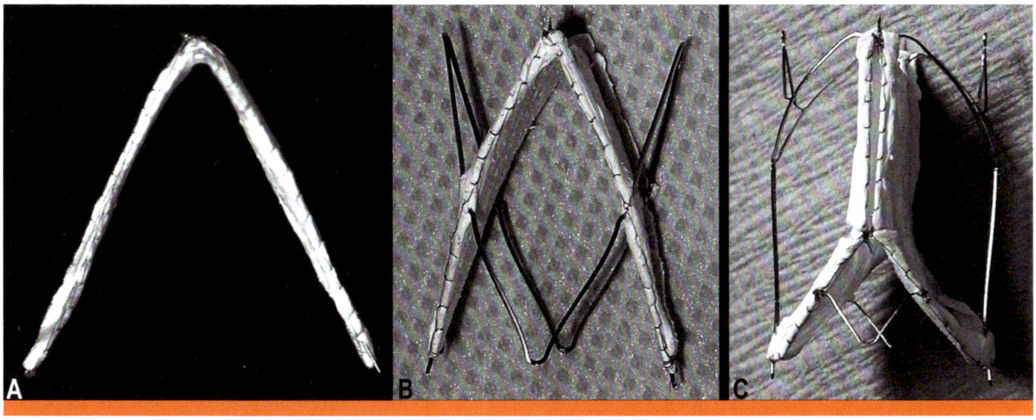

FIGURE 13.1 Three types of bioprosthetic venous valves covered with SIS (BVV). **A.** Side view of the BVV1. **B.** Side view of the BVV2. **C.** Side view of the BVV3.

of bioprosthetic venous valve (BVV2) gave the best results. The BVV2 stent frame was made of nitinol tubing.[18] This frame was similar to the BVV1 frame, except a second square stent without barbs was added to the midpoint of the original valve (Figure 13.1b). The BVV2 was placed through a 10 Fr sheath. Altogether, 28 BVV2s were implanted in JVs of 14 sheep. All implanted valves remained in place, completely centered and functioning well on immediate follow-up venograms. At 6 weeks, follow-up, 26 valves continued to function well. Only 2 oversized valves were incompetent and exhibited reflux. Gross and histologic examination showed similar findings to those for BVV1, namely, partial SIS remodeling and leaflets thickening due to neointimal hyperplasia. In 2 incompetent oversized valves, the leaflets were either partially or completely fused with the vein wall, separated by thick neointima and unable to coapt.[18]

Third Generation of Bioprosthetic Venous Valve

The third-generation valve (BVV3) was designed to prevent potential contact of free leaflet portions with the venous wall and ensure continued leaflet coaptation even with their possible shortening (Figure 13.1c). A 10 Fr sheath was used for the valve placement and altogether 12 BVV3s were implanted into JVs of 6 sheep. Six BVV3s were oriented in the same spatial orientation as the native valves (group A) and the other 6 were rotated circumferentially 90° to the native valve leaflets (group B)[19] to assess the importance of different spatial orientation for valve implantation.

The desired spatial orientation was achieved after deployment in all valves and all remained stable and completely functional as assessed by venography after implantation. At 6 weeks, all valves in group A remained competent, while in group B, one valve was incompetent, exhibiting reflux. On gross examination, the remodeled SIS leaflets were free from the vein wall except at their distal parts, where the SIS was thickened and attached to the vein. Extent of the attachment was significantly smaller and the free leaflet segment was larger in group A than in group B, underlining the importance of valve placement in the same orientation as the native valve[19] (Figure 13.2).

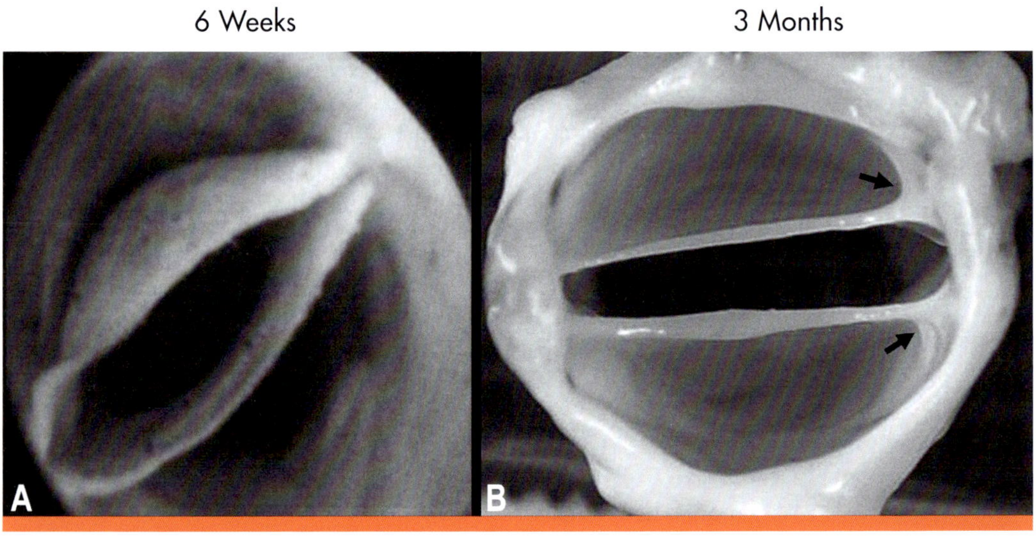

FIGURE 13.2 BVV3 placed into the sheep jugular vein. **A.** The endoscopic image confirms opening and demonstrates valve function at 6 weeks. **B.** At 3 months, an axial view of the specimen from above shows incorporation of the BVV3 into the vein wall. Arrows demonstrate thickened valve leaflets that are spread apart by intimal hyperplasia.

Percutaneous Autologous Venous Valve Transplantation

The limitation of the current techniques in the treatment of CDVI prompted exploration of the feasibility of endovascular transplantation of a stent-supported autologous natural valve as a possible treatment alternative.[22-25] Dalsing et al explored endovascular transplantation of a JV valve supported with a 6- or 8-mm-diameter Z stent in a canine model.[23] They deployed the valve stent assembly through a long 16 Fr sheath into the common or external iliac vein. At 1 to 4 weeks' follow-up, only 1 of 5 valves in an overdilated recipient vein with a relatively high flow remained patent; the other 4 valves were occluded.[23] Ofenloch et al achieved better results in goats with the use of an endoscopically harvested JV segment containing a valve supported by a short 10-mm-diameter WALLSTENT.[24] After venotomy, a 12 Fr sheath was used for placement of the valve stent device into the opposite JV. At 1 week, all 5 tested valves were competent. At 6 weeks, the transplanted vein segment was fully incorporated into the host vein. Angioscopically, 5 of 6 valves were competent and of normal appearance, while only 1 valve was obliterated by recanalized thrombus.[24] Kucher et al achieved similar good results in canines when comparing a standard femoral vein interposition with transplantation of a short, 8-mm-diameter nitinol symphony stent-supported JV segment containing a valve into the femoral vein.[25] An 11 Fr sheath was used for placing the stent device (covered from inside and outside by vein wall) into the contralateral femoral vein. Only 1 of 7 dogs had bilateral femoral vein occlusions at the 2-week follow-up. The remaining 6 had patent and well-functioning valves at 120 days in both the surgical grafts and the transplanted stent-supported JV segments. The surgical grafts exhibited minimal to moderate stenoses at the suture lines, not seen with the stented veins.[25]

Pavčnik et al reported percutaneous autogenous venous valve (PAVV) transplantation in 9 sheep. The PAVV consisted of a vein segment containing a native valve that was attached to a stent template designed and handmade in our research laboratory.[22] The stent template consisted of 2 stainless steel square stents, 13 or 15 mm in diameter to fit the ovine JV. A valve-containing segment of the JV was surgically harvested and fixed with sutures and barbs to the inside of the stent template. The valve device was then manually compressed and front loaded inside a 4-cm-long chamber of the 13 Fr delivery sheath. This was followed by over-the-wire delivery into the contralateral JV by a femoral vein approach. Transplanted PAVVs were studied using immediate and 3-month venograms when JVs were harvested for angioscopic evaluations in vitro. PAVV transplantation was successful in all 9 animals. Good valve function with no reflux was observed on the immediate and 3-month venograms in 8 valves. Venoscopic examination at 3 months revealed intact, flexible, nonthickened valve leaflets in 8 specimens (Figure 13.3).

One PAVV exhibited normal function of one leaflet only; the other cusp was absent, accidentally cut during the transplantation procedure. All transplanted autologous valves were free of thrombus and incorporated into the vein wall of the host vessel.[22]

Valve Implantation—Clinical Study

Clinical Use of BVV1 in 3 Patients

Three patients with severe CDVI, ranging in age from 38 to 64 years, were treated with BVV1s as part of a safety trial (see Figure 13.1a). Patients began warfarin (Coumadin) therapy 4 days prior to the BVV implantation at 5 mg/day to achieve a therapeutic INR of 2 to 3 and were kept on this dose for 3 months. Prior to BVV1 implantation, patients received 5000 units of heparin. The valves were implanted percutaneously by a right internal jugular approach using a previously described over-the-wire delivery system. Descending venograms of the involved

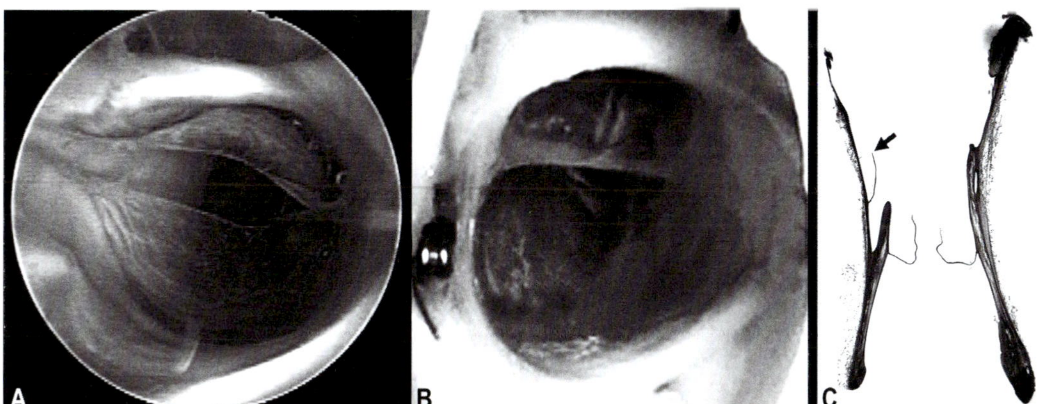

FIGURE 13.3 Percutaneous autologous venous valve transplantation at 3 months. **A.** Venoscopy of the transplanted valve inside a flow model demonstrates thin leaflets in open position. **B.** On explants, the valve is thin and of normal appearance. **C.** Longitudinal microscopic view of both transplanted leaflets. Arrow points to native valve above incompletely incorporated edge of autologous valve.

limb were done first in the upright position without and with Valsalva. The proximal and distal femoral vein (FV) diameter was measured in 2 projections in the location of the intended vein implantation using 0.035-graduate measuring guidewire (Cook Inc.).

The valve was selected using a size similar to the vein diameter measured with the Valsalva's maneuver, about 1 to 2 mm larger than vein diameter without increased pressure. The selected lyophilized BVV was rehydrated with an injection of 10 cc heparinized saline through the side arm of the 11 Fr guide catheter 15 minutes before valve delivery. The BVV was implanted into proximal FV just below bifurcation with PFV. Delivery of the BVV was accomplished by withdrawing the guiding catheter while holding the 9 Fr dilator. As the BVV was deployed, it self-attached to the vein wall. The retention dilator and the 9 Fr (ID) guiding catheter were removed, leaving the 11 Fr sheaths in the internal jugular vein for the follow-up venograms. The BVVs were studied for function and stability in the upright position by injecting contrast medium above the BVV. Follow-up descending venograms were done at 2 months, and then the patients were followed by duplex ultrasonography at 1, 3, 6, and 12 months.

Patient 1

A 38-year-old male with postthrombotic syndrome had severe venous claudication with a CEAP C_6 (active ulcer) secondary to valve insufficiency of the deep veins of the left limb. The disease involved mainly deep veins, and descending venograms showed severe grade IV reflux at the left common femoral vein (CFV), which extended into the profunda femoral vein (PFV) and valveless FV all the way into the calf. There was no significant reflux into the greater saphenous vein and grade I reflux into the lesser saphenous vein. After a 15-mm BVV was deployed, descending venography demonstrated only minimal reflux. Follow-up descending venograms at 2 months and duplex ultrasonography at 1, 3, 6, and 12 months demonstrated no spontaneous reflux through the valve into the femoral vein. A significant grade III leak between vein wall and valve frame was seen only when Valsalva was performed. Clinically, the patient's active ulcer was found healed at 1 month after BVV implantation and did not recur at 1-year follow-up (CEAP C_5). Edema of the left leg improved, the left thigh circumference decreased from 63.8 cm before valve placement to 58.5 cm at 1-year follow-up. Circumferences of the calf and ankle were not significantly changed during follow-ups.

Patient 2

A 64-year-old man had skin changes, edema, and pain of the left leg due to severe pelvic venous incompetence (PVI) at the left femoral and popliteal vein. Placement of an 18- to 19-mm BVV was technically successful, but it was placed 8 to 10 mm lower in the proximal FV than intended. This resulted in an oversized BVV with significant valve leak. During the 1-year follow-up, the BVV stayed patent and did not cause any complication, but there was no change in the patient's clinical symptoms and disability scores.

Patient 3

A 40-year-man with DVIS due to posttraumatic posthrombotic syndrome had severe venous claudication with CEAP C_4 (skin changes, edema, pain) in his left leg. These symptoms were due to severe reflux in the left femoral and valveless popliteal veins. The 11 mm BVV placed into the distal left FV resulted in about 30% valve tilting. The immediate follow-up venogram showed good valve function with minimal leak. The patient had immediate clinical improvement of his symptoms, mainly a decrease of edema and pain in his leg. Follow- ups with duplex ultrasonography documented patency and competency of the valve with minimal leak of the BVV valve at 1, 3, 6, and 12 months. At present, 5 years after BVV placement, the patient's symptoms are significantly decreased, and the BVV is functioning well as a monocusp valve (due to tilting) with a minimal leak.

Percutaneous Valve Implantation—Clinical Safety Pilot Study

Based upon promising experimental studies, a 1-year clinical study was conducted in 4 institutions with approval of their Institutional Review Boards to determine the safety of the BVV3 implantation. Fifteen patients with advanced symptomatic CDVI, including 8 patients with large venous ulcers, received the valve. A single BVV3 (see Figure 13.1c) was deployed into the femoral vein percutaneously via transjugular approach with an over-the-wire delivery catheter system. Pre- and postdeployment examinations included clinical examination, intravascular ultrasonography (IVUS), duplex ultrasonography, and descending venography at 3 and 12 months.

Device and Delivery System

The BVV3 frame (Cook Medical, Bloomington, IN) was made of laser-cut nitinol tubing and had 4 barbs for valve stabilization. The round geometry of BVV3 allowed SIS leaflets to coapt and the larger pockets of the valve improved blood flow and prevented potential thrombus formation. Two gold markers on the nitinol frame facilitated precise anatomical orientation during valve deployment (see Figure 13.1c).

The 110-cm-long 12 Fr delivery system consisted of an introducer sheath with a radiopaque marker tip and Tuohy Borst adapter (Cook Medical) and dilator with a cutout where the BVV3 was loaded. The lyophilized BVV3 was selected and rehydrated at least 10 minutes before implantation by injecting heparinized saline through the side arm of the sheath.

Seven days prior to the BVV3 implantation, patients began warfarin (Coumadin) therapy at 5 mg/day to achieve a therapeutic INR of 2 to 3. Patients also received 5000 units of heparin prior to valve implantation. Descending venograms and IVUS of the involved limb were done in the upright position prior to implantation, and the selected target location of the femoral vein (FV) diameter was measured. The BVV3 was selected using a size similar to the vein diameter measured. The selected lyophilized BVV3 was rehydrated with 10-cc-heparinized saline injected through the side arm of the guide catheter 15 minutes before the BVVs were implanted into proximal, middle, or distal FV.

Successful placement of all 15 BVVs was achieved without tilting or migration, although 3 valves were oversized. Immediate valve competence was seen in 14 limbs (93%). Follow-up studies at 3 and 12 months showed no migration of the implanted valves. Eleven valves (73.4%) were patent and 4 occluded (26.6%). Three valves occluded early (<2 weeks), and one occluded late at 7 months. One valve occluded after placement into a duplicate femoral vein and 3 valves occluded in patients with low level of INR or after discontinuation of Coumadin for spine surgery. At 3 months, only 2 valves remained fully functional. At 12 months, none of the valves remained competent. Thickening and rigidity of the leaflets of the nonthrombosed valves resulted in various degrees of reflux and caused their incompetence (Figure 13.4). Clinically, however, valve implantation gave better results. Twelve of 15 patients (80%) had immediate and 3-month clinical improvement that continued in 9 patients (60%) at the 12-month follow-up (Figure 13.5). Large venous ulcers healed completely in 3 of 8 patients, improved in 4 and only one giant ulcer did not show improvement. None of the 15 patients' clinical symptoms worsened after valve implantation.

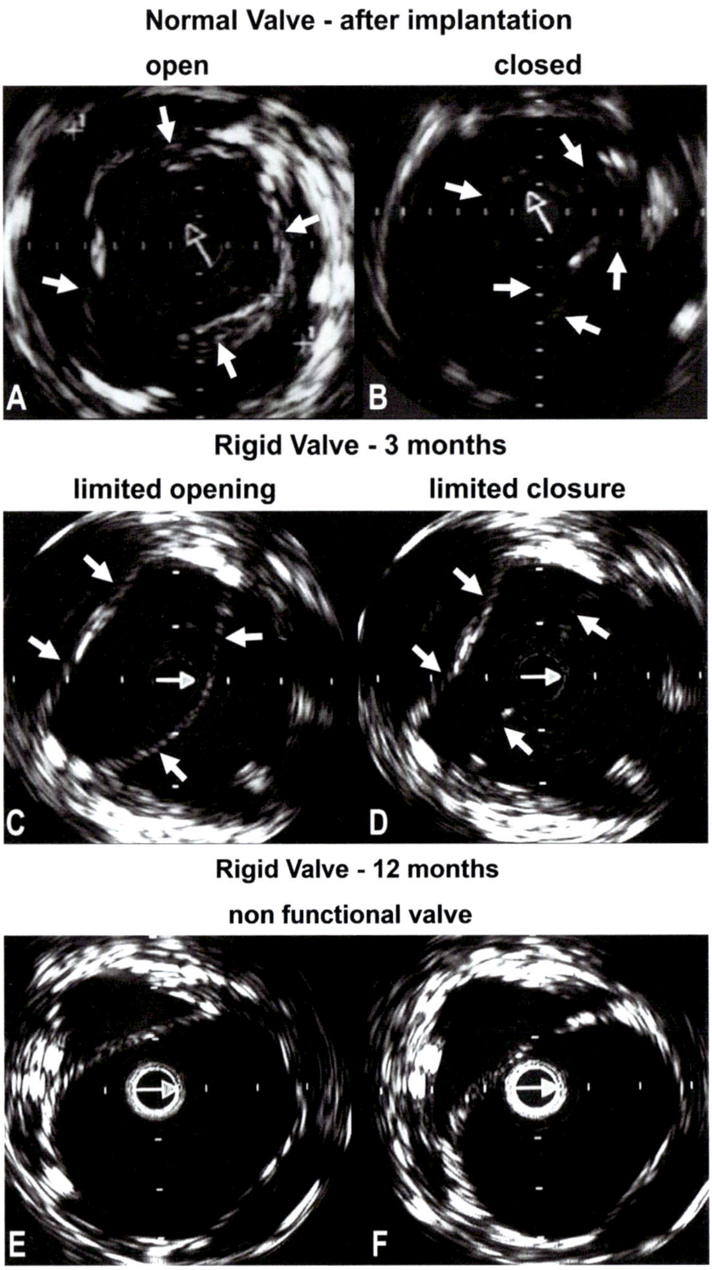

FIGURE 13.4 The intravenous ultrasonography studies of the third-generation valve implanted into the femoral vein of a 79-year-old female with active venous ulcer (CEAP C_6) **(A, B)** the valve exhibits a good flexibility and function. **A.** In open position (arrowheads). **B.** In closed position (arrows). **(C, D)** Rigid, thickened leaflets show limited cusp flexibility (arrows) at 3 months. Central arrow shows the imaging catheter. **(E, F)** Rigid, thickened nonfunctional valve at 1 year. Central arrow shows the imaging catheter.

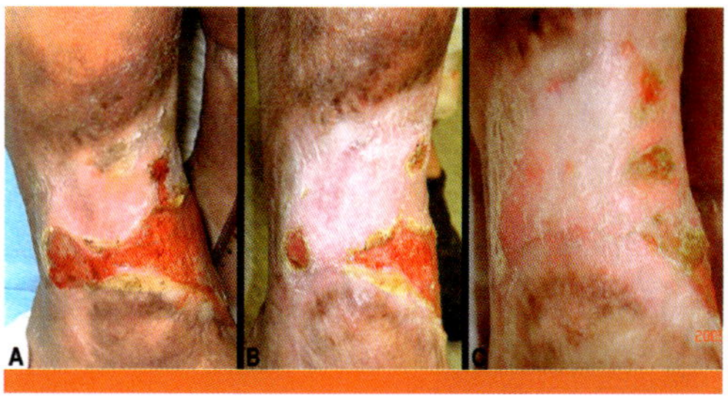

FIGURE 13.5 A 79-year-old female with primary insufficiency who had an active ulcer (CEAP C_6). BVV3 was implanted into femoral vein. **A.** Active ulcer before valve implantation. **B.** Clinically the patient was improved with a decrease in ulcer size at 3 months. **C.** Almost-healed ulcer at the 12-month follow-up.

Conclusion

A very long path with many small steps and tedious experimental research work is usually necessary to take a new idea to a successful clinical reality. At the present time, more steps are still necessary for the percutaneous BVV implantation to become clinically useful. The BVV3 stent frame is, in our opinion, well suited to form a base for a valve. It is easy to deliver and it self-centers and remains stable in the vein. It allows good leaflets coaptation even when the leaflets remodel and shorten and prevents their contact with venous wall. The SIS biomaterial for leaflets showed very promising early results with pliable leaflets and good valve function. In the long term, however, because of the scaffolding nature of SIS with fibrotic transformation and excessive neointimal formation, the SIS leaflets thickened, became rigid, and caused the valves to become incompetent. In our unpublished studies, leaflets treated or coated with cytostatic chemotherapy agents and nonsteroidal anti-inflammatory drugs did not give better results than leaflets with untreated SIS. Potentially, there are a couple of routes to solve this problem. The first option is to bioengineer a method to cover the SIS leaflets with endothelial cells to prevent neointimal hyperplasia and enhance valve functionality. The other option is to use a more compatible biomaterial than SIS. Our experimental and clinical research have brought the final goal of a long-term functional percutaneous artificial venous valve one step closer to reality.

References

1. Raju S. Chronic venous insufficiency of the lower limb and stasis ulceration: changing concept and management. Ann Surg. 1983;197(6):688-97.
2. Sumner DS. Hemodynamic and pathophysiology of venous disease. In: Rutherford RB, ed. Vascular Surgery. Philadelphia: WB Saunders Co.; 1989. p1483-504.
3. Schmidt- Schönbein GW, Takase S, Bergan JJ. New advances in the understanding of the pathophysiology of chronic venous insufficiency. Angiology. 2001;52 (Suppl 1):S27-34.
4. Raju S, Neglen P. High prevalence of nonthrombotic iliac vein lesions in chronic venous disease: a permissive role in pathogenicity. J Vasc Surg. 2006;44:136-43.
5. Raju S, Fredericks RK, Hudson A, Fountain T, Neglén PN. Venous valve station changes in "primary" and postthrombotic reflux: an analysis of 149 cases. Ann Vasc Surg. 2000;14(3):193-9.
6. Sheridan KM, Dalsing MC. The surgical treatment of deep venous valvular incompetence. In: Rutherford RB, ed. Vascular Surgery. 6th ed. Philadelphia: WB Elsevier Saunders Co.; 2005. p2287-302.
7. Dalsing MC. Surgical therapies in chronic venous insufficiency: deep venous surgery valve transplantation/SEPS. In: Labropulos N, Stansby G, eds. Venous and Lymphatic

Diseases. New York, London: Taylor & Frances; 2006. p393-409.

8. Maleti O, Lugli M. Venous valvular reconstruction in post thrombotic syndrome. J Vasc Surg. 2006;43:794-9.
9. Dalsing MC. Artificial venous valves. In: Gloviczki P, ed. Handbook of Venous Disorders. 3rd ed. London: Hodder & Arnold; 2009. p483-9.
10. Uflacker R. Percutaneously introduced artificial venous valve: experimental use in pigs. The 1993 Annual Meeting of the Western Angiographic & Interventional Society; 1993 Sep 29-Oct 3; Portland, OR. 1993. p30.
11. Thorpe PE, Osse FJ, Correa LO. The Valve-stent: development of a percutaneous prosthesis for treatment of valvular insufficiency. The 12th Annual meeting of the American Venous Forum; 2000 Feb 3-6; Phoenix, AZ. 2000; p82.
12. Gomez-Jorge J, Venbrux AC, Magee C. Percutaneous development of a valved bovine jugular vein in the swine venous system: a potential treatment for venous insufficiency. J Vasc Interv Radiol. 2000;11:931-6.
13. de Borst GJ, Teijink JA, Patterson M, Quijano TC, Moll F. A percutaneous approach to deep venous valve insufficiency with a new self-expanding venous frame valve. J Endovasc Ther. 2003;10:341-9.
14. Serino F. Preliminary clinical experiences with VenPro PVVB. The pending matters: updating course in vascular pathology of surgical interest—deep venous surgery and new technologies for varicose veins. 2002 Nov 30-Dec 1; Pisa, Italy.
15. Gale SS, Shurman S, Beebe HG, Pigott JP, Comerota AJ. Percutaneous venous valve bioprosthesis: initial observations. Vasc Endovascular Surg. 2004;38(3):221-4.
16. Badylak SF. Small intestinal submucosa (SIS): a biomaterial conductive to smart tissue remodeling. In: Bell E, ed. Tissue Engineering: Current Prospective. Cambridge, MA: Burkhauser; 1993. p179-89.
17. Pavčnik D, Uchida BT, Timmermans HA, Corless CL, O'Hara M, Toyota N, et al. Percutaneous bioprosthetic venous valve: a long-term study in sheep. J Vasc Surg. 2002;35:598-602.
18. Pavčnik D, Uchida B, Kaufman J, Corea L, Hiraki T, Keller FS, et al. Second generation bioprosthetic venous valve. Short-term study in sheep. J Vasc Surg. 2004:40(6):1223-7.
19. Pavčnik D, Kaufman J, Uchida B, Case B, Corea OL, Hamada A, et al. Significance of spatial orientation of percutaneously placed bioprosthetic valve in an ovine model. J Vasc Interv Radiol. 2005;16(11):1511-6.
20. Pavčnik D, Kaufman JA, Machan L, Uchida B, Keller FS, Rösch J. Percutaneous treatment of deep vein reflux. Seminars in Interventional Therapy. 2005:22 (3):225-32.
21. Pavčnik D. Update on venous valve replacement: long term clinical results. Vascular. 2006;14 (Suppl 1):S106.
22. Pavčnik D, Yin Q, Uchida B, Park WK, Kim MD, Hoppe H, Keller FS, et al. Percutaneous autologous venous valve transplantation: feasibility study in and ovine model. J Vasc Surg. 2007;46(2):338-45.
23. Dalsing MC, Sawchuk AP, Lalka SG, Cikrit DF. An early experience with endovascular venous valve transplantation. Vasc Surg. 1996; 24:903-5.
24. Ofenloch JC, Changyi C, Hughes JD, Lumsden AB. Endoscopic venous valve transplantation with a valve stent device. Ann Vasc Surg.1997;1:62-7.
25. Kucher T, Brenner B, Marak M, Parsonnet V. Endovascular delivery of vein segment with valves versus direct anastomosis. Endovasc Ther. 2005;12:366-70.

CHAPTER

14

Valve Reconstruction Therapy

Indications, Techniques, and Outcomes

Peter Neglén

The first successful internal valve repair by Kistner in 1968 was a seminal event in venous therapy.[1] Although initially controversial, it sparked a resurgence of interest in venous disease. Many of the basic concepts and techniques developed by Kistner and his team still stand.[2-4] Not only did Kistner show that surgery could be performed on delicate valve leaflets and competence achieved, but perhaps more importantly he proved that surgery could be performed on veins without inducing thrombosis. Until then the prevailing belief was that a clamped, incised, and sutured vein would immediately thrombose. Today valve repair and other interventions in the deep system are established treatment of selected patients with chronic venous disease (CVD).

Chronic Venous Insufficiency. Contemporary Endovascular Management series. © 2011 Mark G. Davies MD and Alan B. Lumsden MD, eds. Cardiotext Publishing, ISBN 978-1-935395-09-6.

Indications and Selection of Patients

It is presently not known at what degree a venous stenosis is hemodynamically significant and, consequently, there is no accurate test for obstruction. Similarly, there is currently no method to accurately quantify reflux at a single valve site or the individual contribution of the superficial, perforator, or deep systems to global reflux. Duplex Doppler is a qualitative, not quantitative, test. It is well known that the duration of reflux (sometimes inadequately called valve closure time) does not correlate with clinical severity. Peak reflux velocity is better, but its poor reproducibility prevents clinical use at present.[5] The lack of quantification of reflux impedes the ability to target the optimal site for valve repair and prioritize which system to correct in patients with multilevel and multisystem reflux. Now the therapeutic approach is blind: trial and error. Minimally invasive venous procedures are presently favored, eg, endovenous saphenous ablation and iliac vein stenting. These interventions are not necessarily targeted toward the dominant pathology but are chosen because of their simplicity. It is recognized that clinical outcome of CVD is improved by partial correction, at least initially. Nevertheless, we will not know if such partial therapy is more durable than complete or optimally targeted corrections until we are able to quantify reflux and obstruction.

Patients with suspected chronic venous insufficiency should all be investigated. It is a fundamental mistake to delay any venous investigations until conservative treatment has failed. Treatment should, to the best of our ability, be based on correct verification and classification of the venous dysfunction. Invasive treatment should then be considered in combination with conservative measures such as compression therapy, which is but one aspect of venous therapy. Conceptually, it would appear logical to start with compression therapy with or without local ulcer treatment or less invasive procedures initially, and proceed to open surgery when minimally invasive therapy fails. The following paradigm for invasive treatment has evolved: attempt minimally invasive intervention before open surgery; correct superficial before deep reflux; iliofemoral obstruction should be treated before axial deep reflux in limbs with combined disease; combine iliac venous stenting and endovenous ablation of superficial reflux, even in the presence of axial deep reflux in multisystem disease; and, only when above measures (including conservative treatment) fail, proceed with surgical repair of the deep valves. Since chronic venous disease in general poses little risk to life or limb, this stepwise approach makes sense. This paradigm may change if a durable artificial valve can be safely placed percutanously.

Potential candidates for deep valve reconstruction should have disabling symptoms with leg pain, marked swelling, hyperpigmentation, dermatitis, lipodermatosclerosis, or ulcer (C_3–C_6 in CEAP).[6] Pain is not adequately included in the CEAP classification. About 10% of the patients with deep valve reflux will have severe pain (more than 5 on the visual analog pain scale) unaccompanied by other clinical manifestations. The severity of pain with or without other clinical features is an important consideration in case selection.

Preoperative Assessment

Patients considered for deep valve repair should have an adequate history taken, and a general as well as a detailed venous evaluation. The CEAP classification should be used. Adequate arterial limb perfusion must be ascertained. A thrombophilia test is recommended to provide guidance for the duration and extent of postoperative anticoagulation.

A duplex Doppler study with standardized compression in an erect position will detect the pattern of reflux. Some crude estimation of reflux severity can be estimated by counting the number of refluxing venous segments (segment score) or the distal extent of uninterrupted axial deep reflux in the limb as described by Kistner.[7-9] "Axial reflux" describes a retrograde flow from the groin into the calf. It is frequently (approximately 40%) but not exclusively associated with severe clinical presentation.[5] Deep reflux is found in 60% to 70% of patients with clinical severity C_4 to C_6 (C-class in CEAP). In general, only axial deep reflux should be considered for valve reconstruction.

In addition, a global hemodynamic test such as ambulatory venous pressure (AVP) or air plethysmography (APG) may be of value. Venous filling time (VFT, seconds; an AVP measure) and venous filling index (VFI_{90} mL/s; an APG measure) have been shown to correlate with global severity of reflux and are useful outcome monitors. [7,8,10-13] Several quality-of-life measures specific for venous disease have become available recently. A few of these are easy enough to be employed on a routine basis in venous practice to assess clinical results.

Contrast dye studies are not used to assess reflux and have been replaced by noninvasive ultrasonography. Patients considered for valve reconstruction should have an ascending venography from the foot and a transfemoral antegrade and retrograde (45°–60° semierect inclination and Valsalva's maneuver) venography.[7,14] These studies are useful in detecting iliofemoral venous outflow obstructions, identifying valve stations, and delineating valve anatomy before proceeding to valve repair.

Valve Station Pathology

Roughly half the patient population undergoing valve repairs have "primary" valve reflux, and the remaining have "secondary" or postthrombotic reflux.[15,16] Rarely, congenital anomalies such as tricuspid valves, absent valves, or duplicated refluxing conduits are found. In primary valve reflux, the dissected valve station appears macroscopically free of apparent disease and has normal or slightly enlarged width. The adventitia is rarely dense, so the valve attachment lines can usually be clearly traced on the surface of the vein from the outside. The angle formed by the 2 valve attachment lines converging at the commissure is widened and often obtuse (normally acute) and may involve 1 or both of the commissures.[15] After incising the vein, the valve cusps are found to be redundant, with excessive pleats and folds failing to coapt properly. The texture of the valve cusps appears normal and translucent.

Contrarily, perivenous and wall fibrosis are a typical finding of postthrombotic valve stations, and the valve attachment lines, if present, are not evident. Neovascularisation induced by prior thrombosis is shown to infiltrate the vein wall and valve remnants on microscopy. The type of damage to the valve station varies. The valve cusps may be preserved, but are secondarily redundant due to a tight fibrotic sheath encasing the valve station, preventing the dilation necessary for proper function. These valves are amenable to direct repair or may even become competent when the perivenous sheath is divided. In others, perforation or adhesion of the valve cusps is observed, which makes the valve nonrepairable. In advanced cases, the valve cusps cannot be identified and the valve station houses only trabeculae. These valve stations have to be replaced.

Postthrombotic reflux is observed in some patients caudad to a refluxing valve station with primary valve disease.[11] It is not clear whether a deep venous thrombus was formed due to axial primary reflux disease or whether the primary reflux is a secondary phenomenon. It has been shown that in postthrombotic limbs de novo, reflux may develop in valves remote from the original thrombus site for unknown reasons.[17]

Surgical Exposure and Test of the Valve Station

The preoperative investigations are usually helpful to localize the site of a repairable valve, but not in all instances. Additional explorations may have to be performed. The patient is positioned supine with the femoral or popliteal (medial approach preferred) areas prepared. One arm is abducted on an arm board with the axilla prepared in case an axillary vein transfer is required.

A femoral valve is usually (>90%) present below the confluence of the profunda femoris vein. This is the most common site for repair. A second inconstant femoral valve may be found 2 to 5 cm below the first valve. Infrequently, a common femoral valve may also be present. These valves provide accessible alternative or additional sites for repair. A profunda femoris valve is present in approximately 85% of limbs close to the confluence, with the femoral vein or a valve found 2 to 3 cm distally. A popliteal vein valve is present in approximately 70% of limbs at the adductor tubercle level. Valves in the mid or distal popliteal vein are found in approximately 50% in nonthrombotic cases. One or more valves are invariably present in the adjoining posterior tibial veins.

Identification of the valve attachment lines is crucial to perform internal and external repairs of a valve station. They are usually evident in primary reflux disease, while careful adventitial dissection of postthrombotic valve stations is necessary. By a combination of sharp and blunt dissection, the adventitia is peeled away (Figure 14.1). It is essential to expose and identify the entire valve attachment line. Commissural apices should be clearly visible. Intact valve lines indicate the presence of valve cusps and a direct repair is typically possible. Interrupted or absent valve attachment lines indicate major valve damage. This finding is finite and there is no need to perform a venotomy to search for possible valve cusps. About 4 cm of the valve station and adjoining vein needs to be cleared of branches in preparation for all types of repairs.

Once the valve station is identified and isolated, a strip test is performed to confirm valve incompetence (Figure 14.2). A clamp is placed 2 to 3 cm caudad to the valve, and the infravalvular segment is emptied cephaled through the valve. If the valve is competent, the segment remains collapsed. A refluxing valve allows the segment to fill from above. In addition, the competence of the valve may be tested by gently squeezing the supravalvular segment to put additional pressure on the valve.

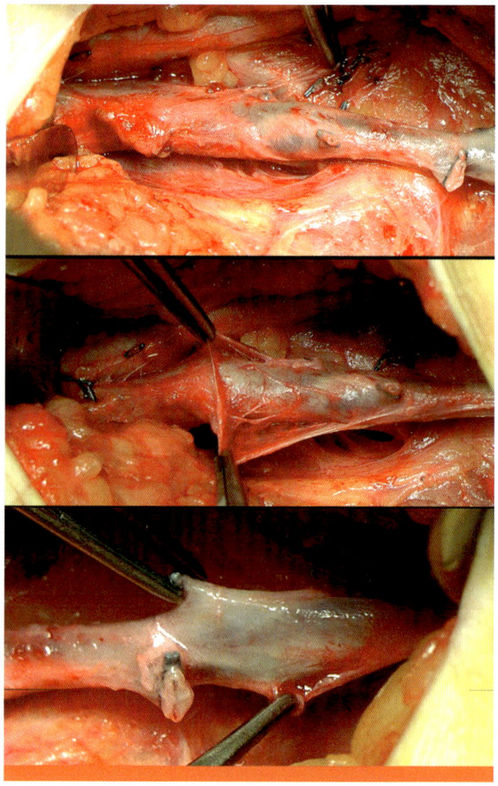

FIGURE 14.1 Careful adventitial dissection of the exposed vein to expose valve attachment lines (shown as thin lines converging toward the left in lower picture).

Specific Valve Reconstruction Techniques

Descriptions of numerous techniques of valve reconstruction can be found in the

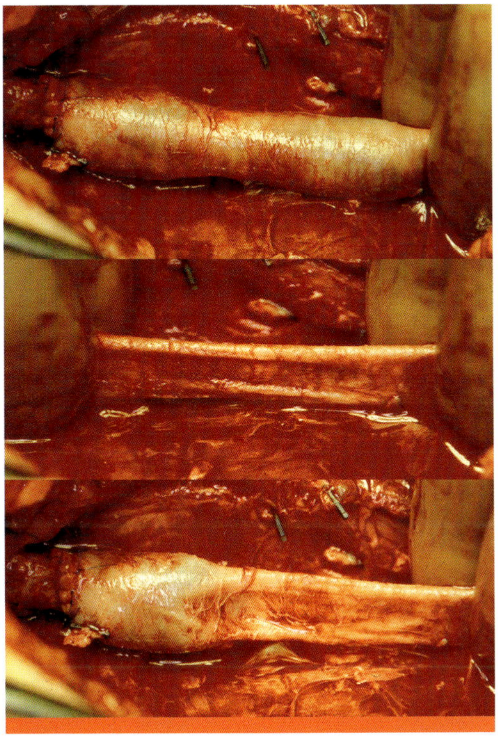

FIGURE 14.2 The strip test. The flow in the vessel is right to left. (Top) The inflow is controlled by the fingers or a clamp placed below the valve; (center) the vein segment above is emptied through the valve; and (bottom) with a competent valve the vein segment will remain collapsed.

literature. Most internal or external valve repair techniques in current use are variations or modifications of the basic techniques originally described by Kistner. Axillary vein transfer is the repair most frequently used when the valves are absent or severely damaged.

Internal Valvuloplasty

The original technique by Kistner[1] places a longitudinal incision between the 2 valve cusps, cutting through the anterior commissural apex after the vein segment has been isolated between clamps. The incision is started 10 to 15 mm below the valve attachment lines and extended upwards through the commissural apex, carefully avoiding damage to the cusps. The incision allows the valve station to be laid open like a book, which provides excellent exposure of the redundant cusps. Frequent irrigation with saline is necessary to visualize the translucent valve cusps and their free edges. Using 7/0 polypropylene sutures, the valve edges are gathered like the pleats of a curtain and tacked to the commissural apex with the knot placed outside. Approximately 20% of the valve edges at each commissure needs to be tacked. Subjective judgment is required in deciding when sufficient valve tightening has been achieved. Unfortunately, the valve competency cannot be tested until the venotomy has been closed and the clamps removed. The venotomy is meticulously closed with everting sutures and good intimal apposition to minimize a potential nidus for thrombus formation.

An alternative approach to the valve is to expose it through a supravalvular transverse incision[18] placed about 5 mm above the commissural apex (Figure 14.3). The main benefit is that the annulus is not traversed, which allows tightening of the valve cusps under direct observation, and the final competence of the repaired valve can often be assessed before closure of the venotomy. The exposure can be further increased by converting the transverse incision into a "T" toward the valve cusps.[19] The "trapdoor" incision provides even greater exposure than the longitudinal incision, but the incision is extensive, increasing the risk of closure complications.[20] The choice of exposure is one of personal preference.

After completing the closure, the valve should be tested for competency by the strip test. Valve competency is readily achieved with some experience. If the valve is not completely competent, the venotomy should be reopened and additional sutures placed.

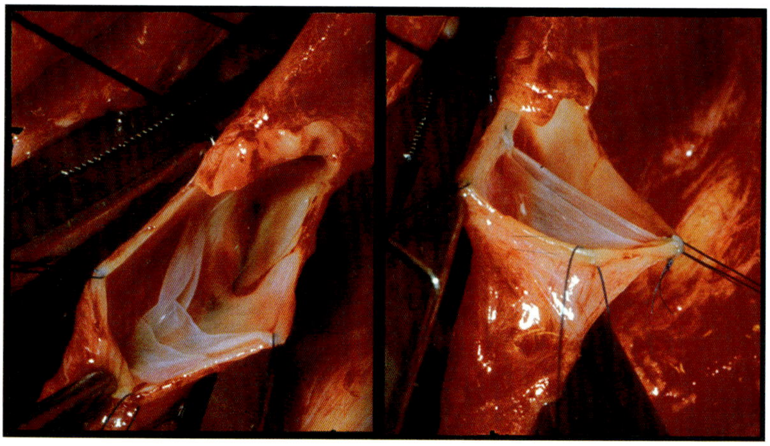

FIGURE 14.3 Internal valvuloplasty through a transverse venotomy as described by Raju. The floppy valve leaflets are seen from above before (left) and after (right) tightening.

An axillary transfer should be performed if reflux cannot be satisfactorily controlled. A precise technique, patience, and absolute control of reflux are essential for success. Re-exploration at the site of a failed repair is rarely successful due to edema, inflammatory response, and scar formation in the wound.

External Valvuloplasty

This technique brings the 2 valve attachment lines together by externally placed sutures at each commissural end (Figure 14.4).[3] The valve redundancy itself is not directly addressed. The vein is not clamped. Starting at the commissural apex, continuous or interrupted transmural sutures are placed along the valve attachment lines to the point where the attachment lines curve sharply away from each other. Additional sutures may be required at one or both commissural sites to achieve competence. A 10% to 20% stenosis is usually created to achieve valve competence, but more severe stenosis at the valve station should be avoided. If excessive narrowing of the lumen is required to achieve valve competence, the technique should be abandoned and replaced by axillary vein transfer.

External Valvuloplasty with Angioscopic Visualization

The use of an angioscope to enhance the external repair technique was first described by Gloviczki et al[21] and subsequently successfully used by others.[22,23] The valve leaflets are visualized with an angioscope, which is introduced through a small venotomy above the valve station. Instead of transmural stitches just apposing the valve attachment lines, transluminal sutures can now be placed to also tighten the valve cusps. Angioscopic irrigation is required for proper visualization of the valve cusps. It may be quite difficult to direct the sutures to catch the valve leaflets under angioscopic visualization. Angioscopic inspection frequently merely confirmed that the valve had been traversed by the sutures after they had been placed. It appeared that transluminal sutures placed along the valve attachment lines usually tacked or tethered the redundant valve cusps. This observation led to the development of the transcommissural valvuloplasty technique.

Transcommissural Valvuloplasty

This technique mimics the angioscopic technique but places transluminal sutures "blindly" without the aid of the angioscope in a nonclamped vein.[24] Initial sutures near the commissural apex are shallow, as the free edges of the valve cusps do not extend far into the lumen at this point. Further down, they do extend gradually more into the lumen, crossing it to the opposite commissure. Each subsequent suture should therefore be placed slightly deeper into the lumen than the previous one to catch the cusp edges. As each repair suture is tied, the slack valve cusps will tighten progressively. Despite the "blind" nature of the technique, valve competency can be consistently achieved, which can be repeatedly checked by the strip test after each suture is placed. Repair is performed at both commissures.

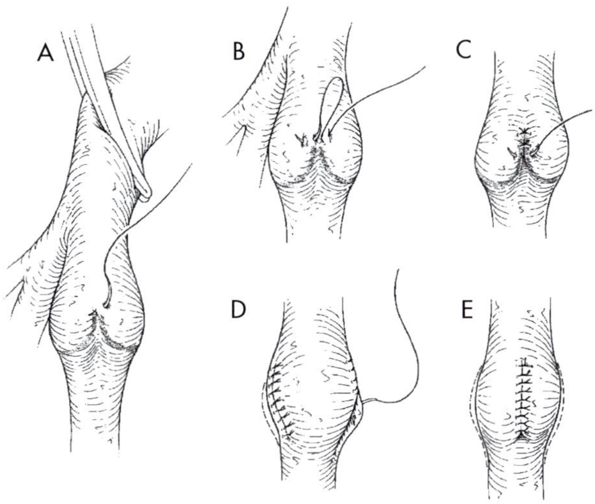

FIGURE 14.4 External valve repair as described by Kistner. The first suture at the commissure engages both cusp margins **(A–B)** and is tied with a knot outside the vein. Multiple sutures are placed coapting the attachments lines **(C)** and performed on both sides **(D)**. After completion, the valve station is slightly narrowed **(E)**. Modified from Bergan JJ, Kister RL. Atlas of Venous Surgery. Philadelphia, PA: WB Saunders; 1992:132. With permission from Elsevier.

Sleeve In Situ

It has been observed that sleeves wrapped around a refluxing valve station may restore valve competence.[25] This technique followed the observation that refluxing valves sometimes became competent when a spasm of the vein was induced by surgical manipulation, ie, the diameter of the vein decreased. A suitably sized prosthetic sleeve of Dacron or polytetrafluoroethylene (PTFE) is wrapped around the slightly constricted valve station to maintain competence. Lane has used the technique more aggressively, using a prosthetic device to constrict valve stations that remained overtly incompetent even after surgical exposure.[26] This technique has attracted lot of clinical interest because of its simplicity. Several short-term series have appeared with good clinical results.[27,28] Substituting reflux for a stenosis or occlusion (which improves symptoms initially) with this technique is a major concern, particularly in postthrombotic cases where there are no valve cusps to coapt with sleeve constriction. Long-term results need to be monitored.

Neovalve

There have been numerous experimental and clinical attempts to create new valve cusps at valve stations where native valves had become destroyed beyond repair. These techniques have obvious appeal for use in postthrombotic cases. Few long-term successes have been reported. A recent technique described by Maleti and colleagues has drawn widespread interest.[29,30] A valve cusp is fashioned out of the thickened intima by sharp dissection. Short-term results with this technique are promising.

Transposition

This technique was first described by Kistner.[2] The femoral vein is divided below the incompetent valve and anastomosed to the adjacent saphenous or profunda femoris vein (Figure 14.5). The receiving veins should have adequate caliber and have competent valve(s) for a successful reconstruction. Such favorable anatomy is rare (2% of all limbs with absent valves). Saphenous and profunda valves are shallower than the femoral and are prone to reflux with dilatation. Long-term competence of this repair after redirection of additional flow is therefore a concern. Perhaps for this reason, published results with this technique appear to be inferior.[11,31,32]

Axillary Vein Transfer

Taheri reported transferring a competent brachial vein valve segment to the femoral vein, later changing it to the popliteal vein because of size considerations.[33] Later reports from others have followed since.[15,16,33-37] The axillary valve is a better-sized match for the femoral vein and has become the standard in valve transfer to the femoral vein (Figure 14.6).

Although the technique may appear simple, attention to detail is important.[12,15,38] The axillary vein is exposed through a transverse incision along the skin crease in the axilla. One or more valves at the distal or mid portion of the vein are usually found, or additional exploration proximally may be necessary by retracting the pectoral muscle. In 14% of explorations no usable valve is found. The valve competence is checked by the strip test. The axillary valve cusps are shallow and even mild rotation or inadequate tension at the transfer site can result in incompetence. Approximately 40% of axillary valves are incompetent in situ before harvest for unknown reasons; and a few are refluxing after transfer despite meticulous technique. The incompetent valve stations are repaired by using an external or transcommissural technique before harvest or after transfer. A 3- to 4-cm length of axillary valve segment should be harvested and the divided ends are ligated. Postharvest arm symptoms are extremely rare (<2%) and transient. The harvested vein segment is kept in a cold, balanced salt solution.

After heparinization and clamping, the dissected recipient vein is divided. The upper end of the axillary valve segment is anastomosed using interrupted sutures. Continuous sutures frequently result in postoperative suture line stenosis after intraop-

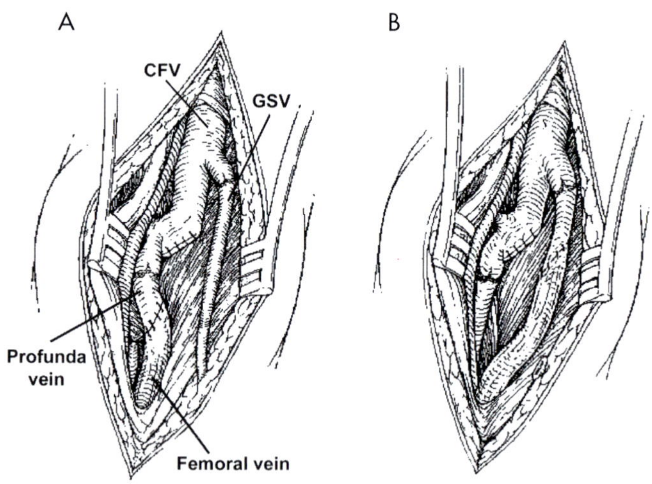

FIGURE 14.5 Vein transposition as described by Kistner. The incompetent femoral vein has been divided and reanastomosed to the profunda femoris **(A)** or great saphenous vein (GSV) **(B)** below a competent valve station. The anastomosis may be fashioned end-to-end or end-to-side. (CFV = common femoral vein). Modified from Bergan JJ, Kister RL. Atlas of Venous Surgery. Philadelphia, PA: WB Saunders; 1992:155. With permission from Elsevier.

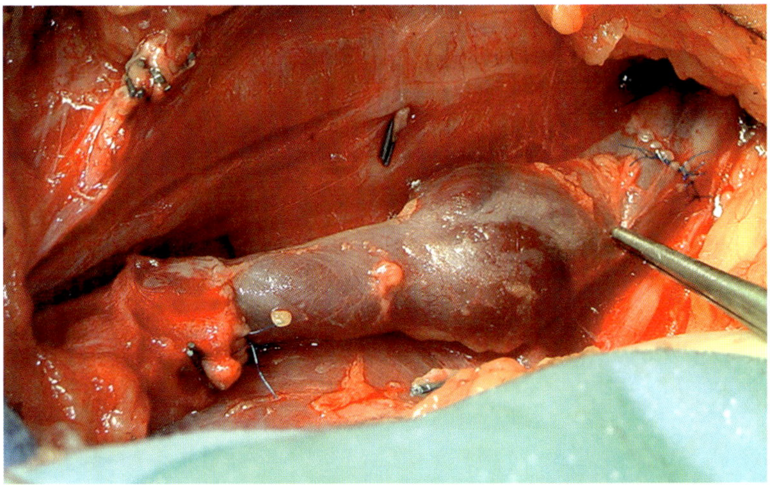

FIGURE 14.6 An axillary vein segment transferred to the proximal femoral vein. The vein wall is thin and the valve station with the slender attachment lines is well seen.

erative spasm of the vein has been relieved. The upper clamp is removed and the transferred valve tested for competence. If refluxing, the valve must be repaired by external technique before completing the lower anastomosis. The level of the lower end of the host vein is determined by placing the transplanted segment under optimal tension. The host vein is divided at that level. Mild over- or understretching or slight torsion of the transferred segment may cause reflux. Leaving the upper clamp off during the lower anastomosis may prevent this from happening. Despite being careful, 16% of transfers remain mildly leaky after insertion. A sleeve of Dacron or PTFE is wrapped around the transferred vein to prevent dilation and incompetence of the valve.

The technique is feasible even in postthrombotic veins with trabeculae.[12] The trabeculae are excised at the cut ends of the host vein to create a single lumen for anastomosis (Figure 14.7). The transplant maintains surprisingly high long-term patency despite the advanced postthrombotic pathology of the host vein. The axillary-basilic complex can be used to reconstruct the entire femoral-profunda confluence in severe postthrombotic cases. Insertion of valve carrying cryopreserved allografts has had poor results with low patency, probably related to immune rejection.[39]

Anticoagulation

Prophylactic or bridge low-molecular-weight heparin (LMWH) is started before surgery and should be continued for at least 5 days postoperatively, initially combined with pneumatic compression. Early ambulation is encouraged. Patients with primary reflux and external repair may not need warfarin anticoagulation beyond the perioperative treatment. The majority of patients will require postoperative warfarin anticoagulation for at least 8 to 12 weeks. Operative endothelial injury is healed by 6 weeks. Longer-term anticoagulation may be considered in patients with known thrombophilia, previous recurrent thrombosis, or other risk factors for developing thrombosis.

Morbidity

Wound hematoma is the most common complication (<15%) and is related to the

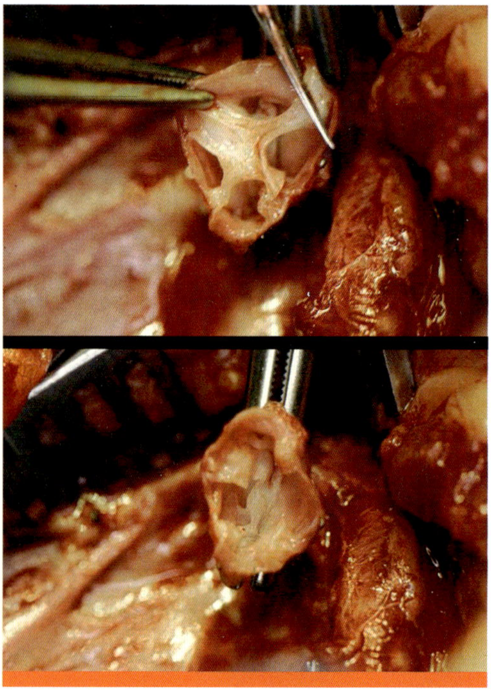

FIGURE 14.7 Trabeculation in femoral vein, which is to receive an axillary vein transfer, is sharply resected to create a single lumen above and below the inserted vein segment.

level of anticoagulation. Seroma formation is rare (1%–2%). Both types of wound collections should be aggressively drained to avoid compression and thrombosis of the repair. Wound infection occurs in 1% to 7% and is related to the presence of active leg ulcers.

The rate of postoperative leg thrombosis (<6 weeks) is the same (approximately 4%) in primary and postthrombotic limbs after valve reconstruction.[12,15,16] The postthrombotic limbs develop late recurrent thromboses from the underlying disease and not related to the surgery per se (cumulative rate of 6% at 10 years). Regardless of the time interval after valve surgery, the thrombus usually does not involve the valve repair itself but occurs at a remote location in the same or opposite limb. Pulmonary embolism and mortality are rare after valve reconstruction.

Clinical and Hemodynamic Outcome

Several long-term clinical results have been published.[11,16,40-43] Only minor differences in ulcer healing have been observed after the different surgical techniques. There is a lag between failure of the repaired valve and recurrence of the ulcer, probably since ulcer formation is a relatively slow process. It is important to emphasize that ulcer recurrence is rare (<10%) when the repaired valve stays competent (duration of reflux less than 0.5 second). In limbs with primary disease, long-term cumulative ulcer healing of 60% to 80% can be expected. Resolution of pain and swelling is also significant. Even though internal valvuloplasty deteriorates in duplex competence over time, like other types of repairs, the rate is less as compared to other valve reconstruction techniques.[40] However, no significant difference in clinical outcome between the various valve reconstruction techniques has been observed, despite variable rates of valve failure over time. In limbs with postthrombotic disease, valve competency is approximately 50% at 5 years, but with longer clinical benefit. Most patients are able to discard or limit the use of compression stockings after successful valve reconstruction.

Normalization of venous hemodynamics is not to be expected when a single-valve reconstruction is performed in an often multilevel and multisystem involvement, especially in limbs with postthrombotic disease. Significant improvement in VFI_{90} (APG) and ambulatory venous pressure should be expected following valve reconstruction; even normalization has been described in some limbs with primary disease.[11,13,24,34,36,42] Clinical failures are associated with nonimprovement in ambulatory venous pressure after valve reconstruction. A decreased ulcer recurrence rate has been observed in limbs with less reflux as measured as VFI_{90} (APG) (limbs with < 4.0 mL/s versus those with > 4.0 mL/s, 28% and 53%, respectively).[44] Similarly, the recurrence rate was only 14% if a VFT (AVP) more than 5 seconds could be maintained as compared to 45% when VFT was less than 5 seconds.[45]

Single vs. Multiple Valve Reconstructions

Whether or not a single valve repair is sufficient to control a multilevel reflux is still controversial. Clinical experience indicates that a single valve repair at the femoral location provides durable clinical relief in approximately 65% of patients (cumulative rate at 6 years), while hemodynamic improvement is often only partial, although significant. Intuitively, multiple valve repairs at more than one location (eg, femoral, popliteal, tibial, profunda femoris) would possibly yield better clinical and hemodynamic outcome. Multivariate analysis of our valve reconstruction database (all cases) showed no advantage for multiple reconstructions.[40] Others have, however, recently shown that multiple repairs (internal, external, or transfer repairs) have increased the rate of valve competency of the venous system of the limb and consequently decreased ulcer recurrence. With multiple valve repairs, one valve is more likely to remain competent.[43,46,47]

A so-called profunda transformation may occur in postthrombotic limbs.[38] With acute thrombotic occlusion of the femoral vein, the frequently preexisting profunda-popliteal connection and the profunda femoris vein may enlarge to compensate. When a transformed profunda vein is incompetent, a valve repair of the femoral vein would be unable to control deep axial reflux since, in reality, the repair is bypassed by reflux in the parallel profunda vein. Valve repair under those circumstances must be performed on both veins. The association of profunda femoris reflux adversely affects ambulatory venous pressure and clinical outcome after femoral valve reconstructions.[11] Eriksson first drew attention to the increasing outflow function assumed by the profunda femoris in postthrombotic disease and successfully repaired profunda valves, with good clinical results.[48] In a selected series from our center, combined femoral and profunda femoris repairs were shown to yield 65% cumulative ulcer healing at 5 years.[38]

Proximal or Distal Site for Valve Repair

The popliteal valve is often considered the "gatekeeper" of the calf venous pump. Attractive in theory, there is no evidence for this concept in hemodynamic data or from any comparative clinical series.[5] In our own material, femoral repairs had a better clinical outcome than repairs at other sites, including the popliteal location.[40] All valve repairs show a steady functional deterioration over time as determined by duplex scanning. One notable exception is a subset of posterior tibial valve repairs that were remarkably durable in function and clinical outcome for unknown reasons beyond 5 years of follow-up. This finding has not been verified by others. The femoral valve showed less deterioration than other repair locations including the popliteal.

Choice of Type and Technique of Repair

The choice of procedure is determined by the absence or presence of valve leaflets, degree of cusp prolapse, long-term results, and surgeon's preference. If a valve is present, the primary choice of valve repair is a sleeve-in-situ in cases of vein wall dilation only; external/transcommissural valvuloplasty in cases with wall dilation and mild/moderate valve prolapse; and internal valve repair in cases of pronounced valve prolapse. Internal valvuloplasty is a precise direct technique with proven long-term efficacy. Clinical outcome appears, as previously discussed, to be similar in a number of clinical series with different direct valve reconstruction techniques. Internal valvuloplasty is a time-consuming technique and not feasible in small-caliber veins. External or transcommissural techniques are quicker, can be performed in small-caliber veins, and are the preferred techniques for multiple valve repairs. Axillary vein transfer is the main repair when valves are absent or a direct repair fails. Transposition is rarely an alternative, but de novo valve creation may be performed in selected postthrombotic patients. Ultimately, the choice of technique is largely governed by personal preference and the experience gained with a certain technique, since there is a considerable learning curve in mastering valve reconstruction techniques.

Valve Reconstruction in Postthrombotic Cases

Valve reconstruction in postthrombotic limbs is controversial. Many avoid performing surgery in these patients for fear of thrombosis. Venographic appearance can be intimidating due to the presence of widespread trabeculation. In some patients, the deep veins may not be visualized at all on venography, as though they were completely "wiped out." However, the majority of such findings are due to anomalous contrast flow and not to absence of deep venous vessels.[12] Our own experience with valve reconstruction in a large cohort of postthrombotic limbs, even those with trabeculated veins, has been surprisingly successful.[12,15,38] There is faster duplex deterioration and lesser degree of hemodynamic improvement in postthrombotic limbs as compared to primary disease, but the clinical outcome is similar. Cumulative ulcer healing in postthrombotic cases with and without trabeculae was similar at 12 years, 61% and 69%, respectively. Thrombotic complications were insignificant. Thrombosis and loss of the transfer vein was rare with a proper anticoagulation protocol. Counterintuitively, trabeculated veins appear resistant to thrombosis after surgical trauma, and direct surgical intervention appears to be safe. Similar good clinical results have been reported by numerous other groups in postthrombotic disease,[28,29,34,36,48,49] using a variety of valve reconstruction techniques. Contrarily, Masuda et al noted good clinical results of 50% at 5 years and 43% at 10 years in 16 postthrombotic cases (cumulative rate); 14 of these utilized segment transfer technique, and axillary vein transplants were used in only 2 patients.[11] This poor outcome as compared to their primary cases (73% at 10 years) was more likely related to the choice of segment transfer technique rather than to the postthrombotic disease. Perrin also noted slightly inferior results in postthrombotic as compared to "primary" limbs, but the long-term cumulative good clinical result was still seen in more than 50% of limbs.[16]

As discussed, valve reconstructions are performed late in the treatment paradigm, more or less after all other forms of conservative or interventional therapy have been exhausted. It is especially a last-ditch procedure in patients with advanced postthrombotic disease with ulcers who are otherwise forced to lifelong compression therapy, often with persistent or recurrent ulcers. Deep venous reconstruction as a salvage effort surely is worthwhile in this group of disabled patients, even if the outcome is not quite as good as in patients with primary reflux.

Is Valve Repair Worthwhile?

There is no doubt that relief of axial deep reflux leads to dramatic clinical improvement. Successful deep valve repair generally results in 95% primary ulcer healing. The patient is provided a 65% possibility of an ulcer recurrence-free interval of more than 6 years using the techniques presently available. One-third of patients who received surgery and were followed for more than 10 years are completely relieved of chronic venous insufficiency symptoms and do not need to wear any compression stockings. It appears that the concept of controlling axial reflux is correct, but the techniques to achieve this goal are suboptimal. Ulcer recurrence is less than 10%, when the repaired valve stays competent. New durable techniques or reliable artificial valves will undoubtedly change the treatment paradigm.

References

1. Kistner RL. Surgical repair of the incompetent femoral vein valve. Arch Surg. 1975;110:1336-42.
2. Ferris EB and Kistner RL. Femoral vein reconstruction in the management of chronic venous insufficiency. A 14-year experience. Arch Surg. 1982;117:1571-9.
3. Kistner RL. Surgical technique: external venous valve repair. Straub Foundation Proc. 1990;55:15-16.
4. Kistner RL, Eklof B, Masuda EM. Deep venous valve reconstruction. Cardiovasc Surg. 1995;3:129-40.
5. Neglen P, Egger JF 3rd, Olivier J, Raju S. Hemodynamic and clinical impact of ultrasound-derived venous reflux parameters. J Vasc Surg. 2004;40:303-10.
6. Eklof B, Rutherford RB, Bergan JJ, Carpentier PH, Gloviczki P, Kistner RL, et al; American Venous Forum International Ad Hoc Committee for Revision of the CEAP Classification. Revision of the CEAP classification for chronic venous disorders: consensus statement. J Vasc Surg. 2004;40:1248-52.
7. Neglen P, Raju S. A comparison between descending phlebography and duplex Doppler investigation in the evaluation of reflux in chronic venous insufficiency: a challenge to phlebography as the "gold standard." J Vasc Surg. 1992;16:687-93.
8. Neglen P, Raju S. A rational approach to detection of significant reflux with duplex Doppler scanning and air plethysmography. J Vasc Surg. 1993;17:590-5.
9. Masuda EM, Kistner RL, Eklof B. Prospective study of duplex scanning for venous reflux: comparison of Valsalva and pneumatic cuff techniques in the reverse Trendelenburg and standing positions. J Vasc Surg. 1994;20:711-20.
10. Gillespie DL, Cordts PR, Hartono C, Woodson J, Obi-Tabot E, LaMorte WW, et al. The role of air plethysmography in monitoring results of venous surgery. J Vasc Surg. 1992; 16:674-8.
11. Masuda EM, Kistner RL. Long-term results of venous valve reconstruction: a four- to twenty-one-year follow-up. J Vasc Surg. 1994;19: 391-403.
12. Raju S, Neglen P, Doolittle J, Meydrech EF. Axillary vein transfer in trabeculated postthrombotic veins. J Vasc Surg. 1999;29:1050-62; discussion 1062-4.
13. Sakuda H, Nakaema M, Matsubara S, Higa N, Kamada Y, Kuniyoshi Y, Koja K. Air plethysmographic assessment of external valvuloplasty in patients with valvular

incompetence of the saphenous and deep veins. J Vasc Surg. 2002;36:922-7.
14. Masuda EM, Kistner RL. Prospective comparison of duplex scanning and descending venography in the assessment of venous insufficiency. Am J Surg. 1992;164:254-9.
15. Raju S, Hardy JD. Technical options in venous valve reconstruction. Am J Surg. 1997;173: 301-7.
16. Perrin M. Reconstructive surgery for deep venous reflux: a report on 144 cases. Cardiovasc Surg. 2000;8:246-55.
17. Caps MT, Manzo RA, Bergelin RO, Meissner MH, Strandness DE Jr. Venous valvular reflux in veins not involved at the time of acute deep vein thrombosis. J Vasc Surg. 1995;22:524-31.
18. Raju S, Fredericks R. Valve reconstruction procedures for nonobstructive venous insufficiency: rationale, techniques, and results in 107 procedures with two- to eight-year follow-up. J Vasc Surg. 1988;7:301-10.
19. Sottiurai VS. Technique in direct venous valvuloplasty. J Vasc Surg. 1988;8:646-8.
20. Tripathi R, Ktenidis KD. Trapdoor internal valvuloplasty—a new technique for primary deep vein valvular incompetence. Eur J Vasc Endovasc Surg. 2001;22:86-9.
21. Gloviczki P, Merrell SW, Bower TC. Femoral vein valve repair under direct vision without venotomy: a modified technique with use of angioscopy. J Vasc Surg. 1991;14:645-8.
22. Welch HJ, McLaughlin RL, O'Donnell TF Jr. Femoral vein valvuloplasty: intraoperative angioscopic evaluation and hemodynamic improvement. J Vasc Surg. 1992;16:694-700.
23. Hoshino S, Satakawa H, Iwaya F, Igari T, Ono T, Takase S. External valvuloplasty under preoperative angioscopic control. [Article in French.] Phlebologie. 1993;46:521-9.
24. Raju S, Berry MA, Neglen P. Transcommissural valvuloplasty: technique and results. J Vasc Surg. 2000;32:969-76.
25. Hallberg D. A method for repairing incompetent valves in deep veins. Acta Chir Scand. 1972;138:143-5.
26. Jessup G, Lane RJ. Repair of incompetent venous valves: a new technique. J Vasc Surg. 1988;8:569-75.
27. Camilli S, Guarnera G. External banding valvuloplasty of the superficial femoral vein in the treatment of primary deep valvular incompetence. Int Angiol. 1994;13:218-22.
28. Akesson H, Risberg B, Bjorgell O. External support valvuloplasty in the treatment of chronic deep vein incompetence of the legs. Int Angiol. 1999;18:233-8.
29. Maleti O, Lugli M. Neovalve construction in postthrombotic syndrome. J Vasc Surg. 2006;43:794-9.
30. Lugli M, Guerzoni S, Garofalo M, Smedile G, Maleti O. Neovalve construction in deep venous incompetence. J Vasc Surg. 2009;49:156-62, 162.e1-2; discussion 162.
31. Cardon JM, Cardon A, Joyeux A, Mangialardi N, Noblet D, Nguyen T, et al. Use of ipsilateral greater saphenous vein as a valved transplant in management of postthrombotic deep venous insufficiency: long-term results. Ann Vasc Surg. 1999;13:284-9.
32. Johnson ND, Queral LA, Flinn WR, Yao JS, Bergan JJ. Late objective assessment of venous valve surgery. Arch Surg. 1981;116:1461-6.
33. Taheri SA, Lazar L, Elias S, Marchand P, Heffner R. Surgical treatment of postphlebitic syndrome with vein valve transplant. Am J Surg. 1982;144:221-4.
34. Bry JD, Muto PA, O'Donnell TF, Isaacson LA. The clinical and hemodynamic results after axillary-to-popliteal vein valve transplantation. J Vasc Surg. 1995;21:110-9.
35. Raju S, Fredericks R. Venous obstruction: an analysis of one hundred thirty-seven cases with hemodynamic, venographic, and clinical correlations. J Vasc Surg. 1991;14:305-13.
36. Nash T. Long term results of vein valve transplants placed in the popliteal vein for intractable post-phlebitic venous ulcers and

pre-ulcer skin changes. J Cardiovasc Surg (Torino). 1988;29:712-6.
37. Jamieson WG, Chinnick B. Clinical results of deep venous valvular repair for chronic venous insufficiency. Can J Surg. 1997;40:294-9.
38. Raju S, Fountain T, Neglen P, Devidas M. Axial transformation of the profunda femoris vein. J Vasc Surg. 1998;27:651-9.
39. Neglen P, Raju S. Venous reflux repair with cryopreserved vein valves. J Vasc Surg. 2003;37:552-7.
40. Raju S, Fredericks RK, Neglen PN, Bass JD. Durability of venous valve reconstruction techniques for "primary" and postthrombotic reflux. J Vasc Surg. 1996;23:357-66; discussion 366-7.
41. Sottiurai VS. Surgical correction of recurrent venous ulcer. J Cardiovasc Surg (Torino). 1991;32:104-9.
42. Wang SM, Hu ZJ, Li SQ, Huang XL, Ye CS. Effect of external valvuloplasty of the deep vein in the treatment of chronic venous insufficiency of the lower extremity. J Vasc Surg. 2006;44:1296-300.
43. Tripathi R, Sieunarine K, Abbas M, Durrani N. Deep venous valve reconstruction for non-healing leg ulcers: techniques and results. Anz J Surg. 2004;74:34-9.
44. McDaniel HB, Marston WA, Farber MA, Mendes RR, Owens LV, Young ML,. Recurrence of chronic venous ulcers on the basis of clinical, etiologic, anatomic, and pathophysiologic criteria and air plethysmography. J Vasc Surg. 2002;35:723-8.
45. Kalra M, Gloviczki P. Surgical treatment of venous ulcers: role of subfascial endoscopic perforator vein ligation. Surg Clin North Am. 2003;83:671-705.
46. Lane RJ, Cuzzilla ML, McMahon CG. Intermediate to long-term results of repairing incompetent multiple deep venous valves using external valvular stenting. Anz J Surg. 2003;73:267-74.
47. Rosales A, Slagsvold CE, Kroese AJ, Stranden E, Risum O, Jorgensen JJ. External venous valve plasty (EVVP) in patients with primary chronic venous insufficiency (PCVI). Eur J Vasc Endovasc Surg. 2006;32:570-6.
48. Eriksson I, Almgren B. Influence of the profunda femoris vein on venous hemodynamics of the limb. Experience from thirty-one deep vein valve reconstructions. J Vasc Surg. 1986;4:390-5.t
49. Taheri SA, Heffner R, Meenaghan MA, Budd T, Pollack LH. Vein valve transplant. Indications and results. Int Angiol. 1985,4: 425-8.

PART

3

Special Circumstances

The conditions of Nutcracker syndrome and pelvic congestion syndrome were relative rarities until the widespread introduction of cross-sectional imaging. In the case of Nutcracker syndrome surgical intervention is the norm; however, the few reports on endovascular therapy raise hopes for a percutaneous option in this condition. In the arena of chronic pelvic pain, pelvic congestion syndrome is treatable endoluminally and is anatomically successful in most cases. Coils currently are the treatment of choice, but whether sclerosants or glue will be of use is unknown. Both syndromes are now more commonly reported; however, reports on therapy remain observational and further work to develop evidence-based approaches is warranted.

CHAPTER 15

Nutcracker Syndrome

Joseph J. Naoum

Vascular compression of the left renal vein (LRV) between the superior mesenteric artery (SMA) and the aorta is an uncommon condition. Diagnosis requires a high degree of suspicion. Helical computed tomography (CT) scans, with the administration of intravenous contrast, and 3-dimensional reconstruction have proven to be a powerful diagnostic tool. Left renal vein venography with pressure gradient measurements is important to confirm the diagnosis. The presence of severe or classic symptoms requires operation. The operative treatment of choice consists of transposition of the LRV; however, left renal autotransplantation has been used with success.

Chronic Venous Insufficiency. Contemporary Endovascular Management series. © 2011 Mark G. Davies MD and Alan B. Lumsden MD, eds. Cardiotext Publishing, ISBN 978-1-935395-09-6.

History

Obstruction of the LRV by the SMA against the aorta was first identified and described in 1944 in autopsy studies.[1] In 1950, El-Sadr and Mina[2] described the first patient with this pathology. However, it was not until 1971 that Chait and colleagues[3] reported the use of venography to demonstrate the vascular impression on the compressed LRV and described the aorta and the SMA as 2 arms of a nutcracker. It appears that in 1972, de Schepper[4] identified the "Nutcracker" compression of the LRV as a syndrome and noted that it resulted in the extensive development of perirenal varicosities. Numerous alternative names to describe this syndrome include Nutcracker syndrome, Nutcracker phenomenon, renal vein entrapment syndrome, vascular compression of the LRV, aortomesenteric compression of the LRV, and mesoaortic compression of the LRV. The latter term seems to best and most accurately describe this disease.

Anatomy

Vascular compression of the LRV between the SMA and the aorta is a real disease with a specific anatomic basis (Figure 15.1). In humans, the SMA arises from the abdominal aorta at the level of the first lumbar vertebra at an angle that averages 42.4°, with a wide range of variation from 18° to 70°. Normally, the LRV crosses the abdomen over the aorta at the level of the second lumbar vertebra to join the inferior vena cava (IVC). Thus, the LRV is fixed at 2 points by the left kidney and the IVC.

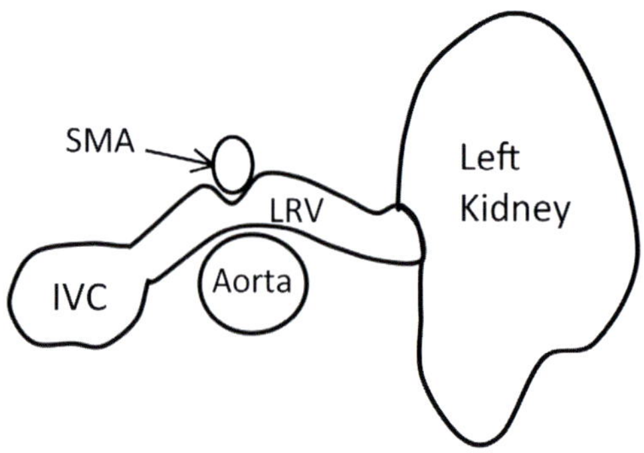

FIGURE 15.1 Axial schematic demonstrating the LRV compressed by the SMA against the aorta.

Minor alterations of the normal anatomic relationships of the SMA, the aorta, the LRV, and the left kidney may lead to this syndrome. A narrow aortomesenteric angle produces extrinsic compression of the LRV by the SMA. Using ultrasonography, Arima and colleagues[5] demonstrated symptomatic compression of the LRV when the angle was less than 6° to 16° compared with 38° to 56° in controls. On the other hand, Ali-El-Dein and associates[6] used magnetic resonance angiography (MRA) to show that symptomatic patients in their series had an average aortomesenteric angle of 54° as compared to 91° in healthy controls. A low origin of the SMA or a high LRV position can also lead to compression. An extensive loss or decrease of retroperitoneal fat pad can contribute to a decrease in the aortomesenteric distance and angle responsible for the development of vascular compression of the LRV. Posterior renal ptosis with concomitant stretching of the left renal vein over the aorta may also be a contributing cause.[7]

Clinical Presentation

Mesoaortic compression of the LRV is an uncommon condition. It can affect children, especially with low body mass index,[8] it is more common in young adults between the ages of 20 and 40 years than in older individuals,[9] and it affects women more often than men.

Symptoms are nonspecific and may include abdominal or left flank pain, pelvic pain of variable intensity that can be aggravated by prolonged standing, and fatigue. Compression of the LRV leads to venous hypertension, which can cause perirenal varicosities and incompetence of the left ovarian or testicular vein. Therefore, men can present with left-sided varicocele while women can have symptoms of pelvic congestion and labial varicosities. It is believed that LRV hypertension may lead to rupture of the thin-walled septum separating the veins and the urinary collecting system and cause unilateral micro- or macroscopic hematuria and proteinuria.[6,10]

Diagnosis

Confirmation of the diagnosis requires a high degree of suspicion and meticulous evaluation. The usual causes for abdominal pain and hematuria need to be considered and evaluated. Laboratory tests to exclude other causes of hematuria are usually followed by cystoscopy or ureteroscopy, which can localize hematuria to the left kidney. A thorough radiographic evaluation is valuable in demonstrating compression of the LRV and confirming the diagnosis. Takebayashi and associates[11] showed that color Doppler sonography was helpful in the diagnosis of Nutcracker syndrome with sensitivity and specificity of 78% and 100%, respectively. Duplex ultrasonography is useful in measuring the peak systolic velocities (PSV) at the site of mesoaortic compression of the LRV and at the renal hilum. The ratio of these 2 PSV in patients with Nutcracker syndrome is usually >4.7 to 7.9 as compared with normal controls in which the ratio is approximately 2.6 to 2.8. [12,13] Contrast CT or MR angiography should be the next diagnostic step to visualize the compression of the LRV between the SMA and the aorta and to delineate other potential causes for a patient's symptoms. Retrograde LRV venography with venous pressure gradient measurements between the prestenotic LRV and the IVC is considered the gold standard. Pressure gradients in mesoaortic compression of the LRV can vary and have been documented between 3.5 and 14.0 mm Hg.[10,14-17]

Management

Patients who present with abdominal or left flank pain, with documented left-sided hematuria or radiographic imaging showing mesoaortic compression of the LRV, and have undergone venography with pressure gradient measurements that confirm the presence of a hemodynamic significant stenosis should undergo treatment (Figure 15.2). The preferred treatment involves transposition of the LRV approximately 5 cm downward with an end-to side primary anastomosis to the IVC.[10,15] The operation is commonly performed through a midline

FIGURE 15.2 Decision-making algorithm for the diagnosis and treatment of mesoaortic compression of the LRV.

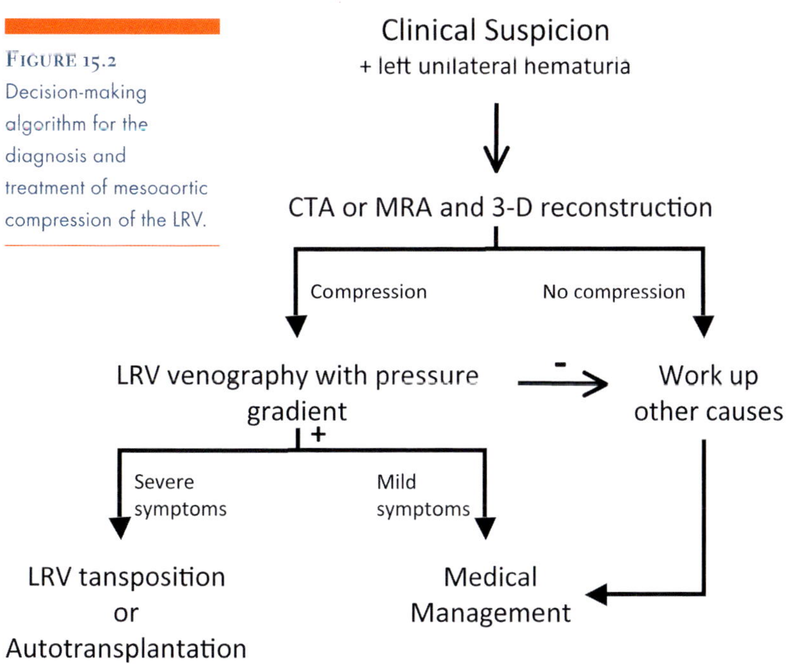

laparotomy incision. To completely mobilize the LRV, it is usually necessary to ligate and divide the left adrenal vein, the ovarian or testicular vein, and the lumbar vein. After the administration of heparin, a vascular clamp is used to control the LRV confluence and allow its excision with a small portion of the IVC. The LRV is mobilized approximately 5 cm downward and reanastomosed to the IVC. The proximal LRV origin at the IVC is then oversewn.

Left renal autotransplatation has also been used with success. It can be performed through a midline or through a left retroperitoneal incision.[6,17] This procedure appears helpful in cases of left renal posterior ptosis. However, Ali-El-Dein and colleagues[6] advocate autotransplantation even for the classic presentation of mesoaortic compression of the LRV.

With the advent of endovascular interventions, mesoaortic compression of the LRV has been treated with the placement of endoluminal stents with variable degrees of success.[15,18,19] In this instance, it is believed that 16 mm in diameter by 60 mm in length self-expanding stents are needed to achieve adequate apposition to the walls of the LRV on either side of the stenosis and avoid dislodgement or migration of the stent into the IVC.[15] Protrusion of the stent into the IVC does not appear to have major consequences.

It is evident that a careful patient evaluation is necessary to establish the diagnosis. However, appropriate patient selection for open or endovascular intervention is necessary to eliminate symptoms and achieve a successful outcome (Table 15.1).

References

1. Grant JCB. A Method of Anatomy, Descriptive and Deductive. 3rd ed. Baltimore, MD: The Williams and Wilkins Company; 1944.
2. El-Sadr AR, Mina E. Anatomical and surgical aspects in the operative management of varicocele. Urol Cutaneous Rev. 1950;54: 257-62.
3. Chait A MK, Fabian CE, Mellins HZ. Vascular impressions on the ureters. Am J Roentgenol Radi. 1971;3:729-49.

TABLE 15.1 **Review of Series results for the Surgical Treatment of the Nutcracker Syndrome**

Source	No. of Patients	Procedure	Symptom Relief (%)
Reed et al,[10] 2009	8	LRV transposition	91.0
Hohenfellner et al,[16] 2002	8	LRV transposition	87.5
Ali-El-Dein et al,[6] 2003	7	LRV transposition (1) Autotransplatation (6)	87.5[a]
Hartung et al,[15] 2005	5	LRV stenting	40.0

[a] An estimated calculation.

4. de Schepper A. "Nutcracker" phenomenon of the renal vein causing left renal vein pathology. J Belg Rad. 1972;55:507.
5. Arima M, Hosokawa S, Ogino T, Ihara H, Terakawa T, Ikoma F. Ultrasonographically demonstrated nutcracker phenomenon: alternative to angiography. Int Urol Nephrol. 1990; 22;3-6.
6. Ali-El-Dein B, Osman Y, Shehab El-Din AB, El-Diasty T, Mansour O, Ghoneim MA. Anterior and posterior nutcracker syndrome: a report on 11 cases. Transplant Proc. 2003;35:851-3.
7. Wendel RG, Crawford ED, Hehman KN. The nutcracker phenomenon: an unusual cause for renal varicosities with hematuria. J Urol. 1980;123:761-3.
8. Shin JI, Park JM, Lee SM, Shin YH, Kim JH, Lee JS, et al. Factors affecting spontaneous resolution of hematuria in childhood nutcracker syndrome. Pediatr Nephrol. 2005;20:609-13.
9. Ahmed K, Sampath R, Khan MS. Current trends in the diagnosis and management of renal nutcracker syndrome: a review. Eur J Vasc Endovasc Surg. 2006;31:410-16.
10. Reed NR, Kalra M, Bower TC, Vrtiska TJ, Ricotta JJ 2nd, Gloviczki P. Left renal vein transposition for nutcracker syndrome J Vasc Surg. 2009;49:386-94.
11. Takebayashi S, Ueki T, Ikeda N, Fujikawa A. Diagnosis of the nutcracker syndrome with color Doppler sonography: correlation with flow patterns on retrograde left renal venography. Am J Roentgenol. 1999;172:39-43.
12. Kim SH, Cho SW, Kim HD, Chung JW, Park JH, Han MC. Nutcracker syndrome: diagnosis with Doppler ultrasound. Radiology. 1996;198:93-7.
13. Cheon JE, Kim WS, Kim IO, Kim SH, Yeon KM, Ha IS, et al. Nutcracker syndrome in children with gross hematuria: Doppler sonographic evaluation of the left renal vein. Pediatr Radiol. 2006;36:682-6.
14. Chen YM, Wang IK, Ng KK, Huang CC. Nutcracker syndrome: an overlooked cause of hematuria. Chang Gung Med. J 2002;25: 700-5.
15. Hartung O, Grisoli D, Boufi M, Marani I, Hakam Z, Barthelemy P, et al. Endovascular stenting in the treatment of pelvic vein congestion caused by nutcracker syndrome: lessons learned from the first five cases. J Vasc Surg. 2005;42:275-80.
16. Hohenfellner M, D'Elia G, Hampel C, Dahms S, Thüroff JW. Transposition of the left renal vein for treatment of the nutcracker phenomenon: long-term follow-up. Urology. 2002;52:354-7.
17. Chuang CK, Chu SH, Lai PC. The nutcracker syndrome managed by autotransplatation. J Urol. 1997;157:1833-4.
18. Segawa N, Azuma H, Iwamoto Y, Sakamoto T, Suzuki T, Ueda H, et al. Expandable metallic stent placement for nutcracker phenomenon Urology. 1999;53:631-3.
19. Wei SM, Chen ZD, Zhou M. Intravenous stent placement for the treatment of the nutcracker syndrome. J Urol. 2003;170:1934-5.

CHAPTER 16

Pelvic Congestion Syndrome

Colleen J. Moore and Robert B. McLafferty

Pelvic congestion syndrome (PCS) is a cause of chronic pelvic pain that typically affects young, multiparous women. It is often characterized by lower abdominal pain exacerbated by long periods of standing or sitting. As with lower extremity varices, the pain can be worse with variations in the menstrual cycle. It is estimated that between 26% and 60% of women with PCS complain of dyspareunia.[1-3]

Anatomy

Before embarking on any evaluation or intervention for pelvic congestion syndrome, it is paramount to understand the venous anatomy of the pelvis. The inferior vena cava (IVC), which begins at the confluence of the common iliac veins, ascends just anterior and to the right of the vertebral column. There are many tributaries of the IVC: paired lumbar veins, renal veins, and hepatic veins. In addition, on the right side the right gonadal (ovarian or spermatic), suprarenal, and inferior phrenic veins drain into the IVC. The left gonadal vein drains into the left renal vein before reaching the IVC.

The internal iliac veins are found posteromedial to the internal iliac arteries. The extrapelvic tributaries include the superior and inferior gluteal veins, internal pudendal, and obturator veins. The obturator veins drain the pelvic wall and perineum and can be an additional source of pelvic congestion syndrome. The intrapelvic tributaries of the internal iliac veins consist of the lateral sacral, visceral veins that drain the presacral and pelvic venous plexuses: rectal, visceral, prostatic, uterine, and vaginal.

Chronic Venous Insufficiency. Contemporary Endovascular Management series. © 2011 Mark G. Davies MD and Alan B. Lumsden MD, eds. Cardiotext Publishing, ISBN 978-1-935395-09-6.

The ovarian vein originates as the confluence of the venous plexus in the broad ligament and is responsible for draining the parametrium, cervix, mesosalpinx, and pampiniform plexus. It communicates with the uterine plexus and courses anterior to the psoas muscle and ureter. The right ovarian vein drains directly into the inferior vena cava, and the left into the left renal vein. There are typically 2 to 3 valves found in this vein, which measures, on average, 3 mm in diameter. The right ovarian vein often has no valves. But if valves are present in the proximal ovarian vein, incompetence can be seen in up to 47% of women.

Incompetence of the saphenofemoral venous junction can also result in symptoms consistent with PCS. The superficial external pudendal vein drains directly into the great saphenous vein. The deep external pudendal vein typically drains into the common femoral vein (CFV) within the fossa ovalis. Reflux into this vein can often lead to labial varices.

Pathophysiology

The etiology of pelvic congestion syndrome remains poorly understood. As with varicose veins, this complex process more than likely involves hormonal, mechanical, and genetic factors. Dilation of the ovarian veins can result in valvular incompetence and retrograde flow into the pelvis. This explains why this syndrome is seen more often in multigravid women. It is postulated that a correlation exists between PCS and ovarian activity, as the syndrome affects premenopausal women almost exclusively.

Varicoceles represent a similar clinical complex of pelvic venous reflux in men. In this type of varicosity, much attention has been given to the etiology being linked to reactive oxygen species. Shiraishi and Nation evaluated 47 testicular biopsies and found the localization and generation of 4-hydroxyl-2-nonenal (4-HNE) proteins. This serves as a marker for oxidative stress. Subsequent evaluations determined that the expression of p53 was also higher in patients with varicocele compared to normal controls. Based on these observations, it was concluded that 4-HNE impairs the proliferation of germ cells through the upregulation of p53.[4] These data in concert with other studies show a link between the generation of reactive oxygen species and the formation of varioceles.[5-8]

Imaging Evaluation

Multiple imaging modalities can be utilized in the investigation of possible PCS.

Lower Extremity Venous Duplex

A lower extremity venous duplex and reflux examination using venous valve closure times in the standing position is an important early step in the evaluation of possible PCS. The symptoms of saphenofemoral reflux and PCS can often overlap with patients also complaining of symptoms such as pain and fatigue in the legs. Varicose veins of the lower extremity that traverse the posterior aspect of the upper thigh and are not in the great saphenous distribution (medial calf and thigh) may be related to pelvic venous insufficiency. Lower extremity ultrasonography can be performed to help identify great saphenous vein insufficiency. If the great saphenous is competent, alternative etiologies should be explored.

Pelvic Ultrasonography

Pelvic ultrasonography can be performed either transvaginally or transabdominally. This is a noninvasive test easily performed in most gynecology offices and can easily exclude other pelvic pathologies that may mimic the symptoms of PCS. Normal pelvic venous plexuses are visualized as 1 or 2 straight tubular structures with a diameter less than 4 mm with the right ovarian vein often being slightly larger than the left.[9] Pelvic or ovarian varicoceles can be seen as multiple dilated venous structures around the ovary and uterus. Any circular or linear venous structure with a diameter greater than 5 mm is indicative of pelvic varices.[5,10-12] Park et al also noted polycystic changes in the ovaries in many patients with PCS. Classic polycystic changes are associated with hirsutism or amennorhea. PCS patients often can have clusters of 4 to 6 cysts of 5 to 15 mm in diameter in bilaterally enlarged ovaries.[12] While no consensus has been reached regarding standard diagnostic criteria for PCS on pelvic ultrasonography, the following are generally considered associative finding in patients with PCS on transvaginal or transabdominal ultrasonography:[9,13,14]

- Tortuous pelvic veins greater than 6 mm in diameter; ovarian veins greater than 8 mm in diameter thought to be those causing symptoms of PCS
- Slow blood flow (3 cm/sec) or reversed caudal flow
- Dilated arcuate veins in the myometrium that communicate across the midline between variceal complexes
- Sonographic appearances of polycystic changes of the ovaries

MRI or CT Venography

Helical computed tomography (CT) scans are often performed to evaluate chronic pelvic pain in women. Rozenblit et al found that 47% of women who underwent CT scanning for planned kidney donation had a dilated ovarian vein on the left. Of these same women, 37.5% had bilateral involvement.[15] Hiromura et al found on CT a 44% incidence of left ovarian vein reflux in multiparous women and in only 5% of nulliparous women. They also demonstrated a significant difference in ovarian vein diameter (8.3 ± 2.1 mm vs. 4.9 ± 1.3 mm).[16] As with pelvic ultrasonography, there are no accepted standard criteria for the diagnosis of PCS on CT-scanning. Proposed criteria include the following:[17]

- Presence of pelvic varicosities >4 mm in diameter and dilated ovarian veins >8mm in diameter.
- Reversed flow in the ovarian vein.

Magnetic resonance venography (MRV) has also been used to evaluate for possible ovarian vein reflux and the presence of PCS. Asciutto et al compared MRV with venography in the detection of ovarian vein reflux. They found satisfactory visualization of the venous anatomy in all patients. In their study, the sensitivity of MRV for detecting ovarian vein congestion was 88%, and the specificity was 67%.[18] The same group proposed that MRV may underestimate venous pathology because the images are obtained in a supine position, and an upright position or increased intra-abdominal pressure can exacerbate the reflux or make it more evident.[14] Criteria for the diagnosis of PCS on MRV are similar to those seen with CT venography.[13]

Varicography

Varicography is a technique employed to visualize the draining veins of perineal and labial varices. These are often the result of saphenofemoral venous reflux but can emanate from any of the pelvic venous complexes implicated in PCS. The technique involves cannulating an accessible varix with a standard intravenous catheter. Contrast media can be injected retrograde to fully delineate the variceal complex and identify the draining veins.

Retrograde Ovarian and Internal Iliac Venography

Ovarian vein venography has been used via the left renal vein since 1965.[19] The initial technique was modified by others specifically to evaluate PCS.[20,21] Venography can be performed from either the jugular or the femoral approach, and remains the standard criterion for the diagnosis of ovarian vein reflux and PCS. It is our preference to access the venous system from the right common femoral vein. With wire guidance, a catheter is then advanced into the left renal vein. Renal vein and ovarian vein venography can then be performed while the patient performs a Valsalva's maneuver. This demonstrates an enlarged ovarian vein and reflux into the pelvis. In some patients, reflux can be demonstrated across the midline and into the right ovarian vein. Reflux can be exacerbated by tilting the table into a semiupright position.

Additional techniques to aid in the diagnosis of ovarian vein reflux include balloon occlusion of the ovarian vein. A balloon catheter is passed into the proximal ovarian vein and gently inflated to occlude the venous outflow. A gentle hand injection is then performed and can often demonstrate subtle reflux. Venography is helpful in the identification of the venous anatomy and internal iliac vein drainage, and can demonstrate any additional reflux into the inguinal, vulval, perivesical, rectal, and lower extremity veins.[11] Venographic features suggestive of PCS include the following:[5]

- Ovarian vein diameter >10 mm
- Uterine venous engorgement
- Congestion of the ovarian plexus
- Filling of the pelvic veins across the midline or filling of vulvovaginal or leg varices

Treatment

The treatment of PCS can be divided into 3 categories: medical, surgical, and percutaneous. To date, few trials exist evaluating the various methods compared to one another. There is little evidence to support any one therapy over another.

Medical Therapy

Hormonal manipulation remains the mainstay of most medical therapy regimens. Two studies demonstrated a reduction of visual analog pain scores in women placed on medroxyprogesterone 50 mg per day.[22,23] The mechanism of medroxyprogesterone is thought to be an increase venous contraction. While initial reports are encouraging, the pain reduction appears to be temporary. Goserelin acetate has been proposed as an alternate therapy for PCS.[24] GnRH antagonist therapy, however, can be complicated by menopausal symptoms such as hot flashes that may limit its usefulness. Other medical therapies include progestins, danazol, oral contraceptive pills, and nonsteroidal anti-inflammatory agents.

Surgical Therapy

Hysterectomy and oopherectomy remain viable options often reserved for those who fail medical management. With the advances in minimally invasive surgical techniques, laparoscopic ovarian vein ligation or oopherectomy has been proposed as a less invasive therapy. Gargiulo et al demonstrated that laparoscopic ligation of the ovarian veins is an effective and viable option for the treatment of PCS.[25] In light of newer percutaneous techniques, surgical intervention is often reserved as a last resort when other modalities have failed.

Percutaneous Interventions

As minimally invasive procedures have evolved in the treatment of arterial disease, the treatment of venous disease has progressed as well. Maleux et al proposed percutaneous intervention as an alternative to hysterectomy in 2000.[3] Percutaneous interventions for PCS can be classified into 2 broad categories: sclerotherapy and transcatheter embolization. Both have been proven successful in the management of symptoms related to PCS.

Performing both procedures begins in similar fashion to retrograde ovarian vein venography. Access is gained to the venous system either from the right internal jugular vein or from the right common femoral vein. In our practice, it is our preference to cannulate the right common femoral vein, as the delivery systems and catheters required for intervention are much smaller. We have also found this to be a much more comfortable approach for the patients. Once access has been obtained and the left renal vein is localized with venography, we place a 6 Fr guiding sheath at the orifice of the left renal vein, and using a Kumpe catheter, perform selective venography of the left renal vein to identify any reflux into the ovarian vein. Some find a cobra-type catheter or a vertebral catheter to be helpful in accessing these left-sided veins. For the right side, it is our practice to use the Kumpe catheter as well. Others recommend the cobra-type or a Simmons catheter with the appropriate curve.

Reflux in the ovarian vein is generally not a subtle finding, as contrast can readily be seen tracking retrograde through the ovarian vein into pelvic varices (Figure 16.1). Using a Glidewire (Terumo Medical Corporation, Somerset, NJ), a 4 Fr glide catheter (Terumo Medical Corporation, Somerset, NJ) can be directed into the ovarian vein for more selective views. These images are helpful in identifying the extent of the pelvic varices and assessing for reflux across the midline and into the contralateral ovarian vein.

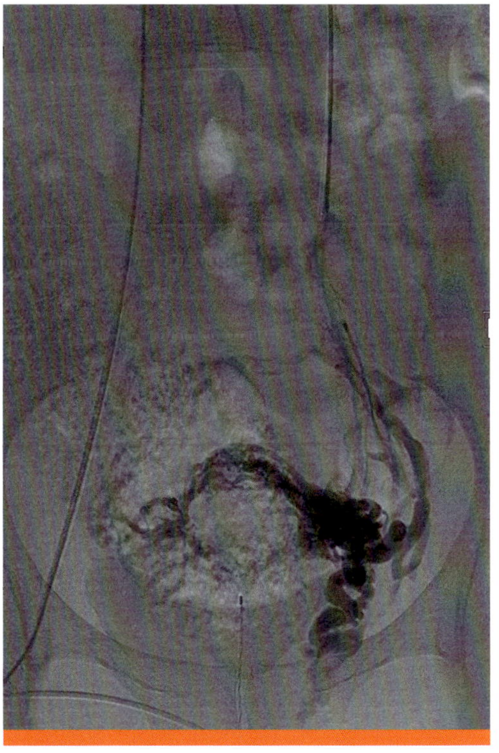

FIGURE 16.1 Venogram of left ovarian vein demonstrates multiple large dilated tributaries with sluggish flow.

Once the reflux has been identified, it is our practice to combine the sclerotherapy and transcatheter embolization techniques. The glide catheter is exchanged over a wire for an appropriately sized balloon. The balloon is gently inflated to occlude the venous outflow. The wire is removed and contrast slowly injected through the wire lumen to fill the varices. The volume of contrast instilled is measured. The balloon is deflated and a sclerosing agent is chosen.

There are many available sclerosing agents for larger pelvic varices. Most physicians who perform these procedures, however, use either sodium morrhuate (Luitpold Pharmaceuticals, Inc., Shirley, NY) or sodium tetradecyl sulfate (AngioDynamics, Queensbury, NY). Sodium morrhuate is a mixture of the sodium salts of saturated and unsaturated fatty acids of cod liver oil. It has a pH of 9.5 and is distributed in a 5% concentration. Upon instillation, it can cause some burning, cramping, or urticaria. Sodium tetradecyl sulfate (Sotradecol) is an anionic surfactant that is manufactured in both 1% and 3% concentrations. It has a pH of 7.9, and in our experience results in less pain and cramping than is seen with sodium morrhuate.

Both agents are diluted with contrast so that during instillation, the agents can be seen filling the varices. It also allows for the amount of "spillage" into the contralateral ovarian vein to be minimized. Sodium tetradecyl sulfate can be instilled as a straight liquid, or can be combined with air to create a foam. It should be noted that the creation of foam is deemed by the US Food and Drug Administration (FDA) as an alteration of the drug and results in creation of a non-FDA-approved drug. Both agents can also be combined with gel foam to create a viscous slurry that mechanically occludes the vein as well as causing a chemical phlebitis.

Coil embolization of the ovarian vein can be done in conjunction with sclerotherapy or as a stand-alone technique. In our practice, we prefer to use sodium tetradecyl sulfate sclerotherapy with or without gel foam as well as coil embolization of the ovarian vein. If coil embolization alone is preferred, it can be done using multiple 0.035-in coils in sizes ranging from 5 to 15 mm and a glide catheter. There is rarely a need for a 3 Fr microcatheter system as the ovarian vein is dilated in these patients. Coils can be placed along the entirety of the ovarian vein from deep in the pelvis to the upper half of the sacroiliac joint. Since we choose to combine both techniques, the sclerosant is instilled to fill the varices and up the ovarian vein to the level of the balloon occlusion. We then place approximately 3 to 4 0.035-in coils through the wire lumen of the balloon to mechanically occlude the ovarian vein outflow (Figure 16.2). Once the coils have been successfully placed, the balloon is deflated and retracted.

Reflux that is identified within the internal iliac vein is treated in a similar manner. Access is often achieved from the contralateral common femoral vein. Once stable catheter placement has been achieved, sclerotherapy and coil embolization can be performed just as with the ovarian vein.

Many of patients will present to a vascular surgeon already having had a CT scan or MRV performed for the evaluation of chronic abdominal and pelvic pain. It has become our standard practice to have the patients follow-up 4 weeks after intervention with an MRV to assess for continued reflux and the resolution of any pelvic varices. If the larger pelvic varices have resolved and the underlying ovarian or internal iliac vein reflux has been successfully treated, there may be smaller cutaneous varices that require intervention.

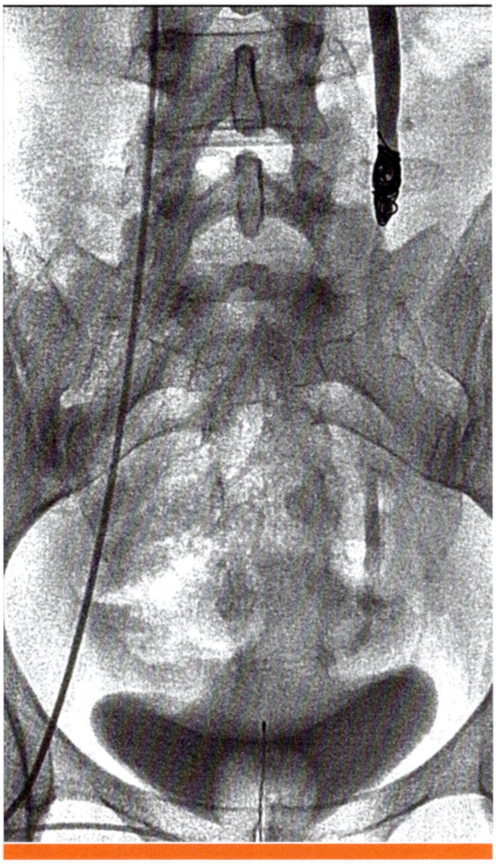

FIGURE 16.2 Venogram shows successful coil embolization of the left ovarian vein.

Varicography can be performed with subsequent "clean-up" sclerotherapy. Varicography is performed by cannulating the perineal, labial, or gluteal varices either under direct vision or using ultrasound guidance. Using a slow-contrast injection as is done with ovarian vein sclerotherapy, the volume of the varices from the sight of cannulation to the level of the broad ligament can be determined. A sclerosant is chosen and the appropriate volume injected to treat the residual veins and their tributaries.

Outcomes of percutaneous intervention have been very encouraging. Maleux reported that 68% of his patients noted marked improvement of their preembolization symptoms.[3] Kim et al reported 100% success in treating 125 patients percutaneously. At follow-up, 83% of patients had an improved clinical outcome at follow-up. A statistically significant reduction in overall pain perception was noted as well.[26]

Premature ovarian failure has been touted as a possible complication following ovarian vein embolization. Kim found that 4 women attempted to conceive after embolization and that 2 were successful. The remaining 2 had fertility issues prior to the embolization.[26]

Conclusion

PCS manifests as chronic pelvic pain and remains a significant healthcare problem resulting in 10% to 40% of all gynecologic referrals a year.[27] Pelvic venous insufficiency has become an increasingly recognized cause of PCS. Better imaging and understanding of the disease result in faster time to intervention and can save many women unnecessary interventions for varicose veins. Through minimally invasive techniques, women can be treated and followed without requiring major disability or surgery.

References

1. Venbrux AC, Chang AH, Kim HS, Montague BJ, Hebert JB, Arepally A, et al. Pelvic congestion syndrome (pelvic venous incompetence): impact of ovarian and internal iliac vein embolotherapy on menstrual cycle and chronic pelvic pain. J Vasc Interv Radiol. 2002;13:171-8.
2. Gandini R, Chiocchi M, Konda D, Pampana E, Fabiano S, Simonetti G. Transcatheter foam sclerotherpay of symptomatic female varicocele with sodium-tetradecyl-sulfate foam. Cardiovasc Inter Rad. 2008; 31(4):778-84.

3. Maleux G, Stockx L, Wilms G, Marchal G. Ovarian vein embolization for the treatment of pelvic congestion syndrome: long-term technical and clinical results. J Vasc Interv Radiol. 2000:11;859-64.
4. Shiraishi K, Naito K. Effects of 4-hydroxyl-2-nonenal, a marker of oxidative stress, on spermatogenesis and expression of p53 protein in male infertility. J Urolology. 2007;178: 1012-7.
5. Cocuzza M, Athayde KS, Agarwal A, Pagani R, Sikka SC, Lucon AM, et al. Impact of clinical varicocele and testis size on seminal reactive oxygen species levels in a fertile population: a prospective controlled study. Fertil Steril. 2008;90(4):1103-8.
6. Saleh RA, Agarwal A, Sharma RK, Said TM, Sikka SC, Thomas AJ Jr. Evaluation of nuclear DNA damage in spermatozoa from infertile men with varicocele. Fertil Steril. 2003;80:1431-6.
7. Allamaneni SS, Naughton CK, Sharma RK, Thomas AJ Jr, Agarwal A. Increased seminal reactive oxygen species levels in patients with varicoceles correlate with varicocele grade but not with testis size. Fertil Steril. 2004;82:1684-6.
8. Chen SS, Huang Wj, Chang LS, Wei YH. Attenuation of oxidative stress after varicocelectomy in subfertile patients with varicocele. J Urolology. 2008;179:639-42.
9. Kennedy A, Hemingway A. Radiology of ovarian varices. Br J Hosp Med. 44;1990: 38-43.
10. Giacchetto C, Cotroneo GB, Marincolo F, Cammisuli F, Caruso G, Catizone F. Ovarian varicocele: ultrasonic and phlebographic evaluation. J Clin Ultrasound. 1990;18:551-5.
11. Adams J, Reginald PW, Franks S, Wadsworth J, Beard RW. Uterine size and endometrial thickness and the significance of cystic ovaries in women with pelvic pain due to congestion. Br J Obstet Gynaecol. 1990;97:583-7.
12. Park SJ, Lim JW, Ko YT, Lee DH, Yoon Y, Oh JH, Lee HK, Huh CY. Diagnosis of pelvic congestion syndrome using transabdominal and transvaginal sonography. Am J Radiol. 2004;182;683-8.
13. Beard RW, Highman JH, Pearce S, Reginald PW. Diagnosis of pelvic varicosities in women with chronic pelvic pain. Lancet. 1984;2:946-9.
14. Ganeshan A, Upponi S, Hon LQ, Uthappa MC, Warakaulle DR, Uberoi R. Chronic pelvic pain due to pelvic congestion syndrome: the role of diagnostic and interventional radiology. Cardiovasc Inter Rad. 2007;30:1105-11.
15. Rozenblit AM, Ricci Z, Tuvia J, Amis ES Jr. Incompetent and dilated ovarian veins: a common CT finding in asymptomatic parous women. Am J Radiol. 2001;176:119-22.
16. Hiromura T, Nishioka T, Nishioka S, Ikeda H, Tomita K. Reflux in the left ovarian vein: ananlysis of MDCT findings in asymptomatic women. Am J Radiol. 2004;183:1411-5.
17. Coakely FV, Varghese SL, Hricak H. CT and MRI of pelvic varices in women. J Comp Assist Tomogr. 1999;73:429-34.
18. Asciutto G, Mumme A, Marpe B, Köster O, Asciutto KC, Geier B. MR venography in the detection of pelvic venous congestion. Eur J Vasc Endovasc Surg. 2008;36:491-6.
19. Tavernier J, Lange D. La phlebograhie utero-ovarienne gauche. Presse Med. 1965;73:863-6.
20. Mayer AL, Machan LS. Correlation of ultrasound and venographic findings in pelvic congestion syndrome. J Vasc Interv Radiol. 2000;suppl:221.
21. Edlundh KO. Pelvic varicosities in women. Acta Obstet Gynaecol Scand. 1964;43: 399-407.
22. Farquhar CM, Rogers V, Franks S, Pearce S, Wadsworth J, Beard RW. A randomized controlled trial of medroxyprogesterone acetate and psychotherapy for the treatment of pelvic congestion. Br J Obstet Gynaecol. 1989:96;1153-62.
23. Walton SM, Batra HK. The use of medroxyprogesterone acetate 50 mg in

the treatment of painful pelvic conditions: prelimary results from a multicentre trial. J Obstet Gynaecol. 1992:12(9) (Suppl 2):550-3.

24. Soysal ME, Soysal S, Vicdan K, Ozer S. A randomized controlled trial of goserelin and medroxyprogesterone acetate in the treatment of pelvic congestion. Hum Reprod. 2001;16:931-9.
25. Gargiulo T, Mais V, Brokaj L, Cossu E, Melis GB. Bilateral laparoscopic transperitoneal ligation of ovarian veins for treatment of pelvic congestion syndrome. J Am Assoc Gynecol Laparoscpy. 2005;10:501-4.
26. Kim HS, Malhotra AD, Rowe PC, Lee JM, Venbrux AC. Embolotherapy for pelvic congestion syndrome: long-term results. J Vasc Interv Radiol. 2006;17:289-97.
27. Ganeshan A, Upponi S, Hon L, Uthappa MC, Warakaulle DR, Uberoi R. Chronic pelvic pain due to pelvic congestion syndrome: the role of diagnosis and interventional radiology. Cardiovasc Inter Rad. 2007;30:1105-11.

PART

4

Venous Malformations

There is a growing realization of the impact that venous malformations have on patients and the complexity of their treatment. Cross-sectional imaging has markedly improved the ability to diagnose and classify these lesions. Considerations are different from interventions for arterial malformations. Venous malformations are low-flow lesions and often truncular in form, with involvement of the lower extremity, and treatment is aimed at controlling the signs and symptoms of chronic venous hypertension. Multimodality imaging and a multidisciplinary management strategy are the norm. Embolization is technically more difficult since the embolization materials are prone to enter the systemic circulation in many variants of venous malformation, and surgery is only reserved for focal lesions and limb salvage situations. Conservative therapy is more common given the anatomic patterns, the relatively benign pathological course of these lesions, and the technical challenges of intervention.

CHAPTER 17

Venous Malformations

Pathophysiology, Classification, and Incidence

Francis Marshalleck and Michael C. Dalsing

Venous malformations (VM) are a subgroup of congenital vascular malformations (CVM), and as the name implies, these malformations are present at birth. The malformation may or may not be evident at birth and may only become important later in life. Symptoms common to all venous disorders may eventually bring the patient to the attention of the clinician. Furthermore, because of an association with congenital venous malformations, symptoms uncommon to more routine venous disorders may be observed.

Chronic Venous Insufficiency. Contemporary Endovascular Management series. © 2011 Mark G. Davies MD and Alan B. Lumsden MD, eds. Cardiotext Publishing, ISBN 978-1-935395-09-6.

Pathophysiology

The etiology of congenital vascular malformations is rooted in changes occurring during embryonic development. In the first 3 weeks of development, 3 stages of vascular system development can be distinguished: stage I is the undifferentiated or capillary network stage; stage II is the retiform stage with the beginning of organization into larger channels; and stage III is the truncular stage in which recognized main vascular trunks are present.[1] Arrested or disturbed development can be a source of vascular malformation, and the stage affected will determine the nature of the malformation. If occurring during the first 2 stages, it stunts the differentiation into main channels such that no true vessels are present but rather primitive vascular channels form the connections present. In terms of the later defined classification category, the defect noted would be an extratruncular malformation. If the process occurs during stage III (the truncular stage), a more refined vascular structure is noted.

The predominant vascular structure affected—arterial, venous, lymphatic, arteriovenous, and combined vascular defects—helps to define the anatomic definition of the current classification system.[2,3] The stage affected also provides some insight into the pathophysiologic consequences of the lesion. Extratruncular lesions retain embryonic tissue remnants of mesodermal origin. Such tissue retains the characteristics of mesenchymal cells (angioblasts) with the potential to proliferate and therefore grow when stimulated. The stimulation can be internal, such as occurs during menarch, pregnancy, or other hormonal stimulus; or external, such as might occur when experiencing trauma or surgery.[3,4] On the contrary, the truncular forms of CVMs have occurred in a later stage of development and lack the growth characteristics of embryonic mesenchymal cells. However, such developed interconnections between vascular structures such as arteries and veins (the arteriovenous malformation) may have more dire hemodynamic consequences for the patient even though it has occurred at a more mature developmental stage. Furthermore, the persistent fetal remnant vessel may not involute normally or may remain as a defective trunk. Consequently, the patient is left with an obstructive or dilated structure sometimes situated in an anatomic location consistent with the fetal state.[3,4]

The histology of vascular malformation demonstrates a lining of quiescent endothelium just like the endothelium of normal vessels, which is different from the endothelial hyperplasia noted in a hemangioma.[5,6] In venous malformations, the walls observed are thin with a normal basement membrane and have sparse, smooth muscle cells present.

Factors that might cause an alternation in vascular development at this stage in embryonic life are many but are not always clearly defined. In reference to venous malformations, there is some indication that genetics may be involved. The absence of venous valves has a familial occurrence.[7] Data show that a sporadic disease may be explained by somatic changes in a gene, causing a rare, inherited form of venous malformation and pinpointing the TIE2 pathways as potential therapeutic targets for venous malformations.[8] Chromosome 9p may be the locus for a dominantly inherited venous malformation.[9] Environmental factors may have an influence in some venous malformations. Fetal diseases have been implicated in truncular venous malformation, namely, allantoic vessel thrombosis or embryonic infection (toxoplasmosis and cytomegalovirus infection).[1] Hemodynamic factors may be a factor in other cases.[10] No matter the cause, the clinician is left with defining the problem (classification) in such a manner that it can be addressed clinically.

Classification

It was recognized in the 1980s that there was confusion surrounding the classification of congenital vascular malformations, a situation not improved by name-based eponyms or traditional terminology. In 1975, Mulliken and Glowacki studied the cellular characteristics of congenital vascular malformations. This resulted in a biological classification separating hemangiomas (endothelial hyperplasia) from vascular malformations that exhibit normal endothelial turnover.[5] Hemangiomas are subdivided into those exhibiting a proliferating phase and an involution phase. Vascular malformations are true structural abnormalities and are further classified into low-flow types (capillary, lymphatic, venous, mixed) and high-flow types (arteriovenous malformations, arteriovenous fistulae). A consensus conference in Hamburg resulted in a more refined classification that offered an anatomic and embryologic basis confirmed by diagnostic studies, which had implications for therapy.[2,3,11] This classification is based on the "predominant component" of the vascular system involved: predominantly arterial, predominantly venous, predominantly lymphatic, predominantly arteriovenous shunting, and a combined vascular defect. Each is further classified into 1 of 2 groups based on the embryonal stage at which the developmental arrest occurred: extratruncular or truncular. The extratruncular form has stopped at an early embryonal stage and retains characteristics of the mesenchymal cells, which allow the lesion to grow when stimulated. It can be further divided into diffuse, infiltrating or limited, or localized. The truncular form has development arrested at a later stage and lacks the ability to rapidly grow when stimulated. It can be further divided into aplasia or obstruction and alternatively dilatation (localized or diffuse).[2,3,12,13] Table 17.1 summarizes this classification system. Depending on the treatment planned, diagnostic studies proceed from noninvasive to more invasive and more costly.[14] Early diagnostic studies should involve magnetic resonance imaging (MRI), which aids in the embryologic staging and anatomic associations. If the diagnosis is in doubt, a venous duplex evaluation will aid in determining anatomy and hemodynamic parameters. It is helpful to note that fast-flow lesions generally have an arterial component while venous and lymphatic defects are slow-flow lesions.

Venous malformations are low-flow lesions and often truncular in form, with involvement of the lower extremity, but they can occur at other locations.[13,15] In the lower extremity, treatment is often aimed at controlling the signs and symptoms of chronic venous hypertension.[12,13,16,17] Some examples

TABLE 17.1 **Hamburg Classification of Congenital Vascular Malformations**

Defect Type	**Anatomical Form**	
	Extratrunucular	***Truncular***
Predominantly arterial	Infiltrating/diffuse Limited/localized	Aplasia or obstruction Dilatation
Predominantly venous	Infiltrating/diffuse Limited/localized	Aplasia or obstruction Dilatation
Predominantly lymphatic	Infiltrating/diffuse Limited/localized	Aplasia or obstruction Dilatation
Predominantly arteriovenous shunting	Infiltrating/diffuse Limited/localized	Deep AV fistula Superficial AV fistula
Combined vascular	Infiltrating hemolymphatic Limited hemolymphatic	Arterial and venous Hemolymphatic

Based on the International Society for the Study of Vascular Anomalies consensus in 1988 with modifications.[2,3,11,12]

of truncular VMs include femoral vein hypoplasia (Figure 17.1), iliac vein agenesis, and the marginal vein, while extratruncular lesions may be localized or infiltrative into muscle or bone (Figure 17.2).[14]

Venous malformations are sometimes amenable to endovascular management, a technique in which venous drainage becomes a very important consideration. A classification introduced to address this specific interventional need was provided by Puig and his associates.[18] The venous drainage is described as absent, into normal veins or into dysplasic veins, or the lesion is described as venous ectasia. The last 2 situations make embolic agents difficult to use since the agents are prone to enter the systemic circulation. However, when large draining veins are accessible, they can be embolized percutaneously to prevent later egress of the liquid sclerosants or embolic agents injected into the venous malformation.

Because symptoms are often due to lower extremity chronic venous hypertension and escalating diagnostic evaluations are obtained based on planned interventions, many VM cases are amenable to reporting standards developed for venous disease. The reporting standards for chronic venous disorders (CVD) must be employed to allow treating clinicians to communicate using objective parameters. It is the opinion of current venous experts that the CEAP method of classifying patients promotes this common language and that the Venous Severity Score (VSS) is a method of determining treatment outcome. This classification and scoring system are meant to be dynamic and improved over time while maintaining basic concepts.

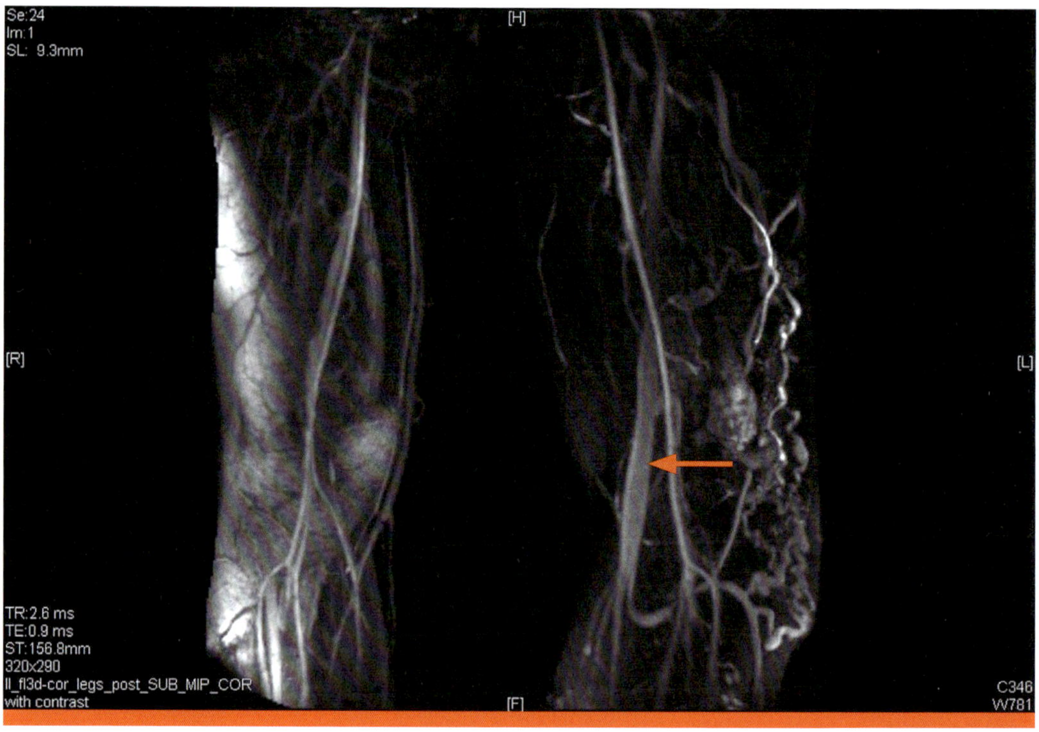

FIGURE 17.1 Example of a truncular venous malformation; a persistent sciatic vein (arrow) is present in the absence of a defined femoral venous system.

In conjunction with the American Venous Forum, an international ad hoc committee developed the first CEAP consensus document, which included a classification and scoring system of the severity of CVD.[19] The CEAP classification system is based on clinical manifestations (C), etiologic factors (E) including a congenital category, anatomic distribution of disease (A), and the underlying pathophysiologic findings (P). It was endorsed by major vascular societies and published as part of venous reporting standards.[20]

Rapid developments and a renewed interest in venous disorders in the 1990s demonstrated a need to upgrade the CEAP classification. Ten years after its introduction, clarification and modifications were agreed to that improve yet do not substantially change the original classification system.[21] In essence, more precise definitions of confusing terms within the clinical classification were provided (eg, reticular veins, corona phlebectatica, eczema, atrophie blanche), a subdivision of C_4 was described ($(_a$ is pigmentation or eczema while $_b$ is lipodermatosclerosis and/or atrophie blanche), and each clinical class is further described as asymptomatic ($(_A)$) or symptomatic ($(_S)$). In each of the E, A, and P categories, n has been added to relate that *no* venous factor is identified. In addition, each CEAP classification is followed by the date of investigation and the level of investigation, which is especially critical when classifying VMs. The level of investigation is 3-tiered: Level 1, H & P =/- hand-held Doppler; level II, noninvasive vascular laboratory (duplex +/- plethysmography); level III, invasive or complex imaging (varicography, venography, venous

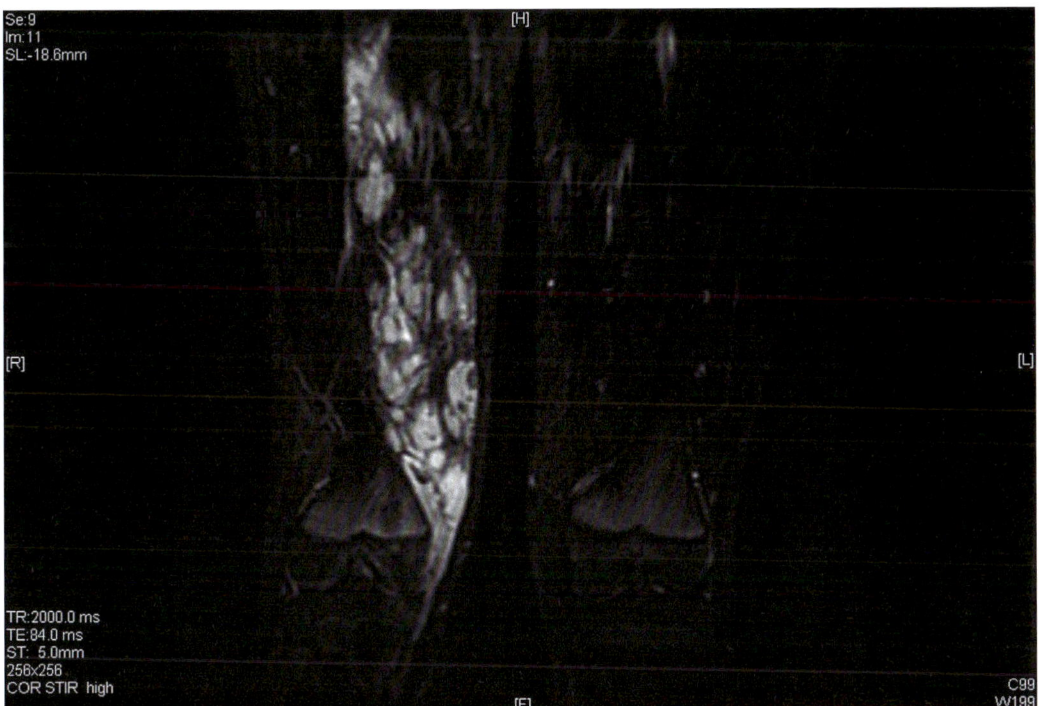

FIGURE 17.2 Extratruncular venous malformation demonstrating the diffuse infiltrating type; medial thigh muscle involvement is quite apparent and widespread.

pressures, computed tomography [CT], or magnetic resonance venography [MRV]). The basic CEAP uses the highest clinical descriptor in the classification and provides anatomic descriptors s (superficial), p (perforator), or d (deep) without providing details for all 18 possible anatomic segments. Full CEAP provides the entire complement of description possible given the level of investigations available.

Venous Severity Scoring is aimed at providing longitudinal outcomes assessment.[22] The aim is to provide objective measures that are quantifiable and capable of promptly reflecting improvement or worsening. There are 2 components to the Venous Severity Score: Venous Clinical Severity Score (based on the C of CEAP) and Venous Segmental Disease Score (a combination of the anatomic and pathophysiologic parts of CEAP). The Venous Clinical Severity Score has 9 clinical descriptors: pain, varicose veins, edema, pigmentation, induration, inflammation, total number of ulcers, duration of active ulceration, and size of largest current ulcer with compression and its compliance as a tenth component. Each descriptor is defined into 1 of 4 categories graded as 0 to 3 for an overall potential total score of 30. The Venous Clinical Severity Score has been validated in clinical studies but may be more suited for the study of moderate to severe disease.[23-26] Within the American Venous Forum, current committee work is aimed at updating the Venous Clinical Severity Scoring to make terms more definite and more inclusive of earlier stages of venous disease. The Venous Segmental Disease Score provides a method to score reflux or obstruction noted on duplex evaluation, with varying points assigned to different veins commensurate with their apparent clinical significance. The maximal score is 20. The last component of this effort is a Venous Disability Score, with 4 levels of disability based on the ability to perform usual activities possible before the onset of disability caused by the venous disorder. Reviewing the work of those dedicated to the treatment of VM, the use of these scoring tools provides a reasonable reflection of the problems these patients face.[13,15,16] Investigators have applied these tools in patients with congenital vascular malformations having a significant venous malformation component demonstrating functionality for such patients.[27]

Generic quality-of-life instruments (Medical Outcomes Study Short Form [SF-36 or SF-12]) in conjunction with venous disease-specific instruments can reflect the impact of therapy. Most of the disease-specific instruments pinpoint a specific population of patients, with less severe disease (CIVIQ, Aberdeen Questionaire)[27-29] or more severe disease such as ulcers (the Charing Cross Venous Ulcer Questionaire),[30] rather than the spectrum of disease. Therefore, the tool chosen must reflect this predilection to provide valid results. The VEINES instrument may be a more inclusive quality-of-life (QOL) tool.[31] These are considered an important element of a properly conducted outcomes study from the patient's point of view. For patients with a VM, QOL can be a relative indication for treatment.[12]

Incidence

Most CVMs are recognized in childhood but may only cause symptoms later in life. Of 1099 neonates examined by Pratt, only 5 demonstrated a CVM, suggesting that these anomalies are rare.[32] Tasnádi examined 3-year-old children looking for signs and symptoms of CVM and found that 43 children that were so afflicted (1.2%).[1] Using the Hamburg classification, Tasnádi documented 432 vascular malformations over a 10-year period at the Heim Pal Hospital for Children and found that nearly 50% (209 cases) were predominantly venous, with 119 extratruncular (57%) and 90 truncular cases.[1] A similar predominance of venous malformations were noted by Lee and his associates while working in South Korea. In their experience, 45% (143 of 318 patients) of their patients had a predominantly venous malformation, but it was even more heavily skewed to those with an extratruncular defect (138).[13]

Venous malformations generally have a slight female over male distribution, with about 60% occurring in females.[1,13] The location of the venous malformation according to the data accumulated by Lee and his associates is lower extremity (35.9%), multiple locations (25.7%), head and neck (22.2%), upper extremity (10.6%), thorax (4.4%), pelvis (0.8%), and abdomen (0.4%).[15] Tasnádi notes that, in general, the truncular forms appear most frequently in the lower extremities while the extratruncular forms (diffuse and localized) are most commonly noted in the head and neck.[1] In the experience of Lee and associates, the mean age was 18.5 years with about 40%, 24%, and 17% of the cases occurring in the first 3 decades of life, respectively.[13]

Conclusion

Venous malformations are a subgroup of congenital vascular malformations. They are further categorized as extratruncular (arrested in an earlier stage of embryonic development) or truncular (arrested at a later stage when defined vascular structures are evident). The extratruncular forms are localized or diffuse (involving muscle or bone) and have the potential to be stimulated by stress or hormonal influences. The truncular form results in aplasia, obstruction, or dilatation (ectasia), with the possibility of an embryonic location of the remaining venous structures. Various factors may play a role in the etiology of the venous malformation. Venous malformations have a slight female predominance, are generally recognized in the first 3 decades of life, and although found throughout the body, have a predilection for the lower extremity. Since the lower extremity is often involved, reporting standards referable to chronic venous disorders can be used to better describe the disorder and demonstrate the effect of any intervention.

References

1. Tasnádi G. Epidemiology and etiology of congenital vascular malformations. Semin Vasc Surg. 1993;6(4):200-3.
2. Belov ST. Anatomophathological classification of congenital vascular defects. Semin Vasc Surg. 1993;6:219-24.
3. Lee BB, Laredo J, Lee TS, Huh S, Neville R. Terminology and classification of congenital vascular malformations. Phlebology. 2007;22:249-52.
4. Bastide G, Lefebvre D. Anatomy and organogenesis and vascular malformations. In: Belov ST, Loose DA, Weber J, eds. Vascular Malformations. Reinbek (Germany): Einhorn-Presse Verlag GmbH, 1989. p20-2.
5. Mulliken JB, Glowacki J. Hemangiomas and vascular malformations in infants and children: a classification based on endothelial characteristics. Plast Reconstr Surg. 1982; 69:412- 22.
6. Mulliken JB. Classification of vascular birthmarks. In: Mulliken JB and Young AE, eds. Vascular Birthmarks: Hemangiomas and Malformations. Philadelphia, PA: W.B. Saunders Company, 1988. p24-37.

7. Lodin A, Lindvall N, Gentell H. Congenital absence of venous valves as a cause of leg ulcers. Acta Chir Scand. 1959;116:256-61.
8. Limaye N, Wouters V, Uebelhoer M, Tuominen M, Wirkkala R, Mulliken JB, et al. Somatic mutations in angiopoietin receptor gene TEK cause solitary and multiple sporadic venous malformations. Nat Genet. 2008;41:118-124.
9. Vikkula M, Boon LM, Mulliken JB. Molecular genetics of vascular malformations. Matrix Biology. 2001;20(5-6):327-35.
10. AE Young. Pathogenesis of vascular malformations. In: Mulliken JB, Young AE, eds. Vascular Birthmarks: Hemangiomas and Malformations. Philadelphia,PA: W.B. Saunders Company, 1988. p.107-13.
11. Belov ST. Classification of congenital vascular defects. Int Angiol. 1990;9:141-6.
12. Lee BB. Critical issues in management of congenital vascular malformation. Ann Vasc Surg. 2004;18(3):380-92.
13. Lee BB, Kim DI, Huh S, Kim HH, Choo IW, Byun HS, Do YS. New experiences with absolute ethanol sclerotherapy in the management of a complex form of congenital venous malformation. J Vasc Surg. 2001;33:764-72.
14. Lee BB, Laredo J, Lee SJ, Huh SH, Joe JH, Neville R. Congenital vascular malformations: general diagnostic principles. Phlebology. 2007;22:253-7.
15. Lee BB, Do YS, Byun HS, Choo IW, Kim DI, Huh SH. Advanced management of venous malformations with ethanol sclerotherapy: mid-term results. J Vasc Surg. 2003;37:533-8.
16. Rosenblatt M. Endovascular management of venous malformations. Phlebology. 2007;22:264-75.
17. Loose DA. Surgical management of venous malformations. Phlebology. 2007;22:276-82.
18. Puig S, Aref H, Chigot V, Bonin B, Brunelle F. Classification of venous malformations in children and implications for sclerotherapy. Pediatr Radiol. 2003;33:99-103.
19. Bergan JJ, Eklof B, Kistner RL, Moneta GL, Nicolaides AN, and the International ad hoc committee of the American Venous Forum. Classification and grading of chronic venous disease in the lower limbs. A consensus statement. Vasc. Surg. 1996;30:5-11.
20. Porter JM, Moneta GL, an International Consensus Committee on Chronic Venous Disease. Reporting standards in venous disease: an update. J Vasc Surg. 1995;21:635-45.
21. Eklöf B, Rutherford RB, Bergan JJ, Carpentier PH, Gloviczki P, Kistner RL, et al and American Venous Forum International Ad Hoc Committee for Revision of the CEAP Classification. Revision of the CEAP classification for chronic venous disorders: consensus statement. J Vasc Surg. 2004;40:1248-52.
22. Rutherford RB, Padberg FT, Comerota AJ, Kistner RL, Meissner MH, Moneta GL. Venous severity scoring: an adjunct to venous outcome assessment. J Vasc Surg. 2000;31:1307-12.
23. Meissner MH, Natiello C, Nicholls SC. Performance characteristics of the venous clinical severity score. J Vasc Surg. 2002;36:889-95
24. Perrin M, Dedieu F, Jessent V, Blanc MP. Evaluation of the new severity scoring in chronic venous disease of the lower limb: an observational survey conducted by French angiologists. Phlebologie. 2003;56: 127-39.
25. Ricci MA, Emmerich J, Callas PW, Rosendaal FR, Stanley AC, Naud S, et al. Evaluating chronic venous disease with a new venous severity scoring system. J Vasc Surg. 2003;38:909-15.
26. Vasquez MA, Wang J, Mahathanaruk M, Buczkowski G, Sprehe E, Dosluoglu HH. The utility of venous clinical severity score in 682 limbs treated by radiofrequency saphenous ablation. J Vasc Surg. 2007;45:1008-15.

27. Delis KT, Gloviczki P, Wennberg PW, Rooke TW, Driscoll DJ. Hemodynamic impairment, venous segmental disease, and clinical severity scoring in limbs with Klippel-Trenaunay syndrome. J Vasc Surg. 2007;45:561-7.
28. Launois R, Reboul-Marty J, Henry B. Construction and validation of a quality of life questionnaire in chronic lower limb venous insufficiency. Qual Life Res. 1996;5:539-54.
29. Garratt AM, Ruta DA, Abdalla MI, Russell IT. Responsiveness of the SF-36 and a condition specific measure of health outcome for patients with varicose veins. Qual Life Res. 1996;5:1-12.
30. Smith JJ, Guest M, Greenhaugh RM, Davies AH. Measuring quality of life in patients with venous ulcer. J Vasc Surg. 2000;31:642-9.
31. Lamping DL, Schroter S, Kurz X, Kahn SR, Abenhaim L. Evaluation of outcomes in chronic venous disorders of the leg: development of a scientifically rigorous, patient-reported measure of symptoms and quality of life. J Vasc Surg. 2003;37:410-19.
32. Pratt AG. Birthmarks in infants. Arch Dermatol Syph. 1967;67:302-5.

CHAPTER 18

Arteriovenous Malformations

Alan B. Lumsden

Arteriovenous malformations (AVMs) are congenital lesions, which consist of a complex of blood vessels and abnormal arteriovenous communications. Although not hereditary, they represent inborn defects in vascular morphogenesis and consist of feeding arteries and draining veins, which communicate through a nidus. The nidus represents a direct communication between the arteries and veins with absence of intervening capillaries. Blood shunts directly through the nidus from the higher-pressure arterial system to the lower-pressure venous system.

AVMs may be mixed (arteriovenous) or predominantly venous (65% of total) in composition, and determination of the major component is an important guide in choice of therapy. Occurring in 1.5% of the population, they are usually isolated but occasionally are associated with identifiable syndromes such as Klippel-Trenaunay or Parkes-Weber syndromes.

The natural history of AVMs is unpredictable. Growth can be stimulated by trauma or hormone exposure, or may become more progressive for no obvious reason. AVMs may be multifocal. Progressive growth requiring multiple interventions is necessary.

Classification of congenital Malformations is confusing because of the multitude of terms. The Hamburg classification of vascular malformations uses criteria that take into account the underlying anatomical, histological, pathophysiological, and hemodynamic status of each malformation (Table 18.1). Congenital vascular malformations (CVMs) include hemangiomas and arteriovenous malformations. The latter behave more aggressively, pursuing a more destruc-

Chronic Venous Insufficiency. Contemporary Endovascular Management series. © 2011 Mark G. Davies MD and Alan B. Lumsden MD, eds. Cardiotext Publishing, ISBN 978-1-935395-09-6.

Table 18.1 **Hamburg Classification of Congenital Vascular Malformation: 1988 with Modification**

Species[a]	Anatomical Form[b]
Predominantly arterial defects	Truncular forms
	Aplasia or obstruction
	Dilatation
	Extratruncular forms
	Infiltrating
	Limited
Predominantly venous defects	Truncular forms
	Aplasia or obstruction
	Dilatation
	Extratruncular forms
	Infiltrating
	Limited
Predominantly AV shunting defects	Truncular forms
	Deep AV fistula
	Superficial AV fistula
	Extratruncular forms
	Infiltrating
	Limited
Combined vascular defects	Truncular forms
	Arterial and venous
	Hemolymphatic
	Extratruncular forms
	Infiltrating hemolymphatic
	Limited hemolymphatic
Predominantly lymphatic defects	Truncular forms
	Aplasia or obstruction
	Dilatation
	Extratruncular forms
	Infiltrating
	Limited

[a] Based on the consensus of the International Society for the Surgery of Vascular Anomalies through the international workshop on congenital vascular malformation held in Hamburg, Germany, 1988.
[b] Based on the embryologic stage at which the developmental arrest has occurred.

tive and locally invasive course. They are a more primitive type of CVM because the majority belongs to the extratruncular form as the residual remnants of a developmental arrest in the early stage of embryonic life.

Venous malformations are differentiated into truncular and extratruncular forms, with the truncular forms (38%) being obstructions or dilations, and the extratruncular forms (62%) being limited or infiltrating.[1] The prevalence of deep venous anomalies associated with venous malformations is approximately 47%.[2]

Presenting Symptoms

Because AVMs can occur anywhere within the body, the potential presenting symptoms are innumerable. Symptoms therefore are highly variable. Most are asymptomatic for long periods of time. Extremity AVMs present with pain, swelling, deformity, limb enlargement (Figure 18.1), and more rarely with skin ulceration and bleeding (Figure 18.2). They may be well circumscribed or locally infiltrative (Figure 18.3), involving adjacent muscles, nerves, and vessels. In venous malformations, dilated superficial veins are usually apparent and numerous. Occasionally AVMs are associated with overlying or synchronous port wine stains, which represent capillary hemangiomas. Limb enlargement may be found in the affected limb.

AVM involving body cavities and solid organs also occur with site-specific symptoms. Pulmonary AVMs present with hemoptysis, renal AVMs with hematuria and flank pain, and pelvic AVMs may have abdominal pain.

Thromboses often occur, especially in venous malformations, and this is often the cause of the sudden appearance of symptoms. Symptoms of progressive venous insufficiency are often seen especially with venous malformations: limb swelling, lipodermatosclerosis, and ulceration. Most peripheral AVMs are suspected based on history and physical examination. However, a variety of imaging modalities are necessary to confirm the diagnosis and then to determine location and degree of involvement of adjacent structures.

Imaging

Ultrasonography is usually our first-line confirmatory imaging test. Duplex scanning can provide information on the structural elements (arteries, veins, venous thromboses) and hemodynamic characteristics of a vascular malformation. However, cross-

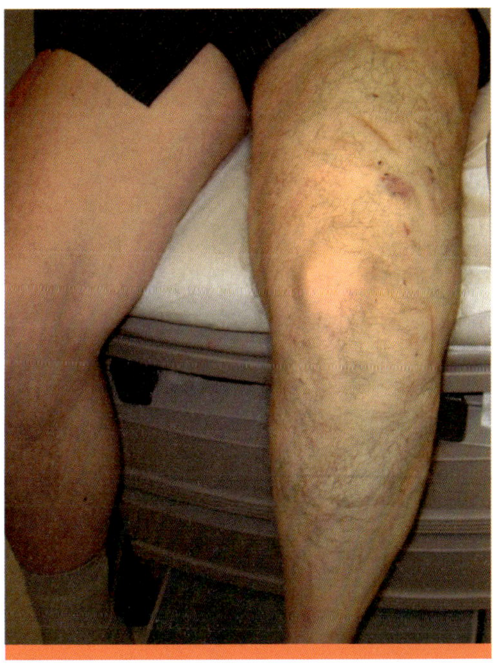

FIGURE 18.1 This patient has Klippel-Trenauny syndrome. The leg is enlarged, and there is diffuse venous malformation causing deformity and pain. Scattered areas of encroachment on the skin are visible. Reprinted with permission from the Department of Cardiovascular Surgery, Methodist DeBakey Heart & Vascular Center.

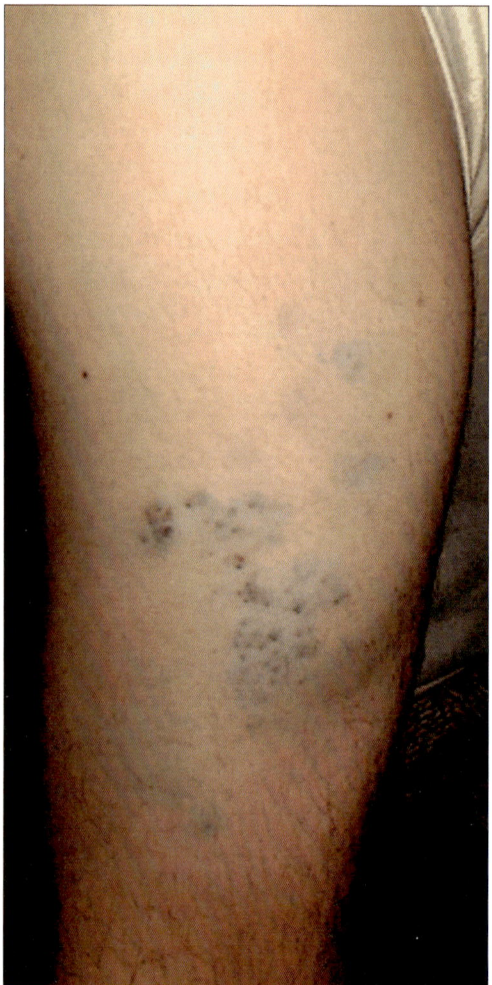

FIGURE 18.2 AVM in lateral thigh with skin involvement and deformity. Reprinted with permission from the Department of Cardiovascular Surgery, Methodist DeBakey Heart & Vascular Center.

sectional imaging and 3-dimensional reconstruction with computed tomography angiography (CTA) or magnetic resonance angiography (MRA) is absolutely required to "stage" the malformation. These techniques provide accurate determination of the size of the AVM, feeding vessels, and involvement or absence of involvement of the adjacent tissue: individual muscles and muscle groups, nerves, axial vasculature. Magnetic resonance imaging (MRI) can characterize the flow pattern of these malformations to guide treatment toward transarterial embolization for vascular malformations and percutaneous embolization for low-flow, venous malformations. MRI (Figure 18.4), like CT scanning, can provide accurate definition of the anatomic extent and involvement of various tissue layers (providing a distinct advantage over ultrasonography [Figure 18.5]). Contrast arteriography and venography are reserved as preinterventional planning tools and are usually utilized as a prelude to immediate intervention (Figure 18.6). Super-selective arterial catheterization techniques are a requirement for embolotherapy in order to ensure access to the nidus. Shunting can be documented with a Technetium-99m labeled human albumen study. However, we do not use this test, as it offers little in terms of diagnosis or therapy.

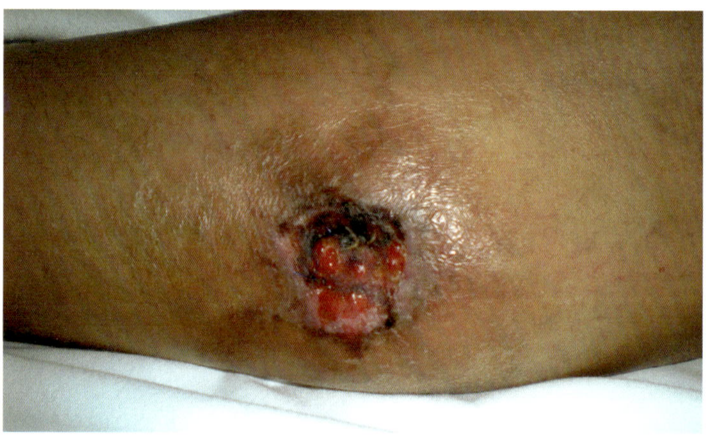

FIGURE 18.3 An absolute indication for intervention is skin erosion and bleeding, which is treated with glue embolization followed by resection and reconstruction. Reprinted with permission from the Department of Cardiovascular Surgery, Methodist DeBakey Heart & Vascular Center.

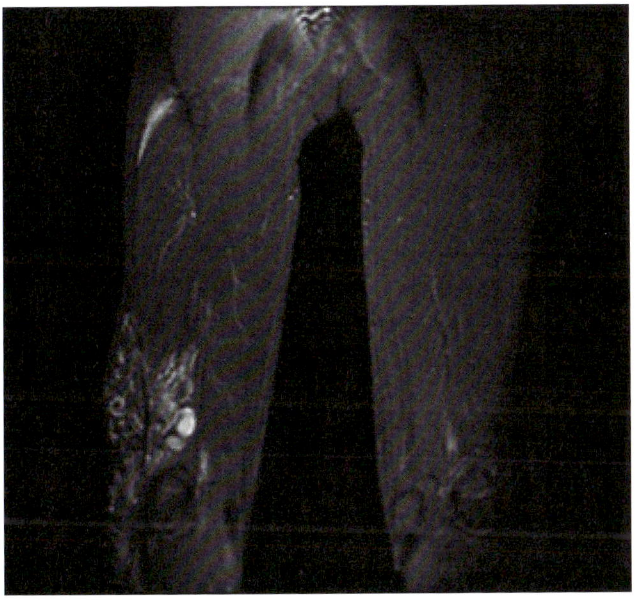

FIGURE 18.4 MRI showing AVM in lower right thigh involving both subcutaneous tissue and underlying muscles. Reprinted with permission from the Department of Cardiovascular Surgery, Methodist DeBakey Heart & Vascular Center.

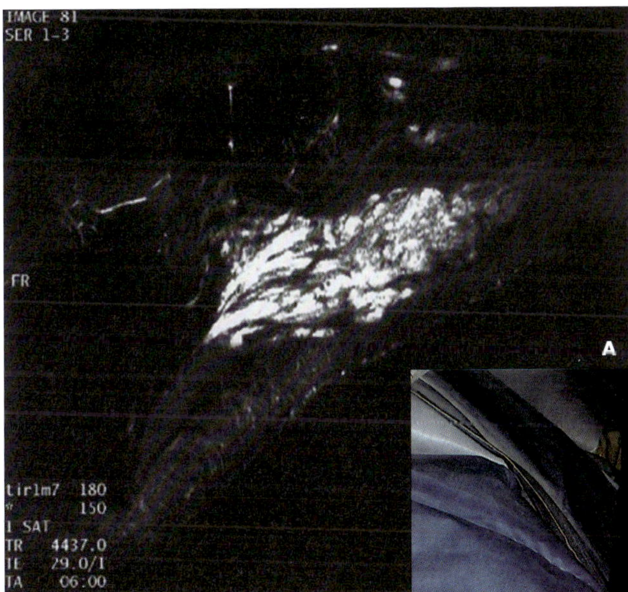

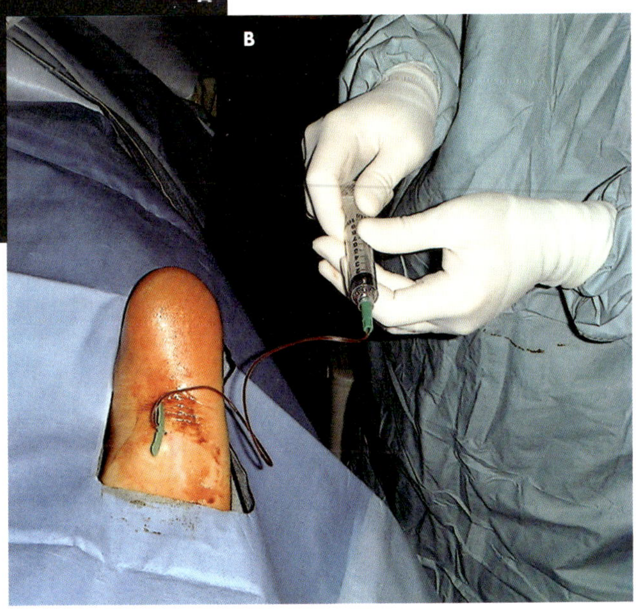

FIGURE 18.5 **A.** MRI showing planter venous malformation. **B.** Malformation treated by injection of sclerofoam. Reprinted with permission from the Department of Cardiovascular Surgery, Methodist DeBakey Heart & Vascular Center.

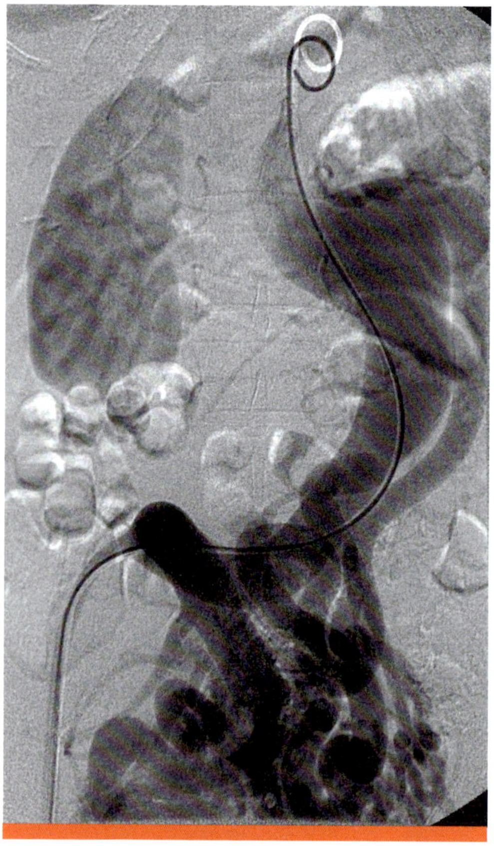

FIGURE 18.6. Angiogram of complex pelvic arteriovenous malformation, which was causing high-output cardiac failure. This was associated with aortic aneurismal changes, a massively hypertrophied inferior mesenteric artery, and venous aneurysms of the internal iliac veins. This was initially treated with coil embolization to slow down the flow followed by glue embolization. Reprinted with permission from the Department of Cardiovascular Surgery, Methodist DeBakey Heart & Vascular Center.

Therapy

Arteriovenous malformations can present very complex management decisions. Since the involvement of underlying structures is often present, and functional impairment a consequence of the AVM, or a possible consequence of therapy, a multidisciplinary team is often used to evaluate the patients: vascular surgery, interventional radiology, plastic surgery, and orthopedic opinions are often necessary. Indications for intervention can be divided into absolute and relative indications, as follows:

Absolute: Hemorrhage, ischemia (steal), ulceration, gangrene, high-flow congestive cardiac failure, intractable pain
Relative: Pain service, impairment of function, deformity, progression, cosmesis, claudication

All AVMs are potentially limb-threatening and even life-threatening. However, what is important is the history of the malformation. Those that have been stable for years are likely to remain so. Consequently, our threshold for aggressive intervention in this situation is high. Many vascular malformations can be managed conservatively with observation, compressive therapy (for chronic venous insufficiency), and orthotics for deformities. For AVMs with a predominantly arterial component, the therapeutic principle is to access and obliterate the nidus, retaining major feeding vessels for future access, as shown in the following list:

Principles for Safe Embolotherapy

- Good preliminary angiography
- Think about collateral pathways
- Stable catheter position
- Use shortest straightest approach
- Use nonheparinized saline to flush and dilute contrast
- Continuous fluoro during embolization
- Intermittent angiograms to evaluate changing flow
- Multiple incremental sessions
- Long-term commitment
- Liberal use of general anesthesia

This is in sharp contradistinction from past strategies where coil embolization or surgical ligation of feeding vessels was employed. This simply results in more vascular growth and is contraindicated as a stand-alone therapy.

Percutaneous Therapy

Catheter-based intervention is the principal therapeutic modality used in arteriovenous malformations. Broadly, venous malformations are treated with direct percutaneous ultrasound-guided access to the malformation and direct inject with alcohol of sclerosing agents (sclerofoam). Arteriovenous malformations, in contrast, are approached by remote arterial access with flow-directed delivery of agents: polyvinyl alcohol (PVA) particles (100–500μm) and cyanoacrylate adhesives. Coils are used in our hands only in very high-flow arteriovenous malformations where they can slow flow sufficiently to permit more controlled delivery of the PVA particles or cyanoacrylate glue.

Particles and liquid occlusive agents are carried by the blood flow distally and induce occlusion at both the arteriolar level and in venular beds. Embolization can achieve 80% occlusion. Complications associated with embolization include access site complications, tissue necrosis, pulmonary embolization, and distal embolization outside the vascular malformations. Risks of embolotherapy include the following:

- Nontarget distal embolic embolization
- Potentially fatal PE from extensive venous thrombosis
- Skin necrosis
- Nerve damage

Our agent of choice is *n*-Butyl cyanoacrylate glue. Features of the glue are shown in the following list:

- Tissue adhesive or "glue"
- Approval for treatment of cerebral AVMs
- Mechanism of action
    - Polymerization contact with ionic fluids
    - Formation of solid cast in vessel
    - Vessel occlusion
- Delivery technique
    - Coaxial super-selective delivery using microcatheter
    - Flushing with nonionic dextrose solution
    - Immediate catheter withdrawal when catheter encroached by glue

Participation in a company-sponsored training course is necessary before the product is shipped. The on-label approval is for cerebral AVMs, but glue is very widely used for peripheral AVMs. The speed of polymerization of the glue is determined by the concentration of the solution utilized. Mixing the glue with ethiodized oil is used to slow the polymerization rate and will result in deeper penetration. Tantalum added to the glue renders it more radio-opaque, increasing visualization and control. Great care must be taken to keep a blood-free delivery system, otherwise premature polymerization will occur. All delivery catheters are purged and their hub irrigated with dextrose to prevent polymerization from occurring. The greatest hazard in infusing glue is failure to appreciate slowing flow, which occurs during glue delivery, with the result that retrograde flow can occur around the catheter and back into the axial arterial tree.

Percutaneous transcatheter or direct puncture sclerotherapy with absolute ethanol is frequently used for predominantly venous malformations. It is very painful and often requires general anesthesia. Absolute ethanol sclerotherapy achieves excellent results in the infiltrating type of the extratruncular forms of vascular malformation.[3] The success of sclerotherapy has been reported to range from 74% to 91%. Absolute alcohol therapy should be used with caution (maximum dose 1 mL/kg body weight), as it is associated with significant side ffects (tissue necrosis, skin sloughing, pulmonary hypertension, deep vein thrombosis [DVT] and nerve injury) in 10% to 30% of cases.[4-6] Although absolute alcohol is very effective in inducing thrombosis, this can be occasionally catastrophic. Consequently, sclerofoam techniques are increasingly being used.

Sotradecol and polidocanol foams (maximum volume 10 mL mixed with 10 cc of air) have also been used as sclerotherapy agents.[7] Use of foam permits small volumes to be used and is associated with less pain and fewer significant side effects (Figure 18.5). Although initial experience with liquid agents relied on arterial injection, direct percutaneous injection is now the preferred approach for venous malformations and has a high reported success rate.

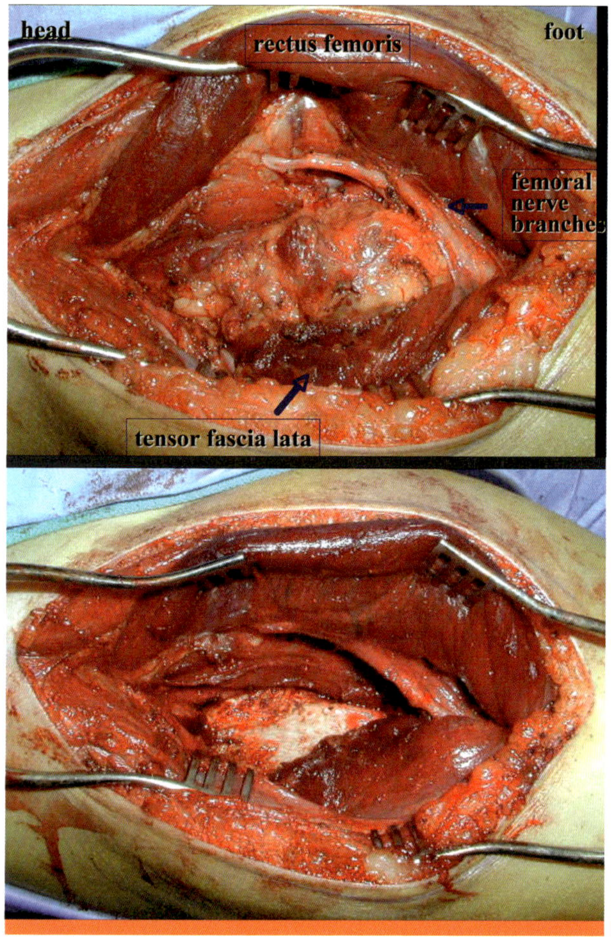

FIGURE 18.7 **A.** Localized AVM in thigh with planned resection. **B.** Postresection with nerves preserved and femur exposed in depths of the wound. Reprinted with permission from the Department of Cardiovascular Surgery, Methodist DeBakey Heart & Vascular Center.

Surgical Therapy

The role of surgical intervention is to accomplish the following objectives:

- Elimination of the lesion
- Reduction of venous hypertension consequences
- Reconstruction
- Amputation

Localized lesions amenable to resection should be removed. This is an uncommon situation but commonly is curative (Figure 18.7). Digit or limb amputation is occasionally required for ulcerating, bleeding, or ischemic lesions. More often, surgical therapy is part of a broader treatment strategy. Patients with diffuse AVMs occasionally develop acutely painful areas, and local resection in our experience has often resulted in symptom relief. A decision for surgical intervention must be carefully considered in terms of bleeding control, healing potential, or need for flap coverage. Large localized AVMs benefit from embolization prior to resection, and this can dramatically reduce bleeding.

Syndromes Associated with Arteriovenous Malformations

Parkes-Weber Syndrome

Parkes-Weber syndrome is a "haemolymphatic malformation," using the Hamburg classification. It is a capillary arteriovenous malformation, which affects the lower limb more often than the upper limb. On MRI, soft tissue overgrowth is noted in the muscle and bony compartments with generalized arterial and venous dilatations. Treatment is tailored to symptoms.

Klippel-Trenaunay Syndrome

Klippel-Trenaunay syndrome (KTS) is a complex congenital anomaly featuring 2 or more of the following: (1) capillary malformations (port-wine stains), (2) soft tissue or bony hypertrophy (or both), and (3) varicose veins or venous malformations. Venous disease in limbs with KTS is a major source of morbidity in affected patients. Limbs with KTS are characterized by complex reflux patterns, severe valvular incompetence, calf muscle pump impairment, and venous hypertension.[8] Imaging shows variable findings in the venous circulation and microcytic features in the lymphatic circulation. The management of patients with KTS continues to be primarily nonoperative, but those patients with patent deep veins can be considered for excision of symptomatic varicose veins and VMs. Although the recurrence rate is high, clinical improvement is significant, and reoperations can be performed if needed. Occasionally, deep vein reconstruction, excision of persistent sciatic veins (PSVs), or subfascial endoscopic perforator surgery is indicated.[9]

References

1. Wassef M, Vanwijck R, Clapuyt P, Boon L, Magalon G. Vascular tumours and malformations, classification, pathology and imaging. Ann Chir Plast Esthet. 2006;51(4-5):263-81.
2. Lee BB, Laredo J, Lee TS, Huh S, Neville R. Terminology and classification of congenital vascular malformations. Phlebology. 2007;22(6):249-52.
3. Lee BB, Do YS, Byun HS, Choo IW, Kim DI, Huh SH. Advanced management of venous malformation with ethanol sclerotherapy: mid-term results. J Vasc Surg. 2003;37(3):533-8.
4. Rimona U, Garniek A, Galili Y, Golan G, Bensaid P, Moraga B. Ethanol sclerotherapy of peripheral venous malformations. Eur J Radiol. 2004;52:283-7.
5. Cho SK, Do YS, Kim DI, Kim YW, Shin SW, Park KB, et al. Peripheral arteriovenous malformations with a dominant outflow vein: results of ethanol embolization. Korean J Radiol. 2008;9(3):258-67.
6. Yakes WF, Luethke JM, Merland JJ, Rak KM, Slater DD, Hollis HW, et al. Ethanol embolization of arteriovenous fistulas: a primary mode of therapy. J Vasc Interv Radiol. 1990;1(1):89-96.
7. Hyodoh H, Hyodoh K. Arteriovenous malformations: ethanolamine oleate sclerotherapy. Acta Chir Iugosl. 2007;54(3):81-6.
8. Delis KT, Gloviczki P, Wennberg PW, Rooke TW, Driscoll DJ. Hemodynamic impairment, venous segmental disease, and clinical severity scoring in limbs with Klippel-Trenaunay syndrome. J Vasc Surg. 2007;45(3):561-7.
9. Noel AA, Gloviczki P, Cherry KJ Jr, Rooke TW, Stanson AW, Driscoll DJ. Surgical treatment of venous malformations in Klippel-Trénaunay syndrome. J Vasc Surg. 2000;32(5):840-7.

Index

Figures are indicated by f *and tables by* t *following the page number.*